THE BRAIN

A Series of Books in Psychology

EDITORS:
Richard C. Atkinson
Gardner Lindzey
Richard F. Thompson

THE BRAIN
A Neuroscience Primer

Second Edition

Richard F. Thompson

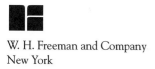

W. H. Freeman and Company
New York

Library of Congress Cataloging-in-Publication Data

Thompson, Richard F.
The brain:a neuroscience primer/Richard F. Thompson.—
2nd ed.

p. c. — (A series of books in psychology)
Includes bibliographical references and index.
ISBN 0-7167-2338-7 (cloth). — ISBN 0-7167-2485-5 (pbk.)

1. Brain. 2. Neurosciences. I. Title. II. Series.
[DNLM: 1. Brain   WL 300 T475b 1993]
QP376.T48 1993
612.8'2—dc20
DNLM/DLC   92-48460
for Library of Congress   CIP

Printed in the United States of America

1 2 3 4 5 6 7 8 9 0 VB 9 9 8 7 6 5 4 3

Contents

To Judith, Kathryn, Elizabeth, Virginia,
Matthew, Kristen, and Grace

Preface

In the few years since the first edition of *The Brain* was published, several major technological developments have changed the face of neuroscience and made imperative the second edition of this book.

* Molecular biology—the basic study of how genes function to make proteins, regulate activities of cells, and program growth and development—is not a new field. But applications of molecular biology are having a profound affect on the study of nerve cells and brain function. The human genome project, mapping all the genes on all the human chromosomes (DNA), is one of the major "big science" projects supported by the United States government in the 1990s.

* Virtually all peptide hormones made in the brain and the pituitary gland have now been characterized and synthesized, and the identities of the genes that express them determined.

* The chemical receptors that control how a neuron responds to hormones, to transmitter chemicals from other neurons, and to drugs are large protein molecules whose identities and gene substrates are just now being determined.

* Noninvasive techniques have been developed for imaging the human brain and identifying regions of the brain that are activated in complex tasks—learning, language, and problem solving. This technology has provided great impetus for current developments in the relatively new field of "cognitive neuroscience."

The success of the first edition of *The Brain* and the many compliments it received were most gratifying. We hope to build on that success in the second edition by keeping readers abreast of major advances in the field.

The second edition of *The Brain* has been extensively revised and updated, and in response to the comments of readers of the first edition, a glossary has been added. The suggested readings at the end of each chapter have been much expanded and updated. These readings range from popular treatments of relevant topics to comprehensive volumes and include a few older classic works. In addition, Chapters 11 and 12 of the second edition are largely new and focus on basic aspects of cognitive neuroscience: learning and memory, language and consciousness. The Appendix—a helpful summary of technical knowledge—has been expanded to include a section on molecular biology.

The research and thought that led to our current understanding of neuron and brain is one of the supreme achievements of science in the twentieth century. And there is far more to be learned than we know now. The United States Congress has declared the 1990s the "Decade of the Brain" with good reason. We are poised on the threshold of a truly deep understanding of the human brain and mind.

As our understanding of how the brain perceives, thinks, and remembers grows, so does our ability to devise machine intelligence much more capable than current computer hardware and software. Indeed, this has already begun to happen. When it was realized that the brain is not a serial processor of information but rather an extraordinarily complex *parallel* system, the field of computer science turned to a new kind of computer—massively parallel processors—that are only now being developed and used. The long-term possibilities have the flavor of science fiction and raise the most basic questions of philosophy and ethics. Can we someday create machine minds as capable, or even more capable, than the human mind in all its ramifications, including the ability to create and evaluate new concepts? (If this happens, the usefulness of scientists becomes problematic.) Can we someday develop instrumentation to "read" the mind? Can thoughts and knowledge someday be implanted in the mind or transferred from one mind to another? Can our intellectual capabilities someday be substantially enhanced by "symbiosis" with machine intelligence? These possibilities need not concern us now, but they may become realities for our grandchildren.

I thank Rosalinda Senaha for her heroic efforts in word-processing, Judith Thompson for preparing the Index, Dragana Ivkovich for preparing the Glossary, Martha Berg for preparing the Test Bank, and Stephanie Hauge for help with the Appendix. Thanks also to my many colleagues around the world who have made the study of the brain the most exciting field in all of the sciences.

R. F. T.
August 1993

THE BRAIN

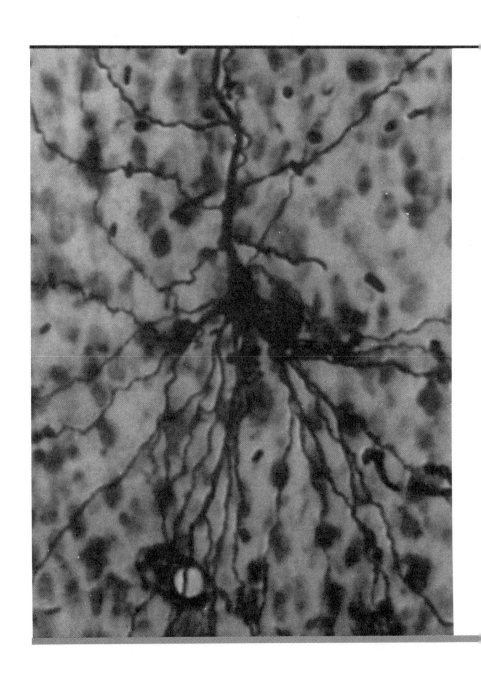

Brain and Neuron

The human brain is by far the most complex structure in the known universe. The extraordinary properties of this three or so pounds of soft tissue have made it possible for *Homo sapiens* to dominate the earth, change the course of evolution through genetic engineering, walk on the moon, and create art and music of surpassing beauty. We do not yet know the limits of the human mind and what it can accomplish.

Neuroscience, the study of the brain, is perhaps the most challenging and exciting field of science. Neuroscientists study all the aspects of the brain: its structure and how it develops, the chemical and electrical phenomena that take place in its nerve cells (neurons) and how they interact, and the brain's unique output, behavior, and experience. The study of the nervous system, particularly of its structure, or anatomy, and of its more elementary functions dates back many centuries, but the field of neuroscience as a unified discipline is only a few years old.

Figure 1-1 *Neuron from the visual cortex of the cat stained to show the cell body and all the fibers of the cell.*

The human brain is thought to consist of perhaps 100 billion (100,000,000,000, or 10^{11}) individual *neurons*. Each neuron is a separate cell. This fact, now taken for granted, only became firmly established at the beginning of the twentieth century. Until then, many anatomists believed that the brain was an exception to the basic biological principle that all tissues are made up of individual cells.

If a piece of brain tissue is stained with a substance that colors all the parts of cells, it will look like a continuous mass of tissue, a tangled web of fibers and processes with cell nuclei scattered throughout. In the late nineteenth century the anatomist Camillo Golgi happened on a special kind of stain that would color only an occasional neuron in brain tissue but would color that one completely. This stain makes it possible to see complete neurons, with all their processes (Figure 1-1). The discovery of the Golgi stain came about, according to the story, when a cleaning woman disposed of a piece of brain tissue from Golgi's desk in a waste bucket that happened to contain silver nitrate solution. Golgi returned and found the tissue, which had undergone the first successful Golgi stain.

Interestingly, Golgi himself did not believe in the "neuron doctrine," which sets forth that the brain is composed of individual neurons. Another anatomist, Ramón y Cajal, applied the Golgi stain systematically to the brain in animal studies and established that all the parts of the brain are composed of individual neurons. Cajal began the immensely complex task of working out the wiring diagram of the brain: the patterns of interconnections among the neurons.

The central character in this book is the neuron. We shall examine it in more detail in Chapter 2, but it is well to become familiar now with some basic features. A typical neuron consists of a *cell body* containing the nucleus and a number of fibers extending from it. The purpose of the neuron is to transmit information to other cells, and it does this by sending activity out just one fiber, the *axon*. All the other fibrous extensions of the cell body, the *dendrites*, receive information from other neurons. The axons of some neurons in the human body are a meter or more in length; other axons are not much longer than dendrites, which are tens to hundreds of micrometers in length.

The neuron is the functional unit of the brain. It receives information at its dendrites and cell body and sends the information out to other neurons and cells along its axon. The axon typically divides into a number of small fibers that end in terminals, each of which forms what is called a *synapse* with another cell. The synapse is the functional connection between the axon terminal and another neuron and is the point where information is transmitted from one neuron to another. A very tiny space, called the *synaptic cleft*, separates the axon terminal and the cell body or dendrite of the cell with which it synapses.

A given neuron in the brain may receive several thousand synaptic connections from other neurons. Hence if the human brain has 10^{11} neurons, then it has at least 10^{14} synapses, or many trillions. The number of possible different combinations of synaptic connections among the neurons in a single human brain is larger than the total number of atomic particles that make up the known universe. Hence the diversity of the interconnections in a human brain seems almost without limit.

The major pathways and systems of synaptic connections that develop in the brain are under genetic control and are formed before birth. However, we now think that many synaptic connections are formed and reformed throughout life. They are shaped and sculpted by experience and may form the structural basis of memory, the topic of Chapter 11.

Animals existed successfully and behaved in adaptive ways long before the neuron came into being. Indeed, some scientists feel that the bacterium can provide a useful model of the basic processes carried on by the brain. It senses stimuli, such as chemicals, and responds to them in ways that enable it, or at least its descendants, to survive.

CELLS, EVOLUTION, AND THE ORIGINS OF LIFE

A brief history of the origins of life and cells as they are thought to have occurred may be helpful to readers who are not familiar with the topic. All living species of animals and plants are made up of an extraordinary entity: the cell. To borrow an example of the diversity and unity of life from neurobiologist Donald Kennedy, consider a spruce and a moose. They are both living creatures, but when one sees them together populating a forest in, say, Montana, they seem very different. The spruce is a plant that can grow to be over 30 meters tall, never moves from its place of birth, and manufactures food from sunlight and carbon dioxide. Although the moose may be large by human standards, it is dwarfed by the spruce. The moose moves about, obtains its food by eating plants, and has a complex social life.

If one took a tiny bit of tissue from both the spruce and the moose and examined it under a microscope, the two creatures would suddenly look much more alike. Both are made up of cells that are similar in structure. Both types of cells have walls, and both contain *organelles*, or little organs. Each cell has a *nucleus*: a central region enclosed in its own membrane that contains the genetic material, the DNA (Figure 1-2). If one proceeds to the laboratory and examines the chemistry of the genetic material in the nucleus of a spruce cell and a moose cell, one would find that they have essentially identical chemical composition.

Cells that have a nucleus are called *eukaryotic* (from the Greek meaning good nucleus) cells. Many single-celled animals, such as the amoeba, and all multicell plants and animals alive today are eukaryotes. The common bacteria

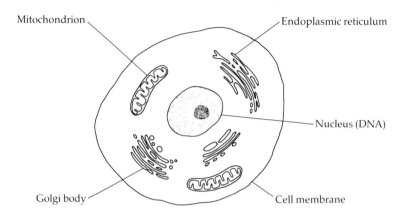

Figure 1-2 Typical eukaryotic ("good nucleus") animal cell. The genetic material (DNA) is contained in the nucleus, and several specialized organelles, or little organs, are present in the material of the cell outside the nucleus, the cytoplasm. The cell is covered by a thin wall, or membrane.

and blue-green algae are examples of about 1800 species of creatures living today that do not have a nucleus or separate organelles within the cell membrane. This type of cell is called a *prokaryotic* (from the Greek meaning before a nucleus) cell. Such cells evolved long before cells with a nucleus. Although there are relatively few species of prokaryotes, their numbers are legion. Twenty-eight grams (a single ounce) of good, fertile soil can contain as many as 70 billion individuals.

The viruses consist of a bit of genetic material (DNA or RNA) surrounded by a protein coat and are in many ways a mystery. They cause a wide range of diseases from the common cold to polio and some forms of cancer. Many biologists do not feel they should even be considered living things. Viruses cannot reproduce by themselves and so invade a host cell and make use of its machinery for the purpose. The biologist S. E. Luria, who won the Nobel prize in 1969 for his work on viruses, has described them as "bits of heredity looking for a chromosome."

The origin of life on earth is a fascinating puzzle. Because no fossil record of the earliest forms of life has yet been found, one can only make educated guesses about what they were like. The fossil record, and thus certain knowledge, begins with very early prokaryotic bacteria. The similarity of the genetic material in all forms of life that exist in the world today, including bacteria, plants, animals, and people, indicates that all living organisms descended from the same single-cell line.

How this cell line, destined for an incredible future, began is still not known. What follows is merely a good guess. Several billion years ago the oceans were filled with a vast array of organic molecules; they were an organic soup. However, these molecules could not reproduce, and the key to life is the ability to reproduce.

At some point a remarkable molecule appeared. It may not have been the most complicated molecule, but it had the unique ability to make copies of itself. This has been called the *replicator molecule*. It is not difficult to see how such a molecule might work. If it were reasonably large, it would consist of a number of smaller units, or building blocks. Suppose each of these blocks is itself a relatively simple compound that exerts a chemical attraction on an identical type of compound that is floating free in the organic soup. If the replicator molecule is a chain of such compounds, it will build up an identical chain attached to it. If they separate, each new replicator molecule can build another, and on and on.

Because the chemical composition of DNA is virtually the same in all living things, it seems likely that all life is descended from one type of replicator molecule. It is even possible that in the early world only one replicator molecule ever developed and developed only once. If other types did develop, their descendants died out.

The earth formed about 4.5 billion years ago. The time frame of the development of life can be likened to a football field, with a goal line representing the beginning. The first life appeared at the 20-yard line about 3.5 billion years ago; humans appeared on the scene at about the 99.99-yard line. The life forms seen in fossil records from very old rocks, for example, those found in Gun Flint, Ontario, were single cells, bacteria. The genetic material, the DNA, formed one long, convoluted molecule within the cell. These early bacteria were inefficient at utilizing energy.

Perhaps half a billion years later, certain bacteria evolved the ability to extract energy from sunlight and carbon dioxide, releasing oxygen. At the time the earth's atmosphere had less oxygen than it does now but much carbon dioxide. For a period of about 2.5 billion years, photosynthetic bacteria flourished and built up the amount of oxygen in the atmosphere. Then the other major cell type appeared: the eukaryotic cell. As we have seen, these cells all have a nucleus, containing the DNA, and several organelles.

Mitochondria (from the Greek for bread and grain) are among the most remarkable organelles in the cell. These small sausage-shaped objects are present in every cell of multicellular animals. They have one primary function, which is simple and essential for the life of the cell: they manufacture energy. All cellular processes require energy, and they obtain it largely from glucose, the form of sugar into which certain food substances are converted by the digestive system. In the mitochondria glucose and other food substances are metabolized to form substances that directly supply the cell with energy.

The internal structure of a mitochondrion is complex. Mitochondria may be the most remarkable organelles in cells because they have a life of their own. When a cell divides, each of the two new cells is allotted some mitochondria from the parent cell. If new cells could only acquire mitochondria in this way, as the cells continued to divide as an animal developed, soon there would not be enough of the original mitochondria to go around. The problem is solved by the mitochondria themselves dividing and forming new mito-chondria within the cell. A mitochondrion can reproduce itself because it has its own genetic material. Mitochondrial DNA is much smaller and simpler than the DNA in the cell nucleus since mitochondrial DNA is charged only with bringing about the division of the mitochondrion and a few relatively uncomplicated tasks, whereas the nuclear DNA must direct all the rest of the business of the cell.

Mitochondria closely resemble prokaryotic bacteria. Both have DNA that is not enclosed in a nucleus. Many biologists now think that the ancestors of mitochondria were free-living bacteria that at some point entered other cells and became symbiotes (from the Greek for living together), entering into a mutually helpful relation with the cell. The cell depends on the mito-chondria to supply it with energy, and mitochondria, which cannot make all the proteins they need to function properly, are provided with them by the host cell's DNA.

An intriguing fact about mitochondria is that all of them in all the cells of your body came from your mother. In sexual reproduction in vertebrates, the egg cell from the female has mitochondria but the sperm cell from the male does not. Hence, when you were first formed as a fertilized egg, all your mitochondria came from your mother's egg cell. As your cells divided and multiplied, so did your maternal mitochondria. And so has it been from the beginning of our species *Homo sapiens*. This fact led molecular geneticists to study the mutation rates of the genes in human mitochondria. An outcome of this work was the "Eve" hypothesis: the original mother of the entire human race lived in Africa about 200,000 years ago! Although this hypothesis is currently a matter of some dispute, it is a striking example of the application of the powerful tools of molecular biology to a question of profound human concern, the origin of our species.

Plant cells have organelles called *chloroplasts* that resemble mitochondria. The chloroplasts contain chlorophyll, which utilizes energy from sunlight and water and carbon dioxide to manufacture foods such as glucose, releasing oxygen in the process. It is thought that the chloroplasts were once free-living bacteria that found their way into the cells that were the ancestors of modern plants, much as the mitochondria did with animal cells.

After the appearance of eukaryotic, or nucleus-containing, cells, the pace of evolution accelerated. The next great step was the appearance of multicel-lular organisms. For the next half-billion years or so green plants and inver-tebrates (animals without backbones) invaded the land, which until that time had been completely empty of life. It provided a vast range of new ecological niches.

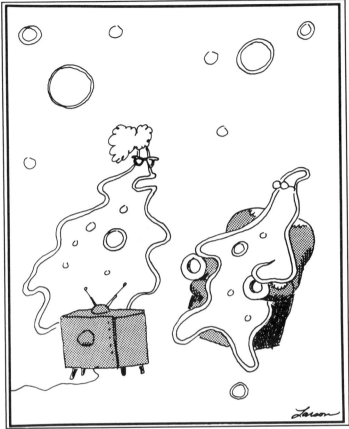

"Stimulus, response! Stimulus, response! Don't you ever *think?*"

EVOLUTION OF THE NERVOUS SYSTEM

Animals such as the sea anemone and the jellyfish developed the first nervous systems, which were simple nerve nets. The sponges, still more primitive animals, have no nervous system at all. A sponge does not behave, it just rests on the bottom of the sea. If nutrients are in the water, it lives; if not, it dies. The jellyfish and the sea anemone represent a great advance over the sponge because they behave; for example, a jellyfish can swim to where nutrients are and capture them. In order for a multicellular animal to move, its cells must somehow be made to move, and some accordingly have become specialized as muscle tissue that can contract. In order for these movements to accomplish anything they must somehow be controlled so that they occur together. Even in the sponge there is a small degree of coordination. If a sponge is prodded in one place, a limited movement of surrounding cells will occur. Hence the cells somehow communicate with one another. This communication is thought to be an electrochemical process that occurs at the cell membranes. Basically the same mechanism became elaborated into a specialized cell, the neuron, or nerve cell, that can communicate over longer distances. Groups of neurons could form larger systems, such as the nerve net of the jellyfish.

So far as is known, neurons in animals from jellyfishes to humans utilize the same basic electrochemical mechanisms for conducting information. The primitive mechanism of the jellyfish neuron worked so well that it became fixed in evolution. In order to progress beyond the jellyfishes' repertoire of behavior and generate more sophisticated and adaptive behaviors, what was primarily needed was more neurons put together in more complicated ways.

If one looks at the general structure of the nervous system in such diverse animals as earthworms, ants, octopuses, and humans, one might feel that nature has experimented endlessly with different kinds of nervous systems. But, as has been said, the basic mechanisms of action of the neurons in all of these creatures are the same. What is enormously different is the organization of the neurons, their patterns of interconnection.

Many invertebrates have relatively simple nervous systems, consisting of only a few thousand neurons. In these animals, many of the neurons can be individually identified by their location and appearance and by their particular functions. The vertebrate nervous system has taken a different track. Each small region of the brain has thousands or millions of neurons. These can be categorized into just a few types on the basis of their appearance, but the number of each type is astronomical. An individual cell cannot be identified, although each type can.

The vast increase in the number of neurons in the vertebrate brain is the ultimate reason for the development of more complex aspects of behavior and experience: the extraordinary increase in "intelligence" that occurred throughout the evolution of the vertebrates. The mind cannot exist in a single neuron; it is the product of the interaction among the myriad of neurons in the vertebrate brain.

The vertebrate brain represents the continuation of a trend already established in the primitive "brains" of worms (Figure 1-3). The nervous system of the worm is a series of collections of neurons, called *ganglia*. Each ganglion is concerned with a local segment of the animal's body. A ganglion has *input fibers* from sensory detectors on the skin of the segment, *interneurons* that run entirely within the ganglion, and *output* or *motor neurons* that control the movement of the segment. The separate ganglia would not be enough of a nervous system for the worm to behave adaptively; the actions of the ganglia must all be coordinated by the nerve pathways that interconnect

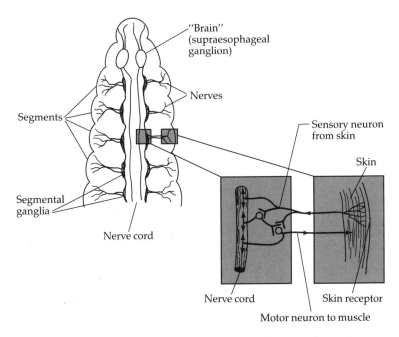

Figure 1-3 Basic plan of a primitive nervous system is shown in the earthworm. The body and nerve cord are made up of segments. Within a segment the nerve cord receives sensory information from skin receptors and sends out motor commands to the muscle cells.

them. The ganglion at the head end of the worm, which is larger than the others, performs this coordinating role and also receives additional sensory input from the "head" of the worm. The head ganglion is the beginning of a brain.

The brains of the most primitive vertebrates were not much more complicated than the brain of a worm. Over the course of evolution, the head ganglion became larger and took more and more command over the other ganglia. The basic plan of the vertebrate brain can be seen most clearly in the stages of embryological development, because the growth and development of the individual animal from the fertilized ovum to the newborn tends to reflect evolutionary history. The growth and development of the brain will be examined in more detail in Chapter 10. In brief, the vertebrate nervous system begins as a relatively straight tube; then at an early stage three enlargements develop at the head end, destined to become the forebrain, the midbrain, and the hindbrain. At the next stage the forebrain and hindbrain differentiate further, and the cerebral hemispheres of the forebrain (in higher vertebrates) grow out and over the lower brain regions.

A BRIEF TOUR OF THE BRAIN

The gross neuroanatomy of the human brain, or its general structural organization, is difficult to learn because it does not seem to make sense. The structure of the nervous systems of such primitive animals as the worm do make sense: there is sensory input, some central processing, and motor output. As the brain evolved, new structures developed and overshadowed older regions. The older regions usually have not disappeared but may have assumed different roles. Evolution tends to be conservative: use continues to be made of what has developed. The overall structure of the human brain makes sense only if it is viewed in the context of evolution.

I shall present here a very brief overview of the major regions and structures of the vertebrate brain; details on important structures and systems will be provided later in the text. It would perhaps be best to read the rest of this chapter without trying to memorize all the new terms, and then refer to this catalogue of brain structures as necessary when reading later chapters.

The brain and spinal cord constitute the *central nervous system* (CNS). The major regions of the brain are shown in Figure 1-4. The *cerebrum* overlies brain stem structures, as does the *cerebellum*. The lower portion of the brain stem is called the *medulla;* the portion just above it with an enlarged ventral region is the *pons,* with the cerebellum overlying it, and the upper portion of the brain stem is called the *midbrain.* Above, or anterior, to the brain stem and midbrain are the *thalamus* and *hypothalamus* and the structures of the cerebrum, including the *cerebral cortex,* the *basal ganglia,* and the *limbic system.* The hindbrain of the human, particularly in the medulla and midbrain, is a continuation of the tubular organization of the spinal cord and resembles the worm's nervous system. However, the forebrain of the higher mammals has so enlarged that it constitutes most of the brain.

In the spinal cord, neuron cell bodies form *nuclei,* or collections of cells, lying in the central core and are surrounded by *fiber tracts* made up of neuron axons. In the cerebellum and cerebrum, however, neuron cell bodies in a layer about two to three millimeters thick surround the more centrally lying fiber tracts. In each case several nuclei are buried within the central core region— the thalamus and basal ganglia within the cerebrum and the cerebellar nuclei within the cerebellum.

Interactions among neurons occur largely in the vicinity of the neuron cell bodies, where axon terminals synapse with the cell bodies, with dendrites, or with other axon terminals. Thus the *gray matter,* which consists of neuron cell bodies and forms the cerebral cortex and subcortical nuclei, is the site of neuronal interactions. *White matter* is made up of fibers that simply connect different regions of gray matter.

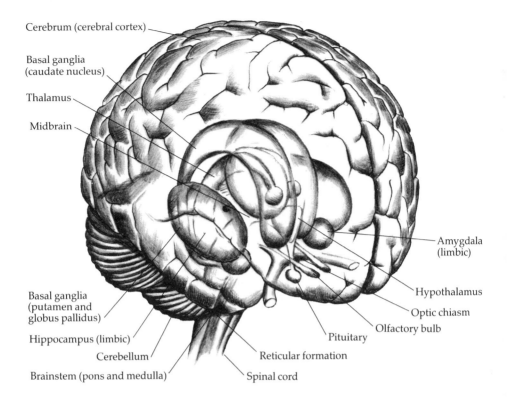

Cerebrum (cerebral cortex)

Basal ganglia (caudate nucleus)

Thalamus

Midbrain

Amygdala (limbic)

Basal ganglia (putamen and globus pallidus)

Hippocampus (limbic)

Cerebellum

Brainstem (pons and medulla)

Hypothalamus

Optic chiasm

Olfactory bulb

Pituitary

Reticular formation

Spinal cord

Figure 1-4 Human brain. Many structures are buried within the vast forebrain or cerebrum, covered by the cerebral cortex. Some of these in the forebrain are the basal ganglia (caudate, putamen, and globus pallidus), the thalamus, the hippocampus, and the amygdala. Lower structures include the hypothalamus, the midbrain, the brain stem (pons and medulla), and the cerebellum. The pituitary gland is just below the hypothalamus and connected to it, but the pineal gland is entirely outside the brain. Other structures shown include the partial crossing of the optic nerves from the eyes (optic chiasm) and the olfactory bulb. The spinal cord is the downward continuation of the nervous system from the brain.

Peripheral Nervous System

Somatic Nerves   Nerves are bundles of neuron fibers. The nerves in the body and head that carry information to and from the central nervous system are called the *peripheral nerves*. The peripheral nerves that connect with the voluntary skeletal muscles and a variety of sensory receptors are called *somatic nerves*. Throughout most of their length in the body the peripheral nerves are mixed: they consist of both incoming (afferent) *sensory fibers* carrying information from receptors of the skin, muscles, and joints to the spinal cord and of outgoing (efferent) *motor fibers* conveying activity from the spinal cord and brain stem motor neurons to muscle fibers (Figure 1-5).

The motor nerve fibers project from cell bodies in the ventral part of the central gray matter within the cord. The axons of these motor neurons go out through the ventral root of the cord, which contains only motor fibers, and then meet up with sensory fibers and form mixed nerves, which travel to various body structures. As the mixed nerves approach the regions where they terminate, the motor and sensory fibers again separate and go to their appropriate locations, for example, a muscle or the skin, respectively.

Autonomic Nerves Autonomic nerves travel to structures such as the internal organs and the glands involved in the autonomic aspects of responding commonly related to emotional behavior, such as crying, sweating, and certain activities of the stomach and heart. The autonomic nervous system is divided into the *sympathetic* ("emergency") and *parasympathetic* ("self-sustaining") systems, each of which has somewhat different connections.

In brief, the motor neurons for the parasympathetic ganglia lie in the brain stem and lower end of the spinal cord. They send motor nerves to their target organs, for example, the heart and the stomach, where they synapse on local ganglia (collections of nerve cell bodies). The local ganglia act on the target organs. In the sympathetic system, on the other hand, motor neurons lie in the spinal cord and send motor nerves to synapse on a chain of local ganglia

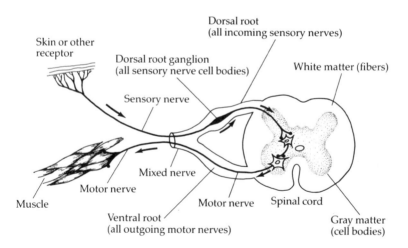

Figure 1-5 Cross section of the spinal cord. Most nerves in the body are mixed, meaning that they contain both sensory and motor fibers, but the two types of fibers separate as they enter the spinal cord into the dorsal sensory nerve or "root" and the ventral motor root.

that lie just outside the spinal cord (the sympathetic ganglia). These in turn send sympathetic neurons to the same target organs innervated (connected) by the parasympathetic neurons. All of the body organs have this dual innervation; they are controlled by both the sympathetic (emergency) and parasympathetic (self-sustaining) parts of the autonomic nervous system. An example of this dual autonomic innervation is shown for the heart in Chapter 5 (Figure 5-7).

Cranial Nerves

The cranial nerves are not really different in principle from the spinal nerves, except that they enter and leave the brain rather than the spinal cord. There are twelve cranial nerves, numbered I to XII from the front to the back of the brain. They convey sensory information from the face and head and commands for motor control of movements of the face and head. The frontmost nerve, the olfactory nerve (I), transmits information about odors from the nose to the brain, and the optic nerve (II) conveys visual information from the eyes. Another sensory nerve of particular importance is the auditory–vestibular nerve (VIII), conveying information about sounds from the ears and about the sense of balance from the vestibular apparatus. Skin sensory information from the face and head is transmitted to the brain via the trigeminal nerve (V). Three cranial nerves are devoted to the control of eye movements, indicative of the importance of this behavior for vertebrates. The vagus cranial nerve (X) plays a major role in the autonomic (parasympathetic) control of the heart and other internal organs.

Spinal Cord

Two general categories of activity are handled by the spinal cord. One is *spinal reflexes:* muscular and autonomic responses to bodily stimuli that occur even after the spinal cord has been severed from the brain, as in a paraplegic accident victim. In addition, a wide variety of *supraspinal activity,* passing up and down between the spinal cord and the brain, is channeled through the spinal cord. The cerebral cortex and other brain structures controlling the movement of the body send information down the spinal cord to motor neurons (which connect to the muscles), and all bodily sensations are conveyed up the spinal cord to the brain. Analogous sensory and motor relations for the head are handled directly by the cranial nerves and brain.

A schematic cross section of the spinal cord was shown in Figure 1-5. The incoming dorsal root fibers and the outgoing ventral root fibers separate each half of the cord into dorsal, lateral, and ventral regions of white matter. Remember that white matter is composed simply of nerve fibers. The dorsal (top) region of white matter is almost entirely taken up by ascending fibers conveying sensory information to the brain, whereas the more lateral (side) and ventral (bottom) portion is taken up almost entirely by descending (motor) fiber systems.

Brain Stem: Medulla and Pons

The medulla is the continuation of the spinal cord in the brain and contains all the ascending and descending fiber tracts interconnecting the brain and spinal cord, together with a number of important neuron cell nuclei. The majority of the cranial nerves enter and leave the brain from the medulla and the bordering region of pons. In addition, several vital autonomic nuclei concerned with respiration, heart action, and gastrointestinal function are in the medulla (Figure 1-4).

The pons is the upward continuation of the brain stem and contains ascending and descending fiber tracts and many additional nuclei. A large bundle of crossing fibers lying on the lower aspect of the pons interconnects the brain stem and cerebellum. Several cranial nerve nuclei found in the pons play a major role in feeding behavior and in facial expression (Figure 1-4).

Midbrain

The midbrain (mesencephalon) is the most anterior continuation of the brain stem that still maintains the basic tubular strucure of the spinal cord. It merges anteriorly into the thalamus and hypothalamus. The top portion of the midbrain (the *tectum*) contains nuclei important for the visual and auditory systems. The bottom portion of the midbrain contains nuclei for the cranial nerves that control eye movement and lower portions of the brain. A large nucleus called the *red nucleus* is found here, as is a collection of dark, heavily pigmented cells, the *substantia nigra*. These structures are involved in the control of movement; Parkinson's disease is associated with degeneration of neurons in the substantia nigra.

The medulla, pons, and midbrain developed early in the course of evolution and are surprisingly uniform in structure and organization from fish to humans, although there are, of course, some variations among species. A general principle of neural organization states that the size and complexity of a structure are related to the behavioral importance of the structure. Among mammals, the bat has a much enlarged inferior colliculus (midbrain auditory relay nucleus), which correlates with its extensive use of auditory information.

(The bat employs a sonarlike system, emitting high-frequency sound pulses to determine the location of objects in space by the echo sounds of the reflected pulses.) The principle of the relation of structure size and complexity to behavioral importance has supplied a number of clues about the possible functions of brain structures.

Cerebellum

The cerebellum is a phylogenetically old structure and was probably the first to be specialized for sensory–motor coordination. It overlies the pons and typically presents a much convoluted appearance, having a large number of lobules separated by fissures (Figure 1-4). As in the cerebral cortex, the neuron cell bodies form a surface layer about two to three millimeters thick that covers the underlying white matter and the cerebellar nuclei. In terms of the organization of neurons, the cerebellar cortex presents a remarkably uniform appearance, in contrast to such structures as the cerebral cortex, which exhibits marked regional characteristics. The cortex and underlying nuclei of the cerebellum receive connections from the *vestibular system* (the balance system in the inner ear), from spinal and cranial sensory fibers, from the auditory and visual systems, from various regions of the cerebral cortex, and from the brain stem. The cerebellum sends motor fibers to the thalamus, brain stem, and several other structures. Although it is probably involved in a number of other functions as well, the cerebellum is primarily concerned with the regulation of motor coordination. Removal of the cerebellum produces a characteristic syndrome (set of symptoms) of jerky, uncoordinated movement. The cerebellum also appears to play an important role in learning.

Thalamus

The thalamus is a large group of nuclei situated just anterior and dorsal to the midbrain (Figure 1-4). In gross appearance it consists of two small ovoids, one within each cerebral hemisphere, or half, of the brain. The thalamus is the final relay station for the major sensory systems that project to the cerebral cortex: the visual, auditory, and somatic sensory systems. It also contains other nuclei, some of which project to still other regions of the cerebral cortex, and receives projections from the cerebral cortex.

Hypothalamus

The hypothalamus is a grouping of small nuclei that lie generally in the lower portion of the cerebrum at the junction of the midbrain and the thalamus

(Figure 1-4). The nuclei lie along the base of the brain (above the roof of the mouth) and are adjacent to the pituitary gland, the master endocrine gland, which is innervated by neurons from the hypothalamus. The hypothalamus interconnects with many regions of the brain. A number of these structures, including the limbic cortex (the part of the cortex that developed first in evolution), portions of the olfactory system, the hippocampus, the septal area, the amygdala, and the hypothalamus itself, are viewed by many anatomists as composing an integrated network of structures called the limbic system.

The *pituitary gland* is under the control of hormones secreted by the near-by hypothalamus. The 1977 Nobel prize in physiology and medicine was awarded to Roger Guillemin and Andrew Schally in part for their discovery of certain critical interrelations between the pituitary gland and the hypo-thalamus. The hypothalamus exerts powerful control over a wide range of body functions, in part by its control over the pituitary gland. The body has two kinds of glands. One type, the *exocrine glands*, secrete onto a body surface (sweat or tear glands) or into body cavities (digestive glands). The other type, the *endocrine glands*, secrete *hormones* directly into the bloodstream, which transports them to act on various body and brain tissues. Hormones strongly affect such diverse events as physical growth, fight or flight reactions, sexual responses, and many other physical expressions of mental states.

The hypothalamus and pituitary act together as a master control system. The hormones they release act on the other endocrine glands to control the hormones that these glands in turn release. The hormones released by the endocrine glands then act back on the pituitary gland and hypothalamus to regulate their activity, an example of feedback control. Chemically, the hor-mones released by the hypothalamus and pituitary and some from other en-docrine glands are *peptides*, or chains of amino acids. Proteins have the same kind of structure but are much larger than the hormone peptides. A hormone peptide, then, is like a relatively small piece of a protein molecule. Many hormones released by the other endocrine glands have a different chemical structure; they are called *steroids* and do not contain amino acids. As we shall see in Chapter 6, hormones act as a type of chemical "transmitter," influenc-ing the activities of neurons and body tissues.

The hypothalamus also seems to be the master control center for emo-tion. Electrical stimulation in one part of the hypothalamus (and in certain regions of the limbic system) can elicit full-blown rage and attack behavior in humans and other animals. Stimulation of a closely adjacent region of the hypothalamus produces a feeling of intense pleasure. This discovery of the brain's "pleasure centers" in 1954 by James Olds and Peter Milner, then at McGill University, was a critical step in understanding brain mechanisms of motivation and reward. Actually, both the hypothalamus and certain other limbic structures seem to form a pleasure system in the brain.

Limbic System

The main structures of the limbic system are the *amygdala,* the *hippocampus,* adjacent regions of the *limbic cortex,* and the *septal area.* These structures form major interconnections with portions of the hypothalamus and with portions of the thalamus and the cerebral cortex (cingulate gyrus).

The general region of the brain that includes the limbic system is shown in Figure 1-6. The limbic system includes structures around the core of the medial (toward the middle) region of the brain and extends down and around to the right into the temporal lobes. During evolution the limbic system was the earliest form of forebrain to develop; for example, essentially the entire forebrain of the crocodile is limbic brain. No negative inferences about the function of the limbic forebrain or of crocodiles are meant, for in addition to being vicious, the crocodile is an intact, functioning organism responsive to sensory stimulation and engaging in a variety of behaviors: feeding, fleeing, fighting, and reproduction.

In relatively primitive beasts, such as the crocodile, much of the limbic forebrain has to do with olfaction, the complex analysis of the intensity, quality, and direction of odors. The limbic forebrain first evolved to provide a

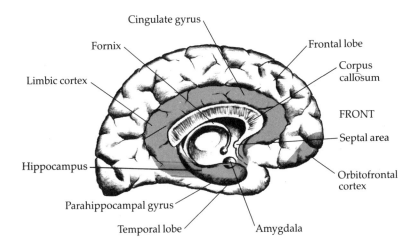

Figure 1-6 Limbic system. The view is of the midline, or medial, wall of the brain. The major parts are the hippocampus and the amygdala, which are buried in the depths of the temporal lobe, the septal area, and several regions of cerebral cortex surrounding the corpus callosum: the cingulate gyrus, the parahippocampal gyrus, and the orbitofrontal cortex. The fornix is a large bundle of nerve fibers interconnecting portions of the limbic system (e.g., hippocampus and septal area).

sophisticated analysis of olfactory stimuli and appropriate responses to those stimuli: approach, attack, mate, or flee. In the course of evolution, much of the specific olfactory function of the limbic system seems to have been lost. Among higher animals, only a portion of the amygdala has direct projections from the olfactory system, although important secondary olfactory projections to the hypothalamus, septal area, and hippocampus remain. However, some structures of the limbic system, such as the hippocampus, have taken on other, quite different functions as well over the course of evolution. The hippocampus, for example, is thought to be involved in learning and memory.

Basal Ganglia

The group of large nuclei lying in the central regions of the cerebral hemispheres are called the basal ganglia (Figure 1-4). They partially surround the thalamus and are themselves enclosed by the cerebral cortex and cerebral white matter. These nuclei, collectively termed the *corpus striatum*, appear to play a role in the control of movement and form the major part of the *extrapyramidal motor system*. The other major motor system, the *pyramidal system*, originates in the cerebral cortex. The two major structures of the basal ganglia are the *caudate nucleus* and the *putamen* and *globus pallidus*, which connect to the cortex, the thalamus, the reticular formation, portions of the midbrain, and the spinal cord. The substantia nigra and the red nucleus of the midbrain, which are usually included in the extrapyramidal motor system, also have connections with the corpus striatum.

Cerebral Cortex

The cerebral cortex is what makes human beings what they are. Within the vast human cortex lies a critical part of the secret of human consciousness, our superb sensory capacities and sensitivities to the external world, our motor skills, our aptitudes for reasoning and imagining, and above all our unique language abilities.

Studies of individuals who had suffered various types of brain damage yielded the first clues that certain regions of the cerebral cortex are specialized for very complex abilities and aspects of consciousness. In right-handed people, damage to a part of the cerebral cortex in the left hemisphere essentially abolishes a person's ability to understand or speak intelligibly. Damage to the corresponding part of the right hemisphere has no effect on language skills. However, right-handed people with right-hemisphere damage have great difficulty in performing spatial tasks. They lose their way, forget well-traveled routes, and have difficulty in understanding complex diagrams and pictures.

Perhaps the most remarkable discovery about the human cerebral cortex came from the work of Roger Sperry and his colleagues at the California Institute of Technology on split-brain patients. In these patients the major pathway that interconnects the cerebral cortex of the two hemispheres of the brain (the *corpus callosum*) had been severed surgically to treat severe epileptic conditions. Sperry found that consciousness and awareness seemed to exist separately and independently in the two cerebral hemispheres in the patients. The left cerebral cortex was found to have awareness that could be expressed with language, whereas the right cerebral cortex had its own form of nonverbal awareness. In normal people, of course, the two hemispheres are interconnected and work closely together. Sperry was awarded the Nobel prize in 1981 for his work.

The cerebral cortex is the brain's outer covering of cells. It is composed of neurons and other kinds of cells and forms a layer about three millimeters thick over the rest of the brain. In pictures of the human brain, the outer surface of the two hemispheres is the cerebral cortex.

If you look at a section of the cortex, going down from the top you will see distinct layers of groupings of cell bodies and fibers (Figure 1-7). There are six layers, starting with layer 1 at the surface and ending with layer 6 at the bottom. A few characteristic neurons are shown in their layers at the left of Figure 1-7. The actual appearance of cell bodies is shown in the middle and the fiber processes are shown at the right. If you look closely at the middle of the diagram you will see columns of cells and at the right fibers running up and down the cortex at right angles to the six layers. It is only in the past few years that we have come to the view that these columns of cells in the cerebral cortex are its basic functional units. In sensory areas of the cerebral cortex the columns seem to correspond to the basic elements of the experience of sensation. We shall return to the columnar organization of the cerebral cortex in Chapter 8.

Looking over the whole surface of the cortex, one can divide it into a number of areas or regions. Perhaps the easiest to identify are the sensory areas. Sensory information coming from sense organs such as the eye and the ear project to specific areas of the cerebral cortex. Visual information projects to the back or *occipital region* (Figure 1-8), information from the skin and body projects to a middle or *parietal region,* and auditory information projects to the *auditory cortex,* buried in the depths of the Sylvian fissure. Just in front of the body region is the motor or *precentral cortex,* the cortical area most concerned with the control of movement.

Each sensory field of the cerebral cortex contains a "map," or spatial layout, of its receptor surface. For the body surface, this is an actual map of it on the cortex. For the eye, a map is formed of the sensory-receptive surface at the back of the eye, the retina. Since the lens of the eye projects a two-dimensional image or map of the external world on the retina, the visual area of the cerebral cortex displays a map of the visual world a person looks at. The

Layers   TOP

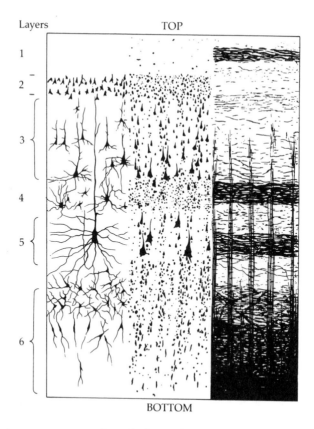

BOTTOM

Figure 1-7 A cross section cut through the cerebral cortex showing the six layers from top to bottom. On the left side of the drawing are a few typical neurons, the center shows the distribution of neuron cell bodies, and the right shows the organization of neuron fibers. Note at the center and right what appear to be columns of cell bodies and fibers running from top to bottom through the layers.

cortical receptor surface from the ear is not so simple; it reflects the sheet of hair-cell receptors along the cochlea, a structure of the inner ear. The frequencies of sounds seem to be coded by places on the cochlea. It appears that there is a spatial sound-frequency map along the auditory area of the cerebral cortex.

Many areas of the cerebral cortex can also be identified in terms of the cross-sectional appearance or architecture of the cells (Figure 1-7). Neurons carrying sensory information that project from below the cortex to cortical sensory areas always project to cells in layer 4, and consequently layer 4 is much enlarged in the visual, body–skin, and auditory areas. The neurons that send axons down from the cerebral cortex to lower regions of the brain and the spinal cord structures are mostly in layers 5 and 6. In layer 5 of the motor cortex, where axons are sent down to the spinal cord to control movements,

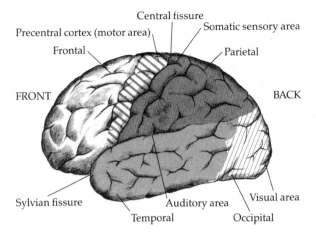

Figure 1-8 Major subdivisions of the cerebral cortex. The central fissure separates the frontal and parietal lobes or areas and the Sylvian fissure separates the temporal lobe from the rest of the cortex. The occipital lobe is at the back of the brain.

many of the neurons have giant cell bodies; these are the Betz cells. Many other areas of the cerebral cortex can also be distinguished on the basis of the appearance of the cells. Authorities disagree on the number of areas in the human cerebral cortex; estimates range from a few to over 200. Everyone agrees, however, on the basic sensory areas and the motor area.

The remainder of the cerebral cortex is arbitrarily called *association cortex*. We are only beginning to understand the functions of some of the association areas, which occupy a great deal of the cerebral cortex in humans and other primates. Interestingly, the basic organization of the primary sensory and motor areas of the cerebral cortex is virtually the same in all mammals, from the rat to the human. As one ascends the mammalian scale of evolution, however, both the brain's absolute size and the relative amount of association cortex increase strikingly (Figure 1-9).

BRAIN SIZE

Humans, incidentally, do not have the largest brains. Porpoises, whales, and elephants have larger ones, although the density of their brain cells may be lower than those of the human brain. Humans do have the greatest brain size relative to the body size. The gorilla, a close relative of humans, is physically larger than a human yet has a brain of only one-fourth the size of the human one.

Figure 1-9 Approximate-scale sketches of the cerebral hemispheres of four mammals. Note the increase in absolute size, the increase in the number of fissures, and the vast increase in association cortex.

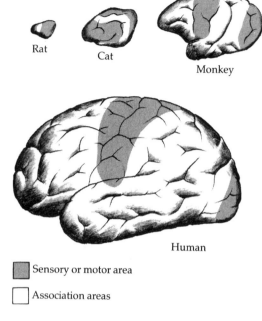

Rat

Cat

Monkey

Human

▨ Sensory or motor area

☐ Association areas

The evolutionary lines leading to humans and the modern great apes began to diverge perhaps 15 million years ago. During most of the ensuing time the increase in brain size of the humans-to-be was not great. Australopithecus, the first creature that could be called an ape-man rather than an ape, lived about 3 to 4 million years ago. It had an upright posture and walked on two legs with the skull balanced above the backbone in human fashion. However, the brain was not much larger than that of the modern chimpanzee.

Fossil evidence indicates that australopithecines were toolmakers. Humans did not develop a large brain by chance and then stand up and start making tools. Upright posture came first, freeing the hands of early ape-men to use rocks and branches as tools and weapons. Upright posture raised their heads above the grasses and presumably helped them to see distant game and enemies. Some 10 million years passed between apes and Australopithecus. However, virtually no increase in brain size occurred over this long span of early human evolution.

The remarkable and still mysterious explosion in brain size of the developing humans took place within the past 3 million years or so, long after our ancestors had become upright ape-men rather than apes. Virtually all of the increase in brain size was due to the extraordinary expansion of the cerebral cortex. As yet we have no very clear understanding of why this happened. The massive change in the human brain over the short span of 3 million years is unprecedented in the evolution of other species.

COMMENT

In this brief tour of the brain, a number of specific structures, such as the basal ganglia, hippocampus, and cerebral cortex, have been mentioned and dia-grammed. It is easy to get the impression that the brain is like a stereo, with various specific components such as a receiver, a tuner, and an amplifier. The brain is not really like that at all. Its various structures were given particular names because they look like particular structures to the naked eye or in a light microscope (the hippocampus looks like what its name means in Greek: sea horse). However, in a sense they are not really structures but simply collec-tions of cell bodies or fibers or both that can be identified by their appearance. The brain is a vast network of connections among neurons.

At each point where a nerve fiber forms a connection or synapse onto another neuron, information is transferred and may be transformed or pro-cessed. Information is continuously flowing through the multitude of synaptic contacts and networks in the brain. During evolution certain regions of cell bodies where these connections occur have expanded enormously, as in the human cerebral cortex. The brain is not simply a collection of special struc-tures but a vast information-processing system.

SUMMARY

The functional elements in the brain are neurons, individual nerve cells that became specialized early in evolution (jellyfish) to transmit information. Neurons are like other cells in the body; they contain a nucleus composed of DNA (the genetic material) and other organelles. The mitochondria are the energy-producing organelles in neurons and all other cells (all your mitochondria came from your mother). The evolution of the nervous system from jellyfish to humans involved primarily vast increases in the numbers and complexity of interconnections of neurons; the basic properties of neurons have not changed much. The major change is the vast increase in the size and complexity of the head ganglion, the brain. The basic plan of the human brain and the nervous system can be seen in the worm. Segments of the body involve sensory input, central processing, and motor output.

The basic organization of the human brain makes sense only if viewed in the context of evolution. The development of the brain in an embryo from conception to birth displays many of the aspects of evolution. The human nervous system begins as a tube, much like the mature nervous system of the worm, that ultimately forms the spinal cord. Enlargements begin at the front of the tube and form the brain stem, midbrain, and forebrain. Somatic nerves carry information to and from the nervous system for skin and muscles; the cranial nerves connect to the brain. The autonomic nerves connect to body organs (heart, stomach) and subserve emergency (sympathetic) and self-sustaining (parasympathetic) functions. The spinal cord controls reflexes and carries information between the body and brain. The brain stem is a tubular continuation of the spinal cord that contains nuclei (collections of nerve cell bodies) for most of the cranial nerves.

The cerebellum (little cerebrum) develops from the brain stem into a large structure with an extensive cortex (layers of nerve cell bodies and connections). It is a very old structure and is primarily involved in the coordination and control of movement. The hypothalamus, at the junction of the brain stem and forebrain, is the key brain structure concerned with motivation and emotion and controls the endocrine (pituitary gland) and autonomic systems.

The forebrain contains a number of recently evolved structures. The thalamus contains the major relay nuclei between the cerebral cortex and sensory and motor systems. The limbic system—the amygdala, the hippocampus, and adjoining regions of cerebral cortex—forms major interconnections with the hypothalamus and the autonomic nervous system. The amygdala seems particularly involved in emotion and the hippocampus plays a key role in memory in higher animals. The basal ganglia are large structures in the depth of the forebrain concerned primarily with movement control. The cerebral cortex, the outer covering of the forebrain, is a vast collection of nerve cell bodies and connections. It has expanded enormously in the course of evolution and is what makes us human. It plays the key role in consciousness, our superb sensory capacities, language, and thought. It is everywhere composed of six layers of neurons, each layer many neurons thick, which show specializations in different regions of the cortex, as in sensory receiving areas, motor control areas, and association areas. The cerebral cortex has evolved incredibly in the past 3 million years, leading to the modern brain of Homo sapiens.

SUGGESTED READINGS AND REFERENCES

Books

Adelman, G. (1987). Encyclopedia of neuroscience. Boston: Birkhauser.

Brodal, A. (1981). Neurological anatomy in relation to clinical medicine. Oxford: Oxford University Press.

Carpenter, M. B. (1985). Neuroanatomy (3rd ed.). Baltimore: Williams & Wilkins.

Changeux, J.-P. (1985). Neuronal man: The biology of man. New York: Pantheon Books.

Granit, R. (1977). The purposive brain. Cambridge, MA: MIT Press.

Heimer, L. (1983). The human brain and spinal cord: Functional neuroanatomy and dissection guide. New York: Springer-Verlag.

Nauta, W. J. H., and Feirtag, M. (Eds.) (1986). Fundamental neuroanatomy. New York: W. H. Freeman.

Ornstein, R., and Thompson, R. F. (1984). *The amazing brain.* Boston: Houghton Mifflin.

Sacks, O. (1987). *The man who mistook his wife for a hat and other clinical tales.* New York: Harper & Row.

Mind and brain (1992). Readings from *Scientific American.* New York: W. H. Freeman.

Young, J. Z. (1978). *Programs of the brain.* London: Oxford University Press.

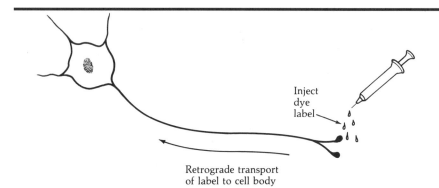

Inject
dye
label

Retrograde transport
of label to cell body

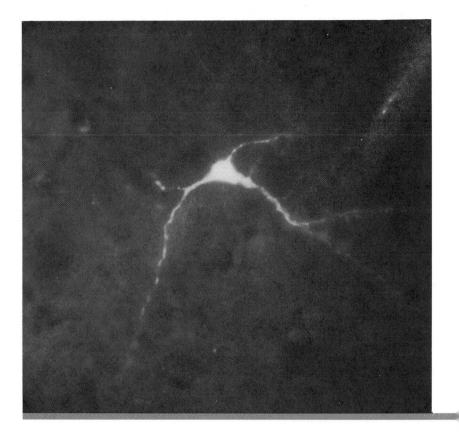

2

Neuron

The brain is made up of individual nerve cells, or neurons. In most ways, neurons are like all other cells in the human body. They have become specialized in only one major way: to transmit information to other neurons or to muscle or gland cells. In order to understand the brain it is necessary to understand the neuron, the basic functional unit in the brain. The brain is what it is because of its structural and functional organization: how the neurons are put together, that is, the brain's wiring diagrams, and how the neurons interact or function together. Understanding the neuron is the first necessary step to understanding the brain.

There have been several important technological developments in the past 50 years or so in the study of the brain (Figure 2-1). The first development came about 50 years ago with the introduction of the microelectrode. A microelectrode is an extremely fine wire or glass tube electrode that makes possible measurement of the electrical activity of single neurons in the brain.

Figure 2-1 Example of a neuron identified by retrograde axoplasmic transport of dyes, a method used to map neuron pathways. A dye or label substance is injected into the region of the axon terminals (above). They take it up and transport it backward to the cell body, where it "lights up" the cell body. The black-and-white photograph (below) shows the dye (fluorogold) in the cell body and dendrites as white.

Much of the current understanding of how the brain works has come from experiments with the microelectrode, for example, how cells communicate at synapses and how the visual part of the brain analyzes visual stimuli to produce the experience of seeing.

A second development has occurred more slowly and is only now in full swing. It has to do with the chemistry of the neuron. Scientists had realized for some time that most neurons in the brain communicate or influence other neurons and muscle and gland cells by releasing tiny amounts of chemicals onto them. These chemicals are termed *neurotransmitter chemicals*, or transmitters. Much of the new knowledge about the brain has come from discoveries about the chemical transmitters of the neuron.

A third development concerns the anatomy, or structures, of neurons and their patterns of interconnection. The electron microscope opened to view a whole new world of microstructures in the neuron. The detailed tracing of nerve pathways in the brain has become possible with the development of labeling techniques: substances that stain neurons or can otherwise be detected are applied to neuron cell bodies or axon terminals, from which the substances are transported out or back on the axons, providing pictures of pathways. With still other techniques, neurons that are more active than others can be labeled.

The most recent development concerns the applications of modern discoveries and technology from molecular biology to the study of neuron and brain. Ultimately, the structures of neurons and the chemicals they make and use derive from the genes. But genes are involved not only in the building of the brain. They actively regulate processes in neurons and other cells throughout life. Study of changes in *gene expression*, resulting in the manufacture of more or less or different proteins that control nerve cell function, is only at its beginning now. It is estimated that there are about 100,000 different genes that make up the chromosomes (DNA) in mammalian cells. The brain utilizes perhaps 50,000 of these genes. Importantly, 30,000 or more of these genes may be unique to the brain. They are of course present in all cells, but they function only in nerve cells.

All of these developments focus primarily on the single neuron, particularly on how it functions electrically, chemically, and metabolically. Fortunately, the basic principles of how the neuron works are quite simple, as we shall see.

CELLS AND NEURONS

Neurons, along with all other cells in multicellular organisms, both plant and animal, have a well-developed cell nucleus that contains the genetic material, DNA, in chromosomes. One major difference between neurons and other cells, however, is that after a certain point neurons never reproduce. As an animal develops from a fertilized egg, neurons of course develop and multiply to form the brain and the rest of the nervous system. In mammals, by the time of birth this process has almost stopped. In fact, in some parts of the brain, there are more cells present at birth than later in life, because some die. However, in contrast to most other cells in the body, after this point, shortly after birth, no neuron will ever divide again: no new neurons are formed.

Particular behaviors and behavior sequences are clearly the result of the development of particular sets of connections, or wiring diagrams, among the neurons in the brain. If the neurons divided and formed new cells, these patterns of connections might be lost.

There are exceptions to this rule. Perhaps the most striking is seen in seasonal songbirds such as the canary. Each year, as mating season approaches, the male canary composes a new song to attract the female. At that time, the part of its brain thought to be the neural basis for the production of songs grows substantially, forming neuron connections and expanding to more than twice its normal size. The song pattern is presumably established in the new neuronal circuits that form in this structure.

After the mating season, the "song structure" in the brain atrophies, or becomes much smaller. As this happens, the song is lost. The next year, as mating season approaches, the song structure begins to grow again and the male canary composes a new song. In this extraordinary and specialized way the canary brain provides a structural basis for learning: it grows an entire new set of circuits. Forgetting occurs because the learning circuits degenerate and disappear.

The situation is very different in mammals. It seems likely that learning involves the establishment of new connections or circuits in the brain. However, once they are established, the new connections seem relatively permanent. Our well-established memories of the sound and use of our native language, for example, last for an entire lifetime. Imagine the quality of life people would have if their brains were like those of male canaries. Each year they would forget their native language and everything else they had learned and would have to start all over again the following year. The growth of new song circuits each year in the canary brain seems to be a very specialized development to accommodate a very special form of learning. The brain circuits responsible for other aspects of the canary's behavior do not grow and disappear. So far as we know, no such specialized process occurs in the mammalian brain. New connections among neurons are presumably formed throughout life, but no new neurons are produced. The physical answer to the question of why neurons do not divide and form new cells after an animal's birth will ultimately be found in the DNA.

The only other major difference between a neuron and other cells is in the neuron's cell membrane: it has become specialized to conduct and transmit information. A typical neuron also looks different from most other cells, in that fibers extend from it. One of these fibers, the axon, has become very specialized to conduct information from the neuron cell body out to other cells. The endings of the axon have also become very specialized as synapses that release chemical transmitters onto other cells.

In the long course of evolution from jellyfishes to humans there has been only one significant change in the nature of the axon. Rapid communication among the cells of an animal provides an adaptive advantage in behavior. How fast an axon conducts information depends on how large its diameter is. The larger the axon is, the faster it conducts. Many invertebrates have developed giant axons for very rapid conduction. In the squid, the giant axon can be as large as a millimeter in diameter. The function of the squid giant axon, incidentally, is to cause contraction of the body mantle, which expels water and squirts the squid rapidly away from danger.

When vertebrates developed, a new kind of axon appeared: the myelinated axon. This is simply an axon surrounded by a thin sheet, or sheath, of a fatty substance called *myelin*. (Myelin is from the Greek meaning full of marrow.) The myelin sheath functions in some ways like the insulation that covers an electrical wire: it serves as an insulator for the axon membrane. If the speed of conduction of information in a naked axon and a myelinated axon of the same size are compared, the myelinated one will be found to conduct information many times faster. The mechanism of how this works will be explained in Chapter 3. The basic electrochemical process of conduction, however, is the same in both naked and myelinated axons.

Vertebrates have made good use of the myelinated axon. In the human brain and the rest of the nervous system, all of the larger axons are myelinated. Interestingly, if an axon is very small in diameter, a point is reached at which myelin is no advantage because both a myelinated and a naked axon of that size conduct at the same speed. Hence all of the axons in the human and other vertebrate nervous systems that are smaller than this critical size have no myelin and resemble invertebrate axons. Examples of unmyelinated axons in the human are the slow-conducting pain fibers that convey information about aches and burns from the skin to the brain and the fibers that carry temperature information.

To give some idea of the advantage of having myelin, consider the human optic nerve, which conveys visual information from the eye to the brain. Each optic nerve consists of about 1 million axons, all of which are myelinated and relatively small. One could design naked axons that would conduct this visual information as fast as the myelinated axons do, but they would be much larger in diameter. The optic nerve made of such fibers would have to be as large as the eye itself and would occupy a significant part of the space inside the skull now occupied by the brain. The actual diameter of the human optic nerve, consisting of myelinated axons, is only about four millimeters. The same functions can be accomplished in a very much smaller space by axons that have myelin.

STRUCTURE OF THE NEURON

A typical neuron is shown in Figure 2-2. A number of fibers extend from the *cell body,* but one and only one fiber per neuron is the *axon.* The axon may branch and send out fibers itself, but only one axon leaves the cell body. As the main axon approaches its target cells, either other neurons or muscle or gland cells, it branches into a number of smaller axons that end in specialized terminals called *synaptic terminals* or knobs. These nerve endings form synapses with other cells. The *synapse* (the word is from the Greek for union) is the place where the neuron transmits information to other cells.

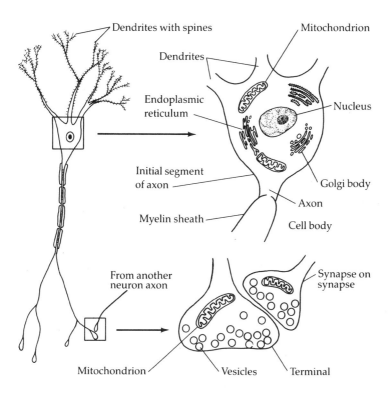

Dendrites with spines
Mitochondrion
Dendrites
Endoplasmic reticulum
Nucleus
Initial segment of axon
Golgi body
Myelin sheath
Axon
Cell body
From another neuron axon
Synapse on synapse
Mitochondrion
Vesicles
Terminal

Figure 2-2 Major parts of a neuron. The cell body contains all the same organelles as other cells (see Figure 1-2). The initial segment of the axon where it leaves the cell body is naked—not covered with myelin. Mitochondria are present in the cell body, the fibers, and the terminals. The terminals also contain small, round vesicles believed to contain neurotransmitter chemicals. Synaptic connections from the fibers of other neurons cover the cell body and dendrites. In many neurons the synapses on dendrites can be seen as little spines. The axon itself has no synapses on it except sometimes at its synaptic terminals, where other neuron axon terminals may form synapses on synapses.

All the other fibers that extend from the neuron cell body are called *dendrites* (from the Greek for tree). The dendrites and the cell body are covered with synapses formed with the axon terminals from other neurons. A typical neuron in the cerebral cortex has literally thousands of synapses from other cells.

Neuron Cell Body and Its Organelles

Mitochondria   The mitochondria, as noted in Chapter 1, have one primary function, which is simple and essential for the life of the cell: they provide biological energy. Mitochondria require glucose and oxygen to manufacture such energy in the form of *ATP* (adenosine triphosphate) molecules. ATP has high-energy chemical bonds, phosphate bonds, which are easily used for almost all of the chemical reactions in the cell requiring energy. In addition to ATP, energy metabolism yields carbon dioxide (CO^2), which is eliminated from the body when we exhale, and water. Oxygen, which we inhale, is essential for the production of energy in the mitochondria. The brain, then, is completely dependent on blood supplies of oxygen and glucose in order to function, since the mitochondria in the neurons cannot make ATP without them.

Almost all of the processes carried out by cells require energy. This is obviously true for muscles, which contract and do work. However, the manufacture of chemicals, cell processes, and other structures in the body all require energy. Interestingly, there is one process in neurons and other cells that in itself requires almost no biological energy: the nerve action potential, the process axons use to carry information from the cell body to the terminals. However, even in the axon unwanted ions (charged chemical particles) must be eliminated by pumping them out through the axon membrane, and the pump does require energy. All of the other tasks undertaken by the neuron require substantial amounts of energy, for example, the manufacture of chemical substances such as transmitters, synapses, and the growth of fibers and other processes. Consequently, mitochondria are found everywhere in the neuron: in the cell body, the axon, the axon terminals, and the dendrites.

Endoplasmic Reticulum and Golgi Apparatus   The endoplasmic reticulum, or ER, is a system of membranes found throughout much of the cytoplasm in the cell. The Golgi apparatus consists of more condensed and discretely structured membranes than the ER and lies between the ER and the outside of the cell.

The ER condenses into clumps of substance in neurons that are particularly sensitive to a chemical called thionine. Franz Nissl, a pioneering neuroanatomist, discovered the thionine stain. The clumps of ER that are stained by thionine are called *Nissl bodies*. They are present only in the cell body of the neuron, and so the Nissl stain shows only the neuron cell bodies and not the fibers that extend from them. The function of the Nissl bodies is believed to be the same as that of the rest of the ER and the Golgi apparatus: the manufacture and release of certain chemical substances. Proteins, peptides, and chemical transmitters are synthesized on the ER and Nissl bodies, packaged in vesicles (little spheres) in the Golgi apparatus, and either released by the cell or transported to other parts of it for later release (Figure 2-3). Both neurons and gland cells release chemical substances via Golgi apparatus. Gland cells of the endocrine glands release the special substances they manufacture, hormones, directly into the bloodstream. Neurons typically release the special chemical substances they manufacture, transmitters, at synaptic terminals.

Axon

The axon has two essential functions in the neuron. One function is to conduct information in the form of the action potential from the neuron cell body to the synaptic terminals in order to trigger synaptic transmission. The other major function is to transport chemical substances from the cell body to the synaptic terminals and back from the synaptic terminals to the cell body. This process is called axoplasmic transport, or simply *axon transport*.

With the development of the electron microscope, the cytoplasm of the cell, which had been thought to be entirely structureless, was found to be filled with structures. The ER is one example; another is the *microtubules*. The neuron axon is filled with microtubules, tiny tubes running the length of the axon from the cell body to the synapses. The microtubules transport a variety of chemical substances both up and down the axon. Certain chemical transmitters are manufactured in the cell body by the ER and then transmitted by means of the microtubules down the axon to be stored in the synaptic terminals. The synaptic terminals themselves take up certain chemical transmitter substances from the synapse and transport them back to the cell body (Figure 2-3).

The details of axon transport are a little complicated, as there are both fast and slow processes. The basic idea behind both processes, however, is straightforward. With fast transport, material moves up and down the axon at a rate of 10 to 20 millimeters per day, and so only a few hours may be required for substances to be moved the length of the axon. In slow transport, substances are moved at a rate of only about a millimeter per day.

Powerful new techniques relying on axon transport have been developed to trace nerve pathways in the brain. One such technique employs fluorescent dyes. Oddly enough, neurons take up many dyes and transport them; if they

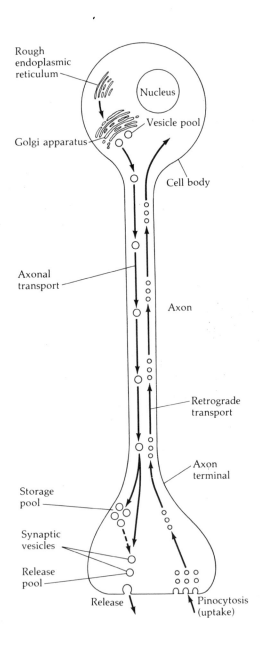

Figure 2-3 Axon transport. Chemicals are moved from the cell body to the terminals (anterograde transport) and from the terminals to the cell body (retrograde transport). It is believed that they move along the axon in tiny tubules that fill the axon.

are injected in the vicinity of a group of neuron cell bodies, the cell bodies will take them up and transport them rapidly down their axons to the terminals. This is technically called *anterograde* (forward) *transport*. If, on the other hand, dyes are injected into a region of the brain containing nerve axon terminals, the terminals will take them up and transport them rapidly back through the axons to the cell bodies. This is called *retrograde* (backward) *transport*. The dyes can then be exposed to light, and they will then "light up" in a microscope (Figure 2-1). Although dyes are transported in both directions, the procedure works better for retrograde transport.

Another new technique employed to trace nerve pathways involves the use of radioactively labeled amino acids. Such amino acids are taken up preferentially by neuron cell bodies and transported out to the axon terminals (anterograde transport). When radioactively labeled amino acids are injected into a region of cell bodies in the brain of an animal, they are transported to the axon terminals after a few hours or a day or two, depending on the length of the axon. The brain is then sectioned into slices that are placed on sensitive photographic x-ray film. These autoradiographs form a picture of where the axon terminals of the cells are.

Synapse

The presence of synapses is characteristic of neural tissue, as only neurons and their target cells form them. Synapses are the points of functional contact between axon terminals and other cells. Under the light microscope, a section of brain tissue appears as a bewildering variety of contacts among neurons. The advent of the electron microscope greatly simplified understanding of the synapse and provided much more detail. There are basically only two types of synapses: *chemical synapses* and *electrical synapses*. Since most synapses in the mammalian brain are chemical, in the following discussion this type will be emphasized.

Chemical synapses have three common features by which they can be identified (Figure 2-4). The most obvious is the presence of a large number of *vesicles* clustered in the *presynaptic* (before the synaptic space) *axon terminal*. The vesicles are believed to contain the chemical synaptic transmitter substance for the particular synapse. The region of the synapse on the *postsynaptic cell* has a dense staining band along the cell membrane that defines the extent of the synapse. (The band is more prominent in some chemical synapses than in others.) In between the pre- and postsynaptic membranes is a space called the *synaptic cleft*. This space is always present and is uniformly about 20 nanometers (20 billionths of a meter) wide; it is a very tiny space but, nonetheless, a space (Figure 2-4).

When a synapse is active and transmits information, the vesicles in the presynaptic terminal are thought to fuse with the presynaptic membrane and release their content of transmitter into the synaptic space (the process of

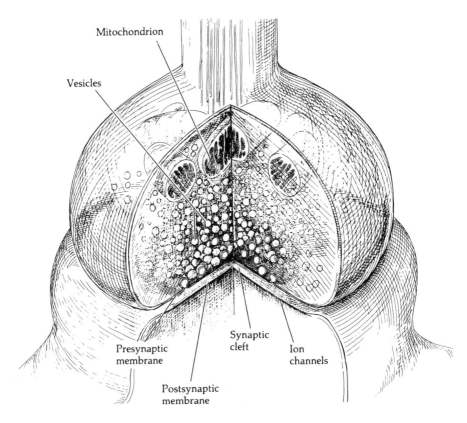

Mitochondrion

Vesicles

Synaptic
Cleft

Presynaptic
membrane

Ion
channels

Postsynaptic
membrane

Figure 2-4 Three-dimensional drawing of a synapse. The axon terminal is the top knoblike structure and the spine of the receiving neuron is the bottom one. Note that there is a space (synaptic cleft) between the presynaptic terminal membrane and the postsynaptic cell membrane.

exocytosis). The transmitter molecules diffuse across the narrow synaptic cleft and attach to specific chemical receptor molecules on the surface of the post-synaptic membrane (Figure 2-5), which activates the postsynaptic target cell.

Three varieties or types of chemical synapses can be seen with the electron microscope. They all have the features described above and all are thought to work in the same way; the main difference may be that the three types involve different transmitters. Thus the *spheroid* (round) *vesicle synapse* is thought to be excitatory, or to increase the activity of the target cell. The *flat vesicle synapse* is thought to be inhibitory, or to decrease the activity of the target cell. The third type, the *dense-core vesicle synapse*, is believed to contain a particular class of transmitter chemicals, the catecholamines, which may be either excitatory or inhibitory. Note that these suggestions for the differences in function of the three varieties of chemical synapse have not yet been proved.

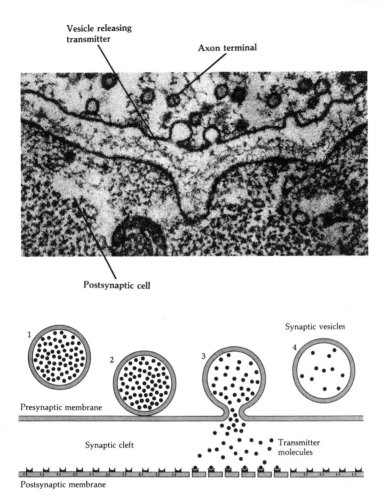

Vesicle releasing transmitter

Axon terminal

Postsynaptic cell

Synaptic vesicles

Presynaptic membrane

Synaptic cleft

Transmitter molecules

Postsynaptic membrane

Figure 2-5 Top: Photomicrograph of a synapse in action taken with the electron microscope. Vesicles are releasing their transmitter chemical into the synaptic cleft. Bottom: Schematic of the process.

Dendrites

The dendrites, which constitute all the fibers extending out from the neuron except the axon, are best thought of as extensions of the cell body. It is the dendrites that give a neuron its characteristic shape; they can range in number and size from a few short fibers to a huge mass of fibers that give it the look of a tree.

The dendrites serve to extend the receptive surface of the neuron, as they are literally covered with synapses. Remember that both the dendrites and the cell body receive information through synaptic connections from other neurons. Information is transmitted from the neuron cell body to target cells, either other neurons or muscle and gland cells, by the one and only axon, as we saw earlier.

In the cerebral cortex, the dendrites of many neurons are covered with thousands of little extensions called *dendritic spines* (Figure 2-6). Each of these spines is a synapse formed with the dendrite by an axon terminal from another neuron. The spine, since it belongs to the dendrite, is the postsynaptic part of the synapse; the presynaptic axon terminal is situated near the spine. Dendritic spine synapses are thought to be excitatory synapses.

Types of Neurons

A section of brain tissue stained so that both the cell body and the processes (dendrites and axon) can be seen, as with the Golgi stain, reveals a multitude of shapes and sizes. Fortunately neurons can, for the most part, be categorized into just a few classes or types, depending in large part on where they go. Remember, though, that such a classification represents a considerable simplification; not all neurons precisely fit a given category.

Perhaps the most easily identified type of neuron is the *motor neuron* (Figure 2-7a). Motor neurons send their fibers out of the nervous system into the body to synapse with muscle fibers or gland cells. The motor neuron has an extensive dendritic tree, a large cell body (the largest in the human nervous system), and a very long myelinated axon. The cell bodies of the motor neurons that innervate the muscles of the body are in the spinal cord, and those that innervate the muscles of the face and head are in the brain stem. The axons exit from the spinal cord or brain stem and travel in groups (nerves) to the muscles. Motor neurons control the activity of skeletal muscles, smooth muscles, and glands. They in turn are controlled by a number of systems in the brain called the motor systems.

Another kind of neuron is the *sensory neuron* (Figure 2-7b). Sensory neurons extend from the body into the nervous system. An example of the action of a sensory neuron is the "touch" you feel when you stroke something lightly with your finger. Receptors in the skin of the finger are activated, and they activate sensory nerve fibers. These nerve fibers run from the finger into the spinal cord to convey touch information to the brain. The cell bodies of sensory neurons lie just outside the spinal cord in groups called *ganglia*. Technically, the sensory nerve fiber from the fingertip to its cell body in the ganglion is a dendrite: it conducts information toward a cell body, whereas axons by definition conduct information away from the cell body. However, such nerve fibers are specialized for fast conduction; they are myelinated, and they should be thought of as axons.

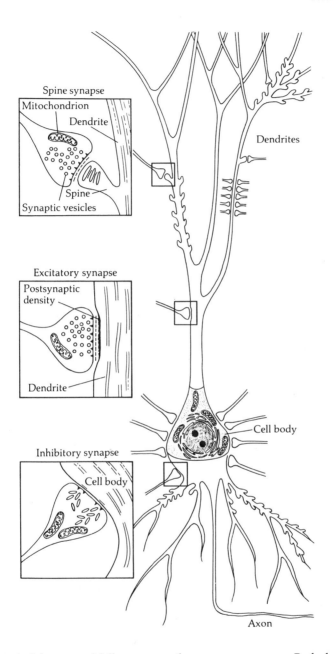

Figure 2-6 Schematic of different types of synapses on a neuron. Both the spine synapse (top) and synapses in which the terminals contain round vesicles (center) are thought to be excitatory; synapses in which the terminals contain flattened vesicles (bottom) may be inhibitory. Inhibitory synapses cluster on the cell body, especially near the initial segment, where the axon leaves the cell body. Synapses on dendrites are generally excitatory.

a

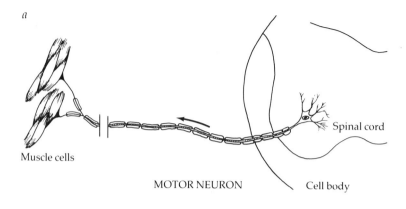

Muscle cells

MOTOR NEURON   Spinal cord   Cell body

b   Cell body in dorsal root ganglion

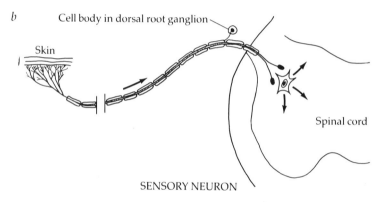

Skin

Spinal cord

SENSORY NEURON

Figure 2-7 (*a*) Typical motor neuron conveying commands from the spinal cord to the muscles to move and (*b*) sensory neuron conveying information from the skin to the spinal cord.

Within the brain we find a large variety of shapes and sizes of neurons. Most brain neurons fit into one of two classes: principal neurons and interneurons. *Principal neurons* are typically the largest neurons in a given structure or region of the brain and are acted on by many other neurons. Principal neurons send the "final message" from their region to other regions through their myelinated axons (Figure 2-2).

Interneurons do not send their axons out from the region where their cell body is. They come in a variety of shapes and sizes. Most interneurons have axons that convey action potentials to nearby neurons (Figure 2-8). Others have no long axon or no axon at all and do not develop action potentials, but they can still influence other neurons at synapses. Our rule that axons trans-

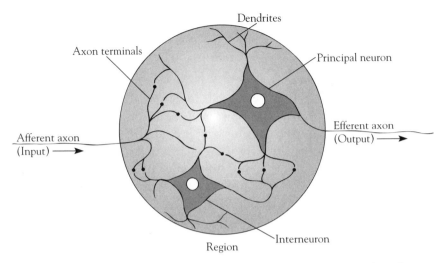

Figure 2-8 Example of the organization of interneurons. They lie entirely within a given region (nucleus, cortex) of the brain and can modify the influence of input afferent axons on the principal neurons that project out from the region (efferent axons).

mit information and dendrites receive information breaks down for some interneurons, where a given dendrite can both receive information from another neuron by a synapse and transmit information to another neuron by a synapse.

In general, a localized region of a given brain structure has only one type of principal neuron but may have several types of interneurons. In addition, nerve fibers come to the structure from other regions. These fibers, called *afferent fibers*, are axons from principal neurons in other regions. Information comes into the structure via afferent fibers and is processed in the structure by the interneurons. The principal neurons then "decide" what kinds of messages they will send out to other regions. Recordings of the activity of the principal neurons in other regions that send information to a particular structure or region and of the activity of the principal neurons that send information out from that structure help us to understand the kind of information processing that occurs in the structure. Using this "input-output" analysis, we can determine in some degree what the interneurons in the structure have done to the information.

Cajal termed principal neurons Golgi type I and interneurons Golgi type II. He noted that the main difference in terms of cell types between the cerebral cortex of a mouse and that of a monkey was that the latter had relatively many more interneurons.

GLIA

The human brain contains perhaps 10^{11} neurons, but it contains even more glia, or glial cells. Glia are nonneural cells, as they do not conduct or transmit information, and in most respects their functions are still not known. The glial cells form a network throughout the brain. Indeed, it was once believed that the main function of the glial cells was to provide structural support for the brain. However, when a clump of glial cells is grown in a petri dish, some types exhibit continuous movement of their processes, which suggests a role other than merely structural.

One of the general functions of glial cells is to take up substances in the brain that are present in excess or not needed. At synapses, they often take up excess chemical transmitter. When a region of the brain is damaged, neurons degenerate and die. At the same time glial cells multiply in the region and clear away the cellular debris. In this regard too, glial cells are very different from neurons, which in the adult brain never increase in number.

Glial cells perform two special functions in the vertebrate brain. One function is the formation of myelin on axons, and the other is the establishment of the blood–brain barrier.

Myelin

We have seen that the larger axons in the nervous system are covered by a sheath of fatty insulating material called myelin. The myelin sheath serves to increase markedly the speed of conduction of the action potential along the axon (which will be discussed in detail in Chapter 3). Myelin sheaths on axons are formed by a particular type of glial cells called *Schwann cells* (Theodor Schwann was the anatomist who first described them). As the brain and nervous system grow and develop in the embryo, Schwann cells send out processes that wrap around and around the axons of the neurons. When an axon is complete, it is covered by the many layers of its Schwann cell sheath, which resemble the layers of an onion.

Blood–Brain Barrier

Another type of glial cells, the *astrocytes*, form what is called the blood–brain barrier. This barrier prevents many substances present in the blood from penetrating the brain. The brain, although it constitutes only about 2 percent of total body weight, receives 16 percent of the blood supply, and per unit mass, brain tissue receives 10 times as much blood as muscle tissue. Hence it is all the more remarkable that in spite of the richness of the blood supply, many substances cannot cross into the brain, whereas the same substances can cross freely into other organs, such as the liver. Many natural substances are poisonous to the brain because they interfere with neuron activity, even though they do not greatly harm other types of cells, such as liver cells, which in any event can divide and regenerate. It would be very adaptive to keep these poisons and other harmful substances out of the brain, and that is exactly what the blood–brain barrier does.

The presumed structural basis of the blood–brain barrier is shown in Figure 2-9. Astrocytes send out processes that form "feet" on the outside, or brain side, of the blood vessels and capillaries. These form a continuous sheet or sheath surrounding all the blood vessels in the brain. The sheet of astrocyte material contains fatty material, and so any substance that is not soluble in fat will have difficulty in dissolving through the barrier into brain tissue. As it happens, many potentially harmful substances are not fat soluble.

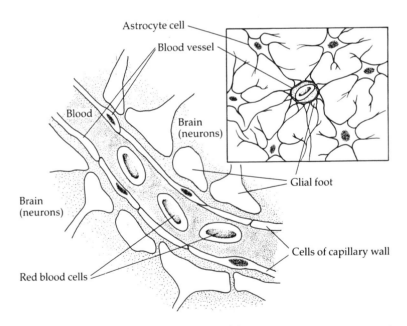

Figure 2-9 Schematic of the blood–brain barrier. A type of glial cell (astrocyte) extends "feet" that form a continuous layer around blood vessels in the brain, thus creating a fatty barrier that prevents substances not soluble in fat from passing from the blood into the brain.

SUMMARY

Neurons are like all other cells in most ways, but they are specialized to transmit and conduct information. An indication of the importance and complexity of neurons is the fact that some 30,000 to 50,000 genes in human DNA, present in all cells, are active only in cells in the brain. Information is conveyed to a given neuron by axons from other neurons, which form thousands of synapses with it. The synapse is formed by the close apposition (but not direct physical contact) between an axon terminal (ending) and the membrane of the target cell (another neuron or muscle or gland cell). As a result of these synaptic actions a neuron "decides" to send or not to send information out its axon to influence other cells. This is the process of synaptic transmission. If the neuron does "decide" to send information out its axon, a nerve impulse exits from the cell body and travels rapidly along the axon to the axon's synaptic terminals on other cells. This is the action potential, the process whereby information is conducted along the nerve axon. A new type of axon evolved in vertebrates, the myelinated axon, a nerve axon membrane that is covered with a fatty insulating sheath. This results in much faster transmission of the nerve impulse along the axon. Synaptic transmission and the action potential are the basic specialized processes of the neuron. To understand these processes one must first learn more about the basic properties of the neuron membrane, the topic of Chapter 3.

The neuron contains the same organelles as all other cells: mitochondria, which manufacture biological energy in the form of ATP from glucose and oxygen; the endoplasmic reticulum and its condensations into Nissl bodies and the Golgi apparatus, where chemical substances are synthesized via instructions from the genes; and microtubules, found in the axon, which transport chemicals up and down the axon. The synapse is a complex structure: the axon terminal (the presynaptic part) is a swelling that contains small vesicles, believed to hold the neurotransmitter chemical. When activated by an action potential, vesicles fuse with the terminal membrane and release the neurotransmitter into the synaptic cleft. The molecules diffuse across the cleft and attach to specialized receptor molecules on the postsynaptic membrane of the target cell. Finally, dendrites are fiber extensions of the cell body that receive thousands of synaptic contacts from other neurons (the cell body also has synaptic contacts but the axon does not).

Neurons are of several basic types. Sensory neurons convey information from the sense organs to the brain and spinal cord and motor neurons convey movement commands from the nervous system to the muscles. Within the nervous system there are two basic types of neurons, principal neurons (Golgi type I), which convey information via their axon to other regions, and interneurons (Golgi type II), whose axons remain with the local region.

The brain also contains several types of nonneural cells, the glia or glial cells. They serve as structural support, for taking up chemicals and debris, for forming the myelin sheaths around axons, and for forming the blood–brain barrier that prevents unwanted chemicals from diffusing from the blood into the brain tissue.

SUGGESTED READINGS AND REFERENCES

Books

Alberts, B., Bray, D., Lewis, J., Raff, M., Roberts, K., and Watson, J. D. (Eds.) (1989). *Molecular biology of the cell* (2nd ed.). New York: Garland.

Bullock, T. H., Orkand, R., and Grinnel, A. (1977). *Introduction to nervous systems.* San Francisco: W. H. Freeman.

Cajal, S. R. (1990). *New ideas on the structure of the nervous system in man and vertebrates* (Swanson, L. W., and Swanson, N., Trs.) Cambridge, MA: MIT Press.

Kandel, E. R., Schwartz, J. H., and Jessell, T. M. (Eds.) (1991). *Principles of neural science* (3rd ed.). New York: Elsevier.

Kuffler, S. W., Nicholls, J. G., and Martin, A. R. (Eds.) (1984). *From neuron to brain: A cellular approach to the function of the nervous system.* Sunderland, MA: Sinauer Associates.

Peters, A., Palay, L., and Webster, H. F. (1990). *The fine structure of the nervous system* (3rd ed.). Oxford: Oxford University Press.

Shepherd, G. M. (1988). *Neurobiology* (2nd ed.). New York: Oxford University Press.

Weiss, L. (1988). *Cell and tissue biology: A textbook of histology* (6th ed.). Baltimore: Urban & Schwarzenberg.

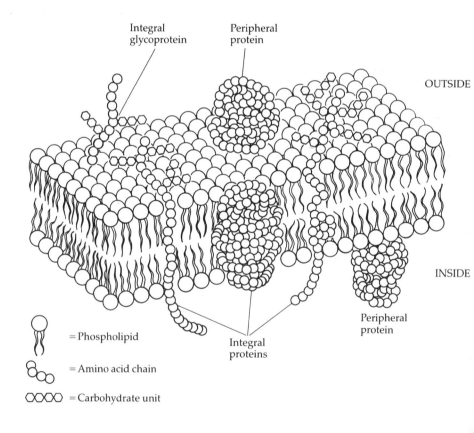

Integral
glycoprotein

Peripheral
protein

OUTSIDE

INSIDE

Peripheral
protein

= Phospholipid

Integral
proteins

= Amino acid chain

= Carbohydrate unit

3

Membranes and Potentials

The neuron can conduct and transmit information to other cells because of the special properties of its cell membrane. The neuron membrane has the same general structure as other cell membranes and it, too, functions to protect the cell and to move chemicals in and out of it (Figure 3-1). Another key property of all cell membranes is the possession of *ion channels*, basically tiny holes through the membrane that allow certain ions to pass in or out. Cells have a resting potential, or voltage difference, across their membrane that is relatively large, nearly one-tenth of a volt. As we shall see, the ion channels create this potential.

When jellyfishlike animals developed the first neurons, certain ion channels became specialized in such a way that a message, in the form of an action potential, could be conducted out the axon of the neuron to influence other cells. In this chapter we shall examine these two basic features of the neuron, the ion channels and how they result in the resting membrane potential and the action potential. The *cell membrane* is a thin, layered sheet that separates the cell from the world outside. Many cells also have other specialized outer

Figure 3-1 *Fluid mosaic model of the cell membrane. Protein molecules associated with chemical receptors and ion channels "float" in the lipid bilayer cell membrane.*

coatings, but the thin cell membrane proper is the functional boundary of the cell. It is quite flexible, indeed fluid, and so can change shape easily. However, it forms a stable and critically important boundary for the cell. All commerce that the cell has with the outside world must somehow penetrate or act through the membrane.

The cell membrane resembles a soap bubble in that it is very thin, about 10 nanometers (10 billionths of a meter) wide, and in that one of its major constituents is fatty acids, which make up the film of a soap bubble. The fatty acids that constitute most of the cell membrane are called phosphoglycerides. A phosphoglyceride consists of phosphoric acid, a strong acid, and the fatty acids called glycerides (Figure 3-2). This molecule has some interesting properties, among them that the phosphoric acid part of the molecule, its

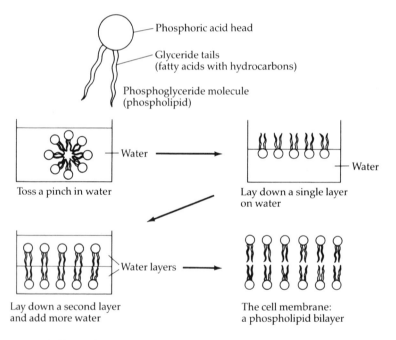

Figure 3-2 Cell membranes are a two-molecule layer (bilayer) of phospholipid molecules. The molecules have a phosphoric acid "head" that is attracted to water (hydrophilic) and fatty, glyceride tails that are repelled by water (hydrophobic). Since both the inside and the outside medium of cells is mostly water, the molecules line up in a bilayer with the heads out into the mediums and the tails inside.

"head," is much attracted to water—strong acids try to combine with water if it is available. The fatty acids are repelled by water for the same reason that oil and water do not mix. The fatty acids have "tails" consisting of hydrocarbons that in particular try to avoid water.

A pinch of fatty acid molecules tossed into water will form little clumps, with the acid heads that are attracted to water on the outside and the hydrocarbon tails that are repelled by water on the inside (Figure 3-2). If one were to very carefully place a layer of these molecules on the surface of water, they would line up with the acid heads in the water and the tails protruding out of it. If another layer of the molecules were added and more water put on top, the molecules would line up with the first layer, forming a layer two molecules wide in which the acid heads protrude into the water on each side and the hydrocarbons line up in between (Figure 3-2). This fatty double layer, or *lipid bilayer*, is the basic structure of the cell membrane.

The molecules of such a lipid bilayer membrane are not connected together in any strong chemical bonding or structural manner. The membrane owes its existence to the fact that water is on both sides and the acid heads prefer water whereas the hydrocarbon tails do not. This means that the membrane is essentially fluid. If there were currents in the water, the membrane would move about with them. The cell membrane seems a rather fragile structure to protect the cell from the outside world, but it does so with great success.

In addition to the fatty acids, or phosphoglycerides, the cell membrane includes various protein molecules scattered throughout it. These large molecules literally float in the lipid bilayer (Figure 3-1).

Some may be large enough to extend all the way across the membrane, but most of them tend to balance closer to the outside or the inside. A protein molecule that is toward the outside generally stays there. It can float laterally, or to the side, along the membrane, but it does not move to the inside or farther to the outside, and the same is true for the proteins that are positioned toward the inside. These protein molecules have carbohydrate side chains, which tend to stick out of the membrane, either on the outside or on the inside. (Sugars and starches are examples of carbohydrates.)

The protein molecules and their carbohydrate side chains are thought to be the *chemical receptors* of the cell membrane. The concept of the receptor molecule has become fundamental in cell biology and for our understanding of the nervous system. Basically, a receptor is a protein molecule that recognizes a particular *chemical messenger*. It recognizes the messenger by its molecular shape and electric charge distribution. A messenger molecule is thought to fit into its receptor like a key fits into a lock. Molecules of messengers attach to the appropriate protein molecules on the cell membrane and may cause various changes in both the membrane and the inner workings of the cell.

ION CHANNELS

The most fundamentally important fact about cell membranes is that tiny, highly selective tunnels go from the inside of a cell membrane to the outside. One type of tunnel, the ion channel, is much too narrow to allow particles as large as a sugar molecule to pass through, but it is wide enough to allow small ions such as sodium, potassium, and chloride to pass through.

Ions are atoms in solution in water that have an electric charge (see Appendix). When sodium chloride—table salt—is dissolved in water, the sodium and chlorine atoms separate as ions, the sodium ions less one electron for a charge of +1, symbolized Na^+, and the chloride ions with an extra electron for a charge of –1, symbolized Cl^-. Another important ion to consider in a discussion of ion channels is the potassium ion, symbolized K^+, which has a charge of +1. Only one other ion need be considered for an understanding of neuron function, namely the calcium ion, which has two positive charges and is symbolized as Ca^{2+}.

The cell membrane provides each kind of ion with its own channels: there are potassium channels, sodium channels, and chloride channels distributed throughout it. Actually, the various ion channels are differentially distributed in different regions of the neuron. Thus calcium channels are present in substantial numbers at axon terminals, where they play a special role in synaptic transmission, to be discussed in Chapter 4.

Figure 3-3 is a highly schematic drawing of the ion channels in a neuron membrane. It shows a portion of a neuron axon that has no myelin covering, like the squid giant axon. The actual density of ion channels is not nearly as great as is shown. For example, it is estimated that there is one sodium channel for every 1 million molecules of membrane. If you were tiny enough to walk along a neuron membrane, you would encounter a channel only now and then. However, over the entire membrane there is a very large number of channels.

The ion channels in cell membranes are of two types: those that are open, or have no lids, or *gates*, and those that are closed off by gates (Figures 3-3 and 3-4). The gates probably do not much resemble actual gates, but the principle is similar.

The channels may not be completely specific for different ion types. In the squid axon, clearly there are open K^+ channels, closed K^+ channels, closed Na^+ channels and probably open Cl^- channels as well. However, it is not clear whether there are some open Na^+ channels or whether Na^+ occasionally leaks through the open K^+ channels. In general, the membrane behaves as if it has specific types of ion channels. The channels are thought to be specific for the size of their particular ion. Water molecules are usually associated with ions (which are then called hydrated ions), causing them to be larger than the corresponding atoms. Different ions form different sizes of hydrated ions.

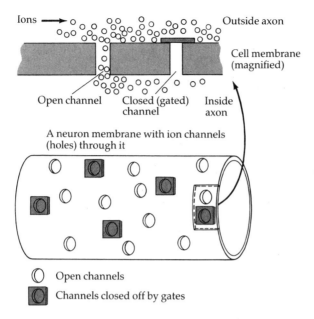

Ions ⟶ Outside axon

Cell membrane (magnified)

Open channel   Closed (gated) channel   Inside axon

A neuron membrane with ion channels (holes) through it

◯ Open channels

▣ Channels closed off by gates

Figure 3-3 Schematic of axon membrane showing both open channels and channels closed by gates.

Potassium channels are mostly without gates (Figure 3-4*a*). This means that a fair number of K^+ ions can pass back and forth across the membrane. When the neuron membrane is at rest, the gated potassium channels remain closed.

The "passive" properties of the cell membrane are determined by the open ion channels, the channels without gates. Neurons and other cells have ion channels that are always open. In particular, the relative numbers of these open ion channels determine the resting membrane potential of the cell and its resistance and capacitance (we shall return to these later).

RESTING CELL MEMBRANE POTENTIAL

Most living cells maintain a *potential difference*, a voltage difference across the cell membrane. Let us first consider an idealized cell that has no fibers. If a microelectrode is used to penetrate the cell membrane and record the voltage difference between the inside and the outside of the cell, the inside of the cell will be found to be about −75 millivolts relative to the outside. This is a very substantial voltage for a tiny cell to maintain, being nearly one-tenth of a volt

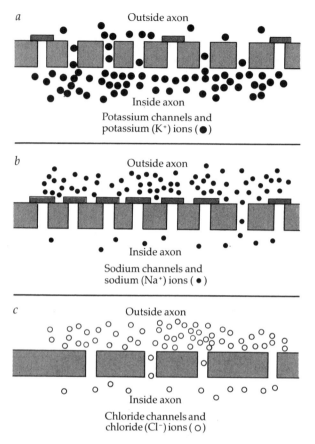

Figure 3-4 Common ion channels in the axon membrane. Most potassium channels are open, and most potassium ions are inside the axon (*a*). Most sodium channels are closed, and most sodium ions are outside the axon (*b*). Chloride channels are open, and most chloride ions are outside, but there are not as many chloride channels as potassium and sodium channels (*c*).

(one volt is 1000 millivolts). Some animals have made special use of this source of voltage; the electric eel has a group of specialized cells arranged in such a way that it can deliver a shock of several hundred volts, enough to stun or kill a fish.

The −75 millivolt potential exists only across the cell membrane. Two electrodes placed outside the cell will record a voltage of zero, or ground level, since the body fluids outside cells are electrically neutral. If both electrodes are placed inside the cell (but not in the nucleus), the voltage recorded will also be zero (Figure 3-5).

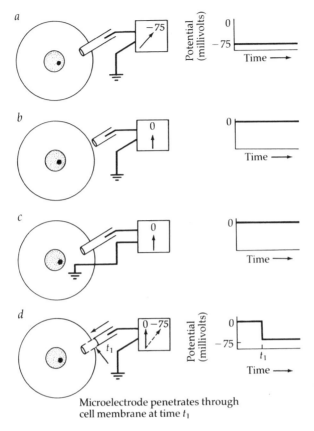

Microelectrode penetrates through
cell membrane at time t_1

Figure 3-5 The resting cell membrane in an idealized cell is -75 millivolts inside relative to outside. The potential exists only across the cell membrane, as shown in (*a*). The outside medium is electrically neutral (*b*), as is the cytoplasm inside. In (*d*) the electrode is shown penetrating the membrane at time t_1, and the measured potential immediately drops from zero to -75 millivolts.

A typical nonneural cell has a resting membrane potential of about -75 millivolts, and it does not develop an action potential. The cell has several types of ion channels, all of the open type, the commonest of which is the potassium channel. There are enough potassium channels so that the K^+ can pass freely back and forth across the membrane.

Cells contain a considerable amount of protein, whereas there is very little protein in the tissue fluid outside the cells. Much of the protein inside cells is in solution as protein ions or charged molecules. The protein ions have a net negative charge, P^{2-}. Since they are much too large to pass through the ion channels in the membrane they remain inside the cell, which is the basic reason why the cell membrane potential is negative inside relative to outside.

Suppose a typical cell is immersed in a solution containing K^+ and Cl^-. Remember that K^+ ions can cross the cell membrane freely: it is permeable to K^+. Assume that the Cl^- ions cannot diffuse as much through the cell membrane. There is a very strong force called the *diffusion force* that acts on ions in solutions to drive them toward equal concentrations throughout the solution. For example, if you drop a pinch of table salt into a glass of water, it will dissolve, and the Na^+ and Cl^- will rapidly be distributed throughout the solution until they are in equal concentrations everywhere.

When the cell is placed in a solution of K^+Cl^-, K^+ will rush into the cell through the open K^+ pores, leaving the negatively charged Cl^- behind. The net charge will then change from neutral. The initial net charge of the K^+Cl^- solution was zero because every K^+ was balanced by a Cl^-. As K^+ ions move into the cell a large *electric force* builds rapidly outside the cell membrane. This force acts in just the opposite direction to the diffusion force; it pulls K^+ outside the cell. In the end, the K^+ is distributed inside and outside the membrane so that the opposing diffusion force and electric force are equal. There is of course constant shuttling of some K^+ back and forth, but the net movement is zero: the system has reached a dynamic equilibrium.

The situation I have described for the cell also applies to artificial nonliving membranes if they are *semipermeable*, meaning that they let some ions such as K^+ pass through freely but not others, such as the larger protein ions, P^{2-}. A semipermeable membrane can function whether it is part of a living cell or not; no biological energy is required for the ions to distribute themselves across the membrane. Indeed, the *Nernst equation* was developed many years ago to describe the function of semipermeable membranes, both living and dead. This equation simply makes possible calculation of the potential difference across the membrane that will exist when a given type of ion has reached equilibrium, that is, has reached stable concentrations on both sides of the membrane. It is assumed that the ion in question can diffuse freely across the membrane.

The Nernst equation is:

$$V = \frac{RT}{kF} \log \frac{[\,I^+\,]_{out}}{[\,I^+\,]_{in}}$$

where k, R, and F are constants, T is the absolute temperature, and $[I^+]$ is the concentration of positive ions. Under standard conditions of pressure with the temperature at 18 degrees Celsius (the temperature appropriate for optimal functioning of the squid axon, by the way, but not for mammalian cells) and the voltage expressed in millivolts, the equation becomes

$$V \text{ (in millivolts)} = 58 \log \frac{[\, I^+ \,]_{out}}{[\, I^+ \,]_{in}}$$

for positively charged ions.

Let us now measure the concentration of K^+ inside and outside the cell. Common values, expressed in concentration units or millimoles per liter (mM/L) might be $[K^+]_{out}$ = 20 mM/L and $[K^+]_{in}$ = 400 mM/L. Putting these values into the Nernst equation gives us

$$V = 58 \log\left[\frac{20}{400}\right] = 58 \log (0.0500)$$

$$= 58 \,(-1.30103) = -75.46 \text{ millivolts or,}$$
rounding, -75 millivolts

Based entirely on the concentration of K^+ inside and outside the cell, the Nernst equation predicts that the membrane potential ought to be -75 millivolts inside relative to the zero level outside. When the actual cell membrane potential is measured with a microelectrode, it turns out in fact to be -75 millivolts inside relative to zero outside. The membrane potential of the cell is determined entirely by the concentration of K^+ inside and outside the cell. Implicit in the Nernst equation is the basic assumption that the ion in question can diffuse freely across the membrane, so we can conclude from our results that for this cell the membrane is freely permeable to K^+.

The mechanism underlying the resting membrane potential in neurons is basically the same as in the idealized cell used earlier as an example; the resting potential is determined mostly by the distribution of K^+ inside and outside the cell. The concentrations of common ions inside and outside the squid giant axon are given in Table 3-1. Most of the K^+ is inside the cell. Application of the Nernst equation to the K^+ concentrations in the squid giant axon gives a resting potential of -75 millivolts, the same as for the ideal cell. However, when a microelectrode is inserted inside the axon to measure the actual resting membrane potential, it turns out to be perhaps -70 millivolts. Hence there is a small but important discrepancy between the actual voltage and the voltage predicted by the Nernst equation applied to K^+ concentrations in the squid giant axon.

Let us reconsider the ion channels in the nerve axon membrane (Figure 3-4). Only the open channels, without gates, are involved in the resting potential; the gated channels remain closed. The K^+ channels are mostly of the permanently open type, but there are also K^+ channels with gates. Potassium cannot cross entirely freely because not all of the channels are open.

TABLE 3-1   Possible ion concentrations inside and outside an axon in millimoles (mM) per liter (l) of axoplasm

Inside axon	Outside axon
K^+ = 400	K^+ = 20
Cl^- = 30	Cl^- = 590
Na^+ = 60	Na^+ = 436
P^{2-} = High	P^{2-} = Very low

Key: K^+ = Potassium ions;
  Cl^- = Chloride ions;
  Na^+ = Sodium ions;
  P^{2-} = Protein ions

The Cl^- channels on the axon membrane are of the open sort. However, there are not as many Cl^- channels as K^+ channels. Cl^- can cross back and forth through the membrane but not as well as K^+; in fact, K^+ can cross about twice as easily as Cl^-. Most of the Cl^- is outside the cell. Typical concentrations would be 30 millimoles per liter inside and 590 millimoles per liter outside (Table 3-1). Application of the Nernst equation to Cl^- concentrations gives a value for the membrane potential of about −75 millivolts, close to the actual value of the resting potential. It should be noted that in the Nernst equation the upper and lower concentration terms are reversed for negative ions such as Cl^-; that is, log $([I^-]_{in})/([I^-]^{out})$. It seems that Cl^- may also play some role in determining the resting membrane potential.

The Na^+ channels in the axon membrane are numerous but almost all of them have gates; they are closed. Only a very few channels are always open. Na^+ can cross the membrane only about one-twentieth as easily as K^+. In essence, Na^+ is kept out of the axon. When the Nernst equation is applied to the concentration of Na^+ inside and outside the cell (Table 3-1), a predicted value for the resting membrane potential of +50 millivolts is obtained, markedly different from the actual level of about −70 millivolts. It seems clear that sodium cannot play an important role in determining the resting membrane potential level.

The Nernst equation gives the right value for the membrane potential only if an ion can diffuse freely across the membrane. Hence the value of +50 millivolts obtained when Na^+ is put into the equation tells us that Na^+ cannot diffuse freely across the membrane. Because a few Na^+ channels are open, we might expect that Na^+ makes some small contribution to the membrane potential, and it does.

Alan Hodgkin and Andrew Huxley and their colleagues at Cambridge University in England did the classic studies that led to much greater understanding of the nerve membrane resting and action potentials, using the squid giant axon as their model of the neuron membrane. They also developed the mathematical equations that explain how ion concentrations and ion movements across the membrane generate the resting and action potentials. They shared the Nobel Prize for this work. Early in their studies they also observed the behavioral function of the giant axon; they stimulated it in an anesthetized squid, whereupon the body mantle contracted and smashed their recording electrodes. Fortunately, the axon can be removed from the animal and kept alive and fully functional in a dish containing appropriate solutions.

In their studies on the resting membrane potential Hodgkin and Huxley varied the concentrations of different ions inside and outside the squid giant axon. This axon is very hardy; the interior substance, the axoplasm, can be squeezed out like toothpaste from a tube and replaced with various solutions of ions without killing the membrane or disturbing its function. Hodgkin and Huxley found that the resting potential of the squid giant axon membrane was determined very closely by the concentration of K^+ inside and out. This relation holds only for K^+; manipulation of Cl^- or Na^+ has much less effect on the membrane potential. The relation between K^+ concentration and membrane potential is not quite perfect, because in fact Cl^- and Na^+ are making small contributions.

The Nernst equation can be expanded to incorporate several ion concentrations rather than just one. This expansion, called the Goldman equation, is also basically quite simple:

$$V = 58 \log \frac{P_K [K^+]_{out} + P_{Na} [Na^+]_{out} + P_{Cl} [Cl^-]_{in}}{P_K [K^+]_{in} + P_{Na} [Na^+]_{in} + P_{Cl} [Cl^-]_{out}}$$

The only new term in the Goldman equation is the *permeability*, P. This is a measure of the degree to which a given ion can diffuse across the membrane. As we noted above, the axon membrane is the most permeable to K^+, only half as permeable to Cl^-, and one-twentieth as permeable to Na^+. Using these permeability values, Hodgkin and Huxley applied the Goldman equation to the squid axon and found that it predicts the resting membrane potential exactly. Remember that the Nernst equation assumes that the membrane is completely freely permeable to the ion in question, for example K^+. In fact, no real membrane is completely permeable to any ion. The Goldman equation takes this into account and uses the actual permeability of the membrane (P) for each type of ion.

The nerve membrane potential will remain constant at about -70 millivolts only if the ion concentrations, particularly that of K^+, remain relatively constant. There is certain to be some leakage. Na^+ is under strong diffusion pressure to leak in since it is present in a much higher concentration outside the cell. Some Na^+ will leak in. Leaking of Na^+ through the membrane will increase the positive charge inside and encourage some K^+ to move out along its diffusion gradient from the high concentration inside to the low one outside.

The system ought to run down eventually. It does not, because a mechanism in the axon membrane actively pumps Na^+ out of and K^+ into the cell across the membrane. The pump requires a significant amount of biological energy, in the form of ATP, to work. It must move the ions against their concentration gradients. The pump does not move the ions fast, but it is always steadily at work. It pumps just enough to maintain the K^+ and Na^+ concentrations at constant values inside and outside the cell.

Hodgkin and Huxley showed the importance of the pump with some simple experiments. They poisoned a squid axon with cyanide, a deadly poison that acts to block the formation of ATP, the source of biological energy that powers the machinery of the cell. At first, nothing happened. The resting potential remained constant and action potentials were conducted normally (the action potential will be considered later). Gradually, however, the axon began to run down and finally ceased to conduct action potentials. Hodgkin and Huxley then added ATP to the axon and found that it returned toward its normal levels of functioning until the ATP was used up.

We can make two important conclusions from the cyanide effect. First, maintenance of the resting potential and conduction of action potentials do not require the immediate use of biological energy. However, the pump does require a constant supply of energy, and in the end it is the pump that maintains the ion concentrations at their constant levels (Figure 3-6). The ion concentrations in turn produce the resting membrane potential and, as we shall see, are the source of energy that drives the action potential. The action potential indirectly runs on biological energy supplied by the pump.

To summarize, the nerve-axon resting membrane potential of about -70 millivolts is due largely to the concentration of K^+ inside and outside the cell (much more K^+ is inside than outside) and involves a passive process of ions moving through permanently open ion channels in the membrane. The distribution of K^+ is due in turn to the presence of negatively charged proteins inside cells. Hence the concentrations of ions are the result of the opposite action of the diffusion force and the electric force. The diffusion of Cl^- and Na^+ is much less important than that of K^+, but these ions do contribute a bit to determining the resting membrane potential level. The ion distributions

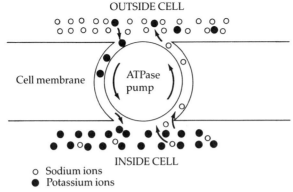

Figure 3-6 The ion pump is coupled: it pumps sodium ions out of the cell and potassium ions in. It uses considerable biological energy in the form of ATP because it must pump both ions against their concentration gradients. Since it is a protein, its activity is determined by the concentration of its "substrate," which is sodium ions inside and potassium ions outside. The more sodium inside the cell, the more active the pump becomes—a perfect example of a self-regulating system.

are maintained at a steady state by a pump that uses biological energy (ATP) to pump Na^+ out of the cell and K^+ in.

ACTION POTENTIAL

The most important fact about the action potential is that it travels down the axon. In a typical neuron, it begins at the point where the axon leaves the call body and travels down to the axon's terminals, which synapse on other neurons or on muscle or gland cells (Figure 3-7). The large and rapid change in voltage across the axon membrane that is the action potential develops at the beginning of the axon and at first involves only a very small tubular length of the membrane. The small region of voltage change then moves along the axon much like a bead moving down a wire. The speed at which the action potential moves down the axon is not extremely high; it varies from less than a meter per second to about 100 meters per second—very much slower than the speed of conduction of electricity in a wire. However, it is fast enough for the brain to function since most axons are quite short, only millimeters to centimeters in length. Distance becomes a factor in special cases, as in how long it takes for a muscle command to travel from the whale's brain to its tail, or even from the tip of your finger to your brain when you touch something.

Figure 3-7 The action potential traveling along the axon. It begins at the point where the axon leaves the cell body and travels at a constant speed out the axon (determined by the diameter of the axon and whether or not it has a myelin sheath; speeds range from a few miles or kilometers per hour to nearly 200 miles or 322 kilometers per hour). When the action potential reaches the terminal it disappears, but first it triggers the release of chemical transmitter molecules from the terminal, the process of synaptic transmission.

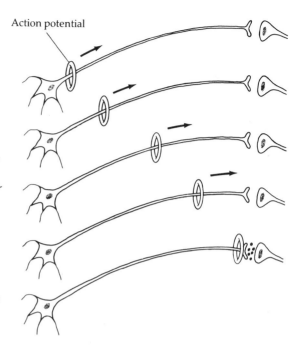

Action potential

Before we examine the mechanism that results in the action potential moving down the axon, it is first necessary to understand how it develops at a given place on the axon membrane. Although an action potential normally begins at the beginning of an axon, it will develop anywhere on the axon if an appropriate electric shock is applied. Thus some aspect of the action potential generating mechanism is sensitive to voltage change. Imagine that a microelectrode has been inserted into an axon at a given place and is recording the voltage across the membrane there. An action potential travels across that place on the membrane (Figure 3-8). A drawing of the action potential recorded by the microelectrode is shown in Figure 3-8a. Voltage change is shown on the ordinate (vertical axis) and time on the abscissa (horizontal axis). Refer also to Figure 3-8b, where the action potential is schematized as a bubble of activity traveling along the axon from the point of electrical stimulation past the place where the recording electrode is. The recording electrode sees what is happening at the one place on the axon over time as the action potential passes over it. Comparing the two figures should help you to visualize more clearly what is displayed on the graph of the action potential.

The first event is an abrupt and rapid increase in the voltage across the membrane from its resting level of −70 millivolts to a peak of +50 millivolts

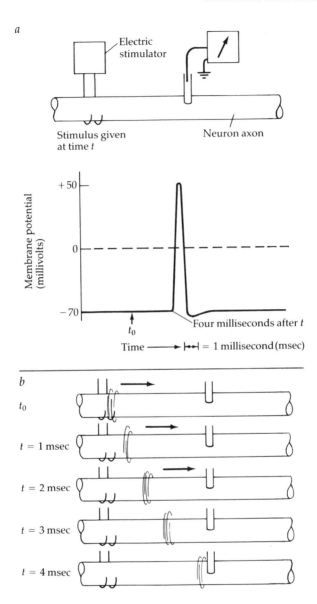

Figure 3-8 An action potential traveling down an axon and passing an electrode that measures the voltage across the axon membrane.

and then a rapid drop in voltage. The drop continues below the resting level and more gradually recovers to the resting level. The initial part of the action potential, the rapid rise and fall of membrane voltage, is often called the *action potential proper*, or the *spike*, and the slower phase, in which the voltage falls below the resting potential and then recovers, is called the *afterpotential*.

The number +50 millivolts, the voltage level the action potential reaches at its peak, might ring a bell. It is the voltage difference between the inside and the outside of the membrane that would exist if the membrane were freely permeable to Na^+. This value was calculated from the Nernst equation in the discussion of the resting potential. When the value for the high concentration of Na^+ outside the membrane and the value for the low concentration inside are substituted into the Nernst equation, the equation predicts a membrane potential of +50 millivolts if the membrane were freely permeable to Na^+.

We saw earlier that the membrane at rest is only slightly permeable to Na^+, about one-twentieth as permeable as to K^+. There are many Na^+ channels in the membrane, but they are mostly gated and most of the gates are closed. When an action potential develops at a place on the membrane, all the Na^+ gates there suddenly pop open and the membrane becomes freely permeable to Na^+ (Figure 3-9). Because the concentration of Na^+ outside the membrane is very much higher than that inside, there is a strong diffusion force pushing the Na^+ in. The resting membrane potential is negative inside (-70 millivolts) relative to the outside, due chiefly to the presence of negatively charged protein molecules. Since Na^+ is positively charged, these ions are attracted inside by the excess negative charge of the proteins. When the Na^+ channel gates are opened, both the diffusion force and the electrical force are working in the same direction to move Na^+ in. This results in a 500-fold increase in membrane permeability to Na^+. The rush of Na^+ into the cell at the site of the action potential is massive, so dominating other ion movements that the membrane potential goes all the way to the Na^+ equilibrium potential of +50 millivolts predicted by the Nernst equation. Because Na^+ is positively charged, at the places where these ions move into the cell the membrane acquires a positive charge inside.

At about the time the membrane potential reaches the Na^+ equilibrium value of +50 millivolts, the Na^+ channel gates pop closed again. The membrane is no longer permeable to Na^+ and its potential rapidly goes back to the resting level of −70 millivolts. (Why this happens will be explained shortly.) One other event also occurs as the Na^+ channel gates open and close. The few K^+ channels that are normally closed at rest open, letting K^+ cross the membrane even more freely than it can when the membrane is at rest. You may remember that the resting membrane potential level predicted by the Nernst equation from the concentrations of K^+ inside (high) and outside (low) is −75 millivolts, a bit more negative than the actual measured level of −70 millivolts. This is partly due to the smaller influences of other ions (Cl^-, Na^+), but it is also due to the fact that the membrane is not completely freely permeable to K^+: some of the K^+ channels have closed gates in the resting state.

The opening of the normally closed K^+ channels allows K^+ to flow freely across the membrane, and the membrane goes to the K^+ equilibrium potential

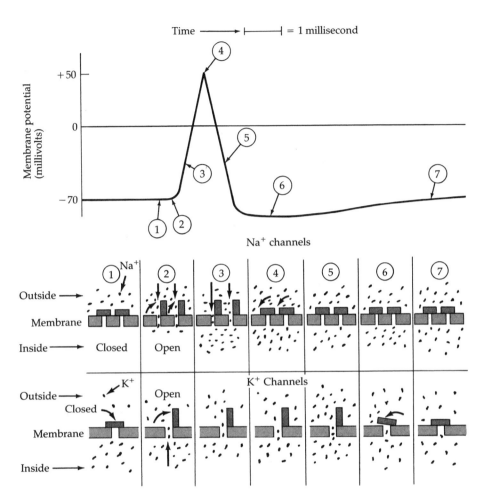

Figure 3-9 When the action potential develops and the membrane potential shifts rapidly from -70 millivolts toward +50 millivolts, the closed sodium channels pop open briefly and then close again. Meanwhile, the many fewer closed potas-sium channels pop open and then close more slowly, producing the afterpotential (at 6).

of −75 millivolts as some K^+ moves out of the cell. The opening and closing of the K^+ gates occurs more slowly than that of the Na^+ gates. Although both sets of gates open at about the same time during an action potential, the effect of the Na^+ gates dominates because the previous concentration of Na^+ on the two sides of the membrane is so much more out of balance; the force moving Na^+ ions in is very much greater than the small force moving K^+ ions out. The Na^+ gates are quickly closed, but the K^+ gates remain open for a while and the membrane potential goes toward −75 millivolts. After the K^+ gates close, the membrane potential returns to its normal resting level of −70 millivolts. The slower K^+ movement out of the cell generates the afterpotential. Remember that K^+ channels with gates that open and close are much less common than the permanently open K^+ channels, which determine the resting level of the membrane potential (Figure 3-9).

To summarize, when an action potential develops at a place on the axon membrane, the Na^+ channel gates open very briefly (for about half a millisecond). Na^+ rushes in and the membrane potential becomes positive inside relative to outside (+50 millivolts). The Na^+ gates close and the potential goes back toward the resting level. Meanwhile, the K^+ gates have opened, so some K^+ moves out and the membrane potential becomes even more negative (-75 millivolts) than at rest for a few milliseconds—this is the afterpotential. The few K^+ channels with gates now close and the membrane returns to its resting potential level of −70 millivolts. The period when the Na^+ gates are open, when the spike of the action potential develops and decays, is often termed the *absolute refractory period* in older texts. During this period the axon cannot be electrically stimulated to generate another action potential. During the period of the afterpotential the axon can be electrically activated, but it requires a stronger than normal electrical stimulus; this is the *relative refractory period*.

We have covered everything about the generation of the action potential except why the gates of the Na^+ and K^+ channels open, when most Na^+ gates and the few K^+ gates are normally closed. The answer turns out to be very simple: the gates are voltage controlled, which is usually termed *voltage gated*. Take the closed Na^+ channels as an example. Think of the gates as having an electrically controlled switch and being spring loaded. A certain voltage change is required to operate the switch. When the switch operates, it releases the gate and the gate springs open. There is in fact a threshold potential shift in the membrane that operates the switch and pops open the channel. In a squid axon, this might be a shift from the normal resting state of −70 millivolts to about −60 millivolts. When the potential difference across the membrane reaches −60 millivolts, the Na^+ channels pop open, Na^+ rushes in, and the action potential develops. When the membrane potential approaches its maximum of +50 millivolts, another switch and spring are activated that closes the Na^+ channels.

This opening of the Na^+ channels is often termed *regenerative*. Once the threshold voltage is reached (for example, −60 millivolts), the channel gates open and the Na^+ rushes in freely until the Na^+ equilibrium potential of +50 millivolts is reached.

The development of an action potential is very much like a chemical reaction that requires a trigger to start it but once started goes all the way to completion. If an explosive gas is heated, when the combustion point is reached, it explodes and the chemical reaction goes to completion; if there is not enough heat to reach the combustion point, nothing happens. So it is with the action potential. If the shift in membrane potential does not reach the threshold level of about −60 millivolts, which springs open the Na^+ channels, nothing happens—the membrane simply returns to its resting level. However, once the threshold is reached and the Na^+ channels open, Na^+ rushes in and the reaction goes to completion—the membrane potential is shifted all the way to +50 millivolts by the inrush of Na^+. Thus the action potential is an all-or-none response; it develops fully or does not develop at all.

The small number of K^+ channels that have gates are also voltage gated. It is believed that they open as the membrane potential becomes positive and close during the afterpotential when the membrane becomes more negative than at resting.

The channel gates are thought to be protein molecules with a net negative electric charge. When the voltage across a membrane is changed toward zero from −70 millivolts with a stimulating electrode, the electrically charged protein gates change their position or shape, thereby opening the ion channel. When a charged particle moves in an electric field, it gives rise to an electric current. If the protein gates actually move, they ought to generate tiny currents, and indeed they do, the so-called *gating currents*. Although the gating currents are much smaller than the large currents generated when Na^+ or K^+ moves across the membrane, it has been possible to measure them in the squid axon.

DIRECT RECORDING OF ION CHANNELS— THE PATCH CLAMP

One of the more remarkable aspects of the early work of Hodgkin and Huxley on the nerve membrane potential has to do with ion channels. At the time (1940s) there was no evidence that ion channels as such existed; Hodgkin and Huxley concluded that it was necessary to postulate their existence in the mathematical formulas they developed to account for the resting and action potentials. Direct evidence of ion channel activities was not actually obtained until the late 1970s. Erwin Neher and Bert Sakmann, working in Germany, developed a new technique called patch-clamp recording that permitted direct measurement of the actions of single ion channels. They shared the Nobel prize in 1991 for this work.

In brief, a glass microelectrode pipette is made with a smooth tip of 1 to 3μ in diameter, somewhat larger than the typical sharp microelectrode used to penetrate nerve cell membranes. The pipette tip is brought to the surface of a cell membrane and slight negative pressure is used to attach the membrane to the tip (Figure 3-10). The glass makes a tight high-resistance seal with the cell membrane. The activity of single channels can thus be studied in the functioning cell. If more suction is applied, the cell membrane is ruptured and the pipette has direct access to the interior of the cell and can record activity of the entire cell. Even more dramatic, if the suction is less than that necessary to rupture the cell wall and the pipette is pulled away from the cell, the membrane tears off from the cell but remains on the pipette tip. The little patch of membrane remains functional and will have one to several ion channels in it. With luck it will have just one functional channel. The current across the isolated patch of membrane can then be measured. The recording reveals a digital event—the channel is either open or closed. This technique has provided us with a great amount of new and precise information about the nature and type of ion channels.

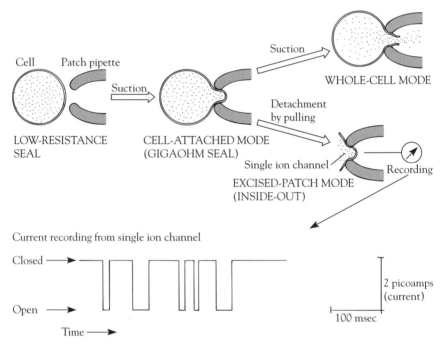

Figure 3-10 Top: Patch-clamp recording. A small glass tube electrode is rounded at the end and attached to the neuron cell membrane by weak suction, making a high-resistance (gigaohm) seal. Increased suction can break the membrane so that the electrode now records from inside the cell (whole-cell mode). But if the electrode is pulled away from the cell, it will pull off a small patch of membrane that might contain only one channel (excised patch mode). Bottom: Current recording from a single ion channel. The channel is either closed or open.

A BIT OF ELECTRICITY

Up to this point we have almost managed to avoid the subject of electricity. The resting membrane potential is in a steady state; there is no net movement of electric charge. The action potential, on the other hand, does involve the movement of charged particles, the ions. You might wish to consult the appendix on electricity at this point. The *potential difference,* or voltage, is the difference in charge between two places, for example, the inside and the outside of a membrane. A simple analogy to potential difference is water pressure. Water under low pressure will not spray very far, but under the high pressure, as in a fire hose, it sprays a long distance. A flashlight battery has a voltage of 1.5 volts, a relatively low voltage that could be obtained by connecting about 20 neurons together in the appropriate way. The "pressure" of the electricity in a flashlight battery, 1.5 volts, is so low that the electricity will pass through only good conductors such as wires, not through skin. You can "taste" the electricity, though, if you connect the wires from the two battery contacts to your tongue, which is wet and thus a better conductor than skin. Many flashlight batteries connected together could give rise to a large voltage, say 500 volts, that could kill a person touching the wires: the electricity is under much greater "pressure."

Electric current is the movement of charged particles and is expressed as *amperes,* or amps. Technically, current is the rate at which charge moves in a conductor. In a fire hose, the water current would be the rate at which the water flows out. This rate is determined by the pressure the water is under and the size of the hose. A small hose has higher resistance to water flow. Water under the same pressure will flow from a large hose faster than from a small hose, because the large hose has lower resistance to flow. In an electrical circuit, the wires and other elements have some *resistance* to the movement of charged particles. Metal wires have low resistance, whereas substances such as glass and fat have high resistance; not much electricity, or amount of charge, can flow in them. Resistance is measured in ohms.

Current, voltage, and resistance are related by the basic equation of Ohm's law: voltage (V) = current (I) × resistance (R): $V = IR$ or $I = V/R$ (see Appendix). For a constant source of voltage, such as a flashlight battery (1.5 volts), the higher the resistance, the less the current.

The resting neuron membrane resembles a battery with a constant voltage of about −70 millivolts, one-twentieth the voltage of a flashlight battery. At rest, the membrane has a relatively fixed resistance. The membrane consists mostly of fatty acids, which have a fairly high resistance. At rest, there is no net movement of charged particles across the membrane and hence no current. When the action potential develops, Na^+ channel gates open and Na^+ moves in; there is an inward current of Na^+. Using Ohm's law, we ought to be able to calculate the current: $I = V/R$. The voltage is changing, but it can easily be measured with a microelectrode. The catch in this is that the resistance of the membrane also changes: it decreases substantially when the Na^+ channels open. The equation has three variables, all changing.

Hodgkin and Huxley solved this dilemma by developing a device called a *voltage clamp*, in essence a feedback device that holds the voltage constant across a membrane. The current needed to do this is automatically changed by the device as the resistance of the membrane changes. It is a simple matter to monitor the feedback current the device is generating, and in this way Hodgkin and Huxley were able to determine the actual magnitude and time course of the ionic currents that underlie the action potential. These are shown in Figure 3-11. Compare these currents with the diagrams of Figure 3-9.

Propagation (Movement) of the Nerve Impulse

Nerve membranes have another electrical property called *capacitance*, the ability to store charge (see Appendix). If two metal plates are placed close

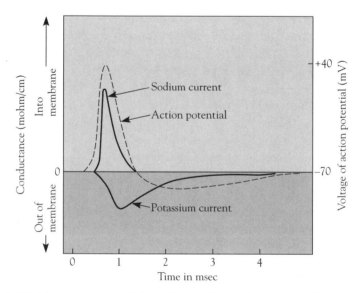

Figure 3-11 The time courses of the sodium and potassium currents that generate the action potential, due to the movement of sodium ions into the membrane and potassium ions out. You can relate these currents to the ion movements shown in Figure 3-9.

together but separated by a glass plate and then connected to a battery, electric charges will accumulate on one of the plates. The rate at which charges accumulate is determined by the resistance of the circuit and the properties of the plates. The neuron membrane is like a condenser in that it has a relatively high resistance, being made of lipids, compared with that of the fluid inside and outside the cell. For condensers, including neuron membranes, the rate at which charge accumulates is very slow compared with the speed at which electricity is conducted in a wire; charge accumulates in thousandths of a second, whereas electricity requires only billionths of a second to travel a fraction of a millimeter in a wire.

As Na^+ moves into the axon at the site of the action potential, the region of axon membrane immediately next to the site begins to depolarize and become somewhat less negative than the resting level of −70 millivolts. The rate at which this occurs is determined by the capacitance of the membrane. Perhaps the easiest way to think about this capacitance is to consider what happens when Na^+ moves into the cell. The positive charge of the ion depolarizes the membrane at that point (to the action potential peak of +50 millivolts). This positive inward current must somehow get back out of the membrane again to complete the electric circuit. The positive charges accumulate on the inner side of the membrane near the open gates, and the membrane potential there becomes less negative (Figure 3-12). Eventually it will reach the threshold for its Na^+ channels to open, Na^+ rushes in, and the action potential develops there. The patch of membrane immediately next to the place where the Na^+ gates are open will then reach the Na^+ gate-opening threshold. In this way the action potential moves continuously down the axon. Its speed is determined by such properties of the axon as its size and resistance, which in turn determine how fast charge can accumulate (its capacitance). The larger the axon, the faster the action potential travels down it.

Does an action potential produced by electrical stimulation of an axon at some point travel in only one direction or in both directions from the stimulating electrode? The mechanisms that generate the action potential are not direction specific and so an action potential can travel both up and down the axon from the point of stimulation. Because action potentials normally begin where the axon leaves the cell body, they usually travel down the axon away from the cell body. How this occurs will be explored in Chapter 4.

Conduction in Myelinated Axons

The larger, faster-conducting axons in the vertebrate nervous system are covered with a fatty insulating sheath of myelin, as we saw in Chapter 2. A

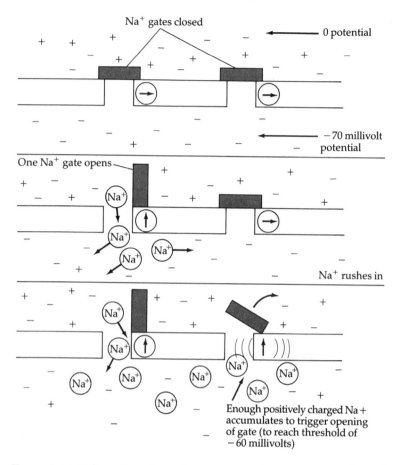

Figure 3-12 Why sodium channels pop open as the action potential develops. Their closed gates are voltage controlled and have a threshold a few millivolts less negative than the resting potential. In the figure an Na^+ gate just to the left of a closed Na^+ gate opens; Na^+ rushes in and, because it carries positive charge, makes the voltage at the inside of the membrane at the next closed Na^+ channel less negative until the threshold is reached. The closed channel pops open, and so on along the membrane (see Appendix).

myelin-covered axon can conduct an action potential much faster than a nonmyelinated axon of the same size.

The myelin sheath of an axon is interrupted every millimeter or so by a brief space with no myelin, called a *node*. If an axon is electrically stimulated at a given node, an action potential develops at the node and Na^+ rushes in. Next to the node is myelin, which is a very good insulator, and so charge cannot accumulate or cross the neuron membrane except at the nodes. The inward sodium current is distributed rapidly inside the axon, since the interior axoplasm is a relatively good conductor. The current spreads almost instantaneously (at the speed of electricity) but weakens with distance from the node where the Na^+ current is moving in. The current is often termed the *electrotonic current* (see Appendix). It causes the positive charge inside the membrane at the next node to increase, and since once again at the new node there is no myelin and the membrane resistance is only that of the membrane itself, the increased positive charge inside the membrane is enough to open the Na^+ gates at this node and cause an action potential to develop there. And so it goes down the axon, skipping from one node to the next.

In an unmyelinated axon the membrane capacitors must be charged by the accumulation of positive charge inside the membrane at each point along it, which takes time. In a myelinated axon, the charge need develop only at each node. Consequently, much less time is required for the action potential to skip down the axon.

The evolution of myelinated nerve fibers in the vertebrates was a tremendous advance. Axons could be fast, yet small. Myelin is probably the primary factor that made possible the greatly increased complexity of the vertebrate brain. Invertebrates typically have many fewer neurons that form specialized circuits that do particular things. If the circuits have to be fast, and some do so that the animal can eat and avoid being eaten, the neurons must be very large. With myelin the vertebrate brain could develop many more neurons that have less specialized functions because myelinated neurons are fast but still small in size. We have the lowly glial cell, which forms the myelin sheath around the nerve fiber, to thank for the ultimate development of the human brain.

At birth, the human brain has only a minimal degree of myelination. The reader might think about the implications of this for the functioning of the infant brain.

SUMMARY

Nerve cells and all other cells have an outer limiting membrane, the cell membrane. It is formed of a lipid bilayer containing phosphoric "heads" that like water and hence form the inner and outer boundaries of the membrane and a central core of hydrocarbon "tails" that do not like water. This membrane resembles the film of a soap bubble and is fluid or very flexible. Within the membrane are many complex protein molecules that serve as chemical receptors and ion channels and for other purposes. Like all other cells, neurons have ion channels, small tunnels through the membrane that allow certain ions to pass through the membrane. In neurons, the key ion channels are for potassium (K^+) sodium (Na^+), chloride (Cl^-) and calcium (Ca^{2+}).

Neurons and all other cells have resting membrane potentials (voltage); for a neuron the resting potential is about −70 millivolts, nearly a tenth of a volt. The body fluid outside cells, including blood, is electrically neutral and the insides of cells have a negative voltage of −70 millivolts. Each cell is a tiny battery. This electrical potential exists only across the cell membrane. The resting potential exists because the cell membrane is freely permeable to K⁺ ions and is passive—it can also be generated across a cellophane bag in a solution with the proper chemicals. The actual value can be calculated from the Nernst equation. The basic reason the nerve cell resting potential is negative inside relative to outside is that the membrane is semipermeable; it lets K⁺ ions pass freely but keeps negatively charged protein ions inside.

The nerve cell membrane has developed special properties to conduct action potentials. It has a great many closed or gated sodium channels, particularly in the axon. When the electrical potential across the membrane becomes a little less negative, the voltage-gated sodium channels pop open, sodium rushes in, and the membrane goes to +50 millivolts. This triggers a chain reaction: neighboring sodium channels pop open, and the action potential travels down the axon to the axon terminals. When the sodium ions rush in, the few closed potassium channels pop open and potassium ions move out, making the nerve membrane potential more negative, which creates the afterpotential. The membrane potential then returns to its resting level, ready to conduct another action potential. Recently, the patch-clamp method has made it possible to record the opening and closing of single ion channels. In vertebrate myelinated axons, the fatty insulating myelin sheath is interrupted every millimeter or so by a region (node) of no myelin. Here, the action potential skips from node to node and hence travels down the axon much faster than in nonmyelinated axons.

SUGGESTED READINGS AND REFERENCES

Books

Dowling, J. E. (1992). *Neurons and networks: An introduction to neuroscience.* Cambridge, MA: Belknap Press of Harvard University Press.

Hille, B. (1991). *Ionic channels of excitable membrane* (2nd ed.). Sunderland, MA: Sinauer Associates.

Hodgkin, A. L. (1964). *The conduction of the nervous impulse.* Springfield, IL: Charles C Thomas.

Kandel, E. F., Schwartz, J. H., and Jessell, T. J. (1991). *Principles of neural science* (3rd ed.). New York: Elsevier.

Kuffler, S. W., Nicholls, J. G., and Martin, A. R. (1984). *From neuron to brain: A cellular approach to the function of the nervous system* (2nd ed.). Sunderland, MA: Sinauer Associates.

Matthews, G. G. (1991). *Cellular physiology of nerve and muscle* (2nd ed.). Palo Alto, CA: Blackwell Scientific Publications.

Sakmann, B., and Neher, E. (1983). *Single-channel recording.* New York: Plenum Press.

Shepherd, G. M. (1988). *Neurobiology* (2nd ed.). New York: Oxford University Press.

Articles

Hodgkin, A. L. (1976). Chance and design in electrophysiology: An informal account of certain experiments on nerves carried out between 1934 and 1952. *Journal of Physiology, 263*:1–21.

Mitochondria

Synaptic terminal

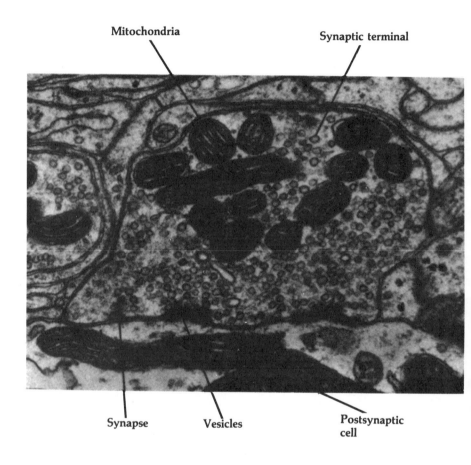

Synapse

Vesicles

Postsynaptic
cell

4

Synaptic Transmission

The event behind all the doings of the nervous system, from planning an evening to orchestrating a sneeze, is *synaptic transmission*: the communication of neurons with other cells at synapses. The human brain, with perhaps 100 billion neurons, has at least 10 trillion synapses, and a typical neuron in the mammalian brain alone may have several thousand. In spite of the vast complexity implied by these numbers, synapses seem to work in only a few different ways. Almost all of the synapses in the mammalian nervous system are chemical in nature, and so in what follows I shall focus on this type (Figure 4-1).

Much knowledge about synaptic transmission has come from studies of the *neuromuscular junction*, the synapse formed between the terminal of a motor nerve axon and a skeletal muscle fiber. In vertebrates, these synapses all use the chemical transmitter *acetylcholine* (ACh). We shall be concerned with the neuromuscular synapse as an example of chemical synapses in general and

Figure 4-1 *Electron photomicrograph of a synaptic terminal forming a synapse on another neuron.*

as an example in particular of one type of chemical synapse, the fast excitatory synapse. In this chapter we will focus on fast synaptic transmission, both excitatory and inhibitory, on examples of synaptic plasticity, and on a type of neurosis, anxiety neurosis, that seems to involve a form of fast synaptic inhibition.

FAST SYNAPTIC EXCITATION

A generalized *neuromuscular synapse* is shown in Figure 4-2. As we have seen, in chemical synapses a tiny space, or *synaptic cleft*, about 20 nanometers wide separates the axon terminal, referred to as the *presynaptic terminal,* and the target-cell membrane, or *postsynaptic membrane.* The presynaptic terminal has many small vesicles clustered near the membrane that are thought to contain the chemical neurotransmitter, ACh in the case of the neuromuscular synapse.

The basic process of chemical synaptic transmission is straightforward. An action potential is conducted down the axon to the presynaptic terminal. When it arrives there, it triggers the release of the transmitter (ACh) from the terminal by opening calcium ion (Ca^{2+}) channels, ion channels we have not yet discussed. These channels are present in axon terminal membranes, are normally closed and are voltage gated. The action potential shifts the voltage at the terminal membranes, causing the Ca^{2+} channels to open briefly. Calcium ions rush into the cell because there are fewer of them inside the cell than outside (the concentration gradient is high outside, low inside). The arrival of the Ca^{2+} inside the axon then triggers the release of neurotransmitters.

The transmitter that is released, ACh at neuromuscular junctions, diffuses across the small synaptic space and attaches to receptor molecules on the postsynaptic membrane. For the neuromuscular synapse this in turn causes Na^+ channels to open, and Na^+ rushes in. The target postsynaptic cell becomes slightly *depolarized* (its membrane potential becomes slightly less negative) for a few milliseconds. During this period the cell is more excitable than before.

Note that the ion channels on the postsynaptic membrane are activated by a chemical: they are *chemically gated* rather than voltage gated. The protein gates of these ion channels are chemical receptors that are selectively sensitive to a chemical transmitter (such as ACh). Here we encounter a third type of ion channel. In the axon membrane we saw that there are both permanently open ion channels and voltage-gated channels, which can be opened by a shift in membrane potential. Because the synaptic gates are chemically activated rather than voltage activated, they are not regenerative: there is no threshold point beyond which they all open. Instead, the number of gates that open depends on the amount of chemical transmitter present and the length of time

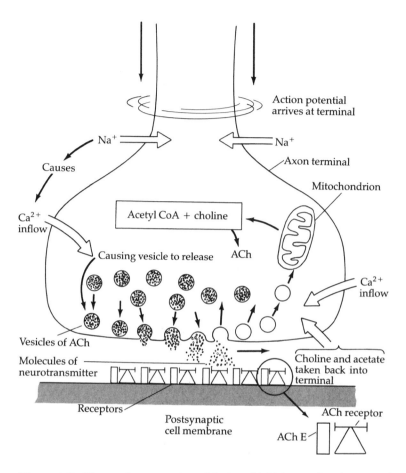

Figure 4-2 Chemical synapse. Acetylcholine (ACh) is used as the example. It is made in the axon terminal from acetyl coenzyme A (acetyl CoA) and choline, stored in vesicles, and released. When the action potential arrives at the terminal, closed calcium channels in the terminal are opened and Ca^{2+} rushes into the terminal, triggering vesicles to fuse with the membrane and release ACh molecules into the synaptic cleft. They attach to ACh receptors on the postsynaptic membrane and trigger the opening of Na^+ channels. ACh is immediately broken down at the receptors by acetylcholine-terase (AChE) into choline and acetate, which are taken back up by the terminal and reused.

they are open depends on how long the transmitter remains attached to the receptor and acts.

It might sound as if the process of synaptic transmission takes a rather long time to occur. The action potential arrives at the terminal; Ca^{2+} rushes in; transmitter is released into the synaptic cleft, diffuses across the space, and attaches to receptor molecules; and the Na^+ channel gates in the postsynaptic membrane are opened, letting Na^+ rush in and depolarize the postsynaptic cell. Actually, the process is quite fast. The time from the arrival of the action potential at the axon presynaptic terminal to the beginning of the depolarization of the postsynaptic cell can be as little as 0.2 millisecond. Part of the reason the process is so fast is that the synaptic cleft, the distance from the presynaptic terminal membrane to the postsynaptic membrane, is very small.

How is the chemical transmitter released from the presynaptic axon terminal? It is not yet known exactly what mechanism is triggered by the inrush of Ca^{2+}. The actual release of the transmitter, however, is generally believed to occur through the process of *exocytosis* (the word is from the Greek for out of the cell); see Figure 2-5, which includes actual electron microscope pictures of the process. A vesicle containing the transmitter substance attaches to the terminal membrane. Its membrane fuses with the terminal membrane and opens to the outside, spilling out the transmitter. The vesicle membrane is then thought to re-form a vesicle. If it remained in the terminal membrane, the terminal would get progressively larger, which does not happen. It should be noted that not all neuroscientists believe that the process of exocytosis is the way transmitter is in fact released at all types of synapses. However, it is a very useful model of how transmitter is released and it is easy to visualize and remember; there are no clear alternative models.

The first evidence that chemical transmitters are released at terminals as *packets*, the contents of vesicles of about equal size, came long before the development of the electron microscope. The work was done by Bernard Katz at the University of London and others using the neuromuscular junction. Katz received the Nobel prize for his work. The neuromuscular junction makes a very convenient experimental preparation. It can be removed from an animal and kept alive in a dish. It is a pure culture of motor nerve terminals forming synapses on muscle cells; no other kinds of synapses are present. In contrast, even a tiny piece of brain tissue includes many different kinds of synapses.

The neuromuscular junction can be examined by inserting a microelectrode into a postsynaptic muscle cell and stimulating the axon fiber that forms a simple synaptic terminal on it. Let us look first at the situation when the synapse is at rest. There are no action potentials in the axon terminal and so no synaptic transmission occurs. Nonetheless, a microelectrode would record some activity; small changes in the postsynaptic membrane potential seem to occur randomly over time. All of these small changes are depolarizations of the muscle membrane; it becomes slightly more positive for very brief periods (Figure 4-3).

If you look closely at these *miniature synaptic potentials*, as they are called, you will see that they are never smaller than a certain size. The potentials that are larger than the smallest size are twice as large, three times as large, and so on. The simplest way to explain this is to assume that packets of transmitter

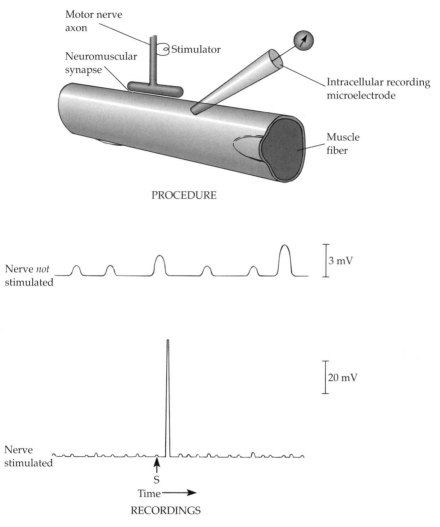

Figure 4-3 Recording of spontaneous miniature postsynaptic potentials from the muscle fiber membrane in the absence of any action potentials in the axon (upper trace) and a unitary potential evoked by an action potential in the axon (lower trace). The miniature potentials are due to random release of quanta (vesicles) of transmitter molecules. The action potential causes release of about 100 vesicles and the unitary synaptic response is about 100 times larger than the smallest miniature potentials.

are being released spontaneously by the presynaptic terminal. The smallest miniature potential would represent the arrival at the postsynaptic muscle membrane of one packet of transmitter. Katz, who discovered the miniature potentials, termed the smallest amount one *quantum* of transmitter. It was estimated that one quantum consisted of about 10,000 molecules of ACh.

Later, with the electron microscope, the size of the vesicles in the ACh terminals at neuromuscular synapses was found to be about large enough to hold 10,000 molecules of ACh. Hence the spontaneous miniature potentials are either the minimum size or some multiple of that size because they represent the emptying of one vesicle, or two at a time, or three, and so on.

The distribution of the sizes of the miniature potentials at the neuromuscular junction is random over time, and they apparently occur all the time at all chemical synapses, in the absence of synaptic transmission. As far as is known, this spontaneous release of transmitter has no function; it is simply noise in a somewhat imperfect system.

Suppose now that the axon leading to the synapse on the muscle cell is stimulated. An action potential will travel down to the terminal and the terminal will release ACh. This simple event, transmission at a single synapse, is called a *unitary synaptic potential*. The unitary synaptic potential is about 100 times larger than the smallest miniature synaptic potential (Figure 4-3). Thus, about 100 quanta, or vesicles, of ACh are released at a single synapse per activation, that is, when synaptic transmission occurs.

At the neuromuscular junction a single activation of one synapse is enough to cause the muscle cell to contract. However, in the vertebrate central nervous system this is virtually never the case: activation of a single synapse on a neuron will not cause it to develop an action potential. A number of synapses have to act together in order for this to occur.

Let us now look at a generalized example of fast excitatory transmission by a neuron in the brain. A recording microelectrode can be inserted into the neuron. Axon terminals from other neurons form excitatory synapses with it, and these can be electrically stimulated. Here it is not possible to study the spontaneous miniature potentials. There are thousands of synapses on the neuron, and some of them are likely to be activated at any given time by action potentials in their axon terminals. Suppose the neuron under study is not developing action potentials. The recording microelectrode in the cell body would show almost continuous small changes in its membrane potential. Many of these changes are likely to be spontaneous miniature potentials, but many others are likely to be actual synaptic potentials resulting from action potentials arriving at synaptic terminals. In the neuromuscular junction, the muscle cell has only one synapse, and a microelectrode can be placed directly under it. In a brain neuron, synaptic potentials can be generated anywhere on the cell body or the dendrites. A recording electrode put in the cell body of a brain neuron will show that the farther away from the electrode a synapse is on a dendrite the smaller the synaptic potential measured by the electrode will be. Hence it is impossible to say whether the small fluctuations in the membrane potential are due to the spontaneous release of quanta of transmitter at synapses (miniature potentials) or to actual occurrences of synaptic transmission (unitary synaptic potentials). It is likely that both occur.

In certain circuits in the central nervous system, it is possible to stimulate a single axon terminal that synapses with the cell body of a neuron under study. In such cases a unitary synaptic potential can be recorded, and it has been found to have the same basic properties as the unitary synaptic potential at the neuromuscular junction.

The basic mechanism of the fast excitatory synapse is an opening of the Na^+ gates at the postsynaptic membrane by the action of the chemical transmitter on the receptor molecules. As we noted earlier, this opening is brief (usually only a few milliseconds) and self-limited and causes only a small depolarization in the cell membrane. The sum of these brief depolarizations is called the *excitatory postsynaptic potential* (EPSP). How do EPSPs cause the cell to generate an action potential? The first thing to note is that the size of the EPSP is graded. The more synapses activated at a cell at the same time, the larger the EPSP. Eventually, the EPSP of the cell membrane can become large enough to cross the action potential-generating threshold, and an action potential occurs at the beginning of the axon, where it leaves the cell body.

This initial segment of the axon has a much lower action potential threshold than the cell body. In fact, its threshold is characteristic of axon membrane in unmyelinated axons. Even in myelinated axons the initial segment is unmyelinated; it is simple axon membrane like that of the squid axon. It has the usual voltage-gated Na^+ and K^+ channels. When the potential inside the initial segment of the axon reaches threshold (say, -60 millivolts), the voltage-controlled ion gates open and an action potential develops and travels down the axon.

The fact that the action potential begins at the initial segment of the axon explains why the action potential is always conducted from the cell body out of the axon to the axon terminals. We saw in Chapter 3 that the action potential can go in either direction in the axon. The reason that it normally does not is that it always starts at the beginning of the axon, as a result of excitatory synaptic actions on the cell body and the dendrites.

The basic mechanism by which EPSPs cause an action potential to develop at the initial segment of an axon is *electrotonic conduction*, the same mechanism that causes an action potential to move along an axon. In fact, the situation is essentially identical to the conduction of an action potential in a myelinated axon. A single excitatory synapse is shown in Figure 4-4 between two central neurons (that is, in the brain). The Na^+ gates on the postsynaptic membrane open momentarily at the synapse and Na^+ rushes in, producing a brief positive shift in the membrane potential there. Since positive charges have moved into the cell, positive charges must also leave the cell for the circuit to be complete. The membrane of the cell body and dendrites has very high resistance, much like myelinated axon, because they are covered with synapses. This is true everywhere except where the axon leaves the cell body, the initial segment. As we have seen, it has the much lower resistance typical

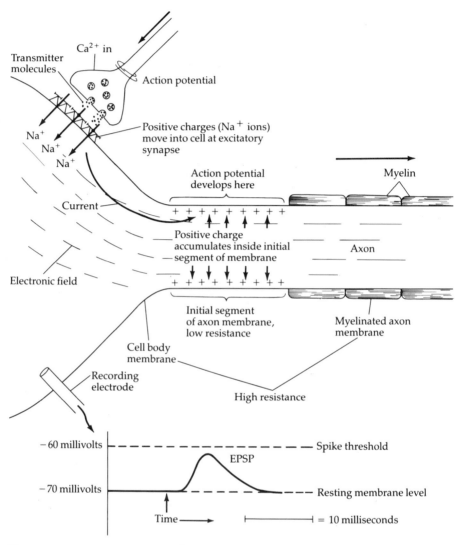

Figure 4-4 Excitatory synapse. When an action potential arrives at the terminal and causes relapse of excitatory transmitters, Na^+ channels are opened briefly in the postsynaptic membrane and NA^+ rushes in, causing an increase in internal positive charge and an electrical charge to flow (current). The initial segment of the axon membrane has a much lower resistance than that of the cell body or myelinated axon, and the spike threshold is reached there first, triggering the beginning of an action potential.

of bare axon membrane. In addition, it is thought that there are fewer voltage-gated sodium channels in the membrane of the cell body and dendrites than in the axon membrane. As positive charge moves out at this low-resistance point and charges the membrane capacitance, the membrane will become more positive inside than its normal resting level of −70 millivolts and may eventually reach the action potential threshold of −60 millivolts. Then the voltage-controlled Na^+ and K^+ gates open, and the action potential goes down the axon.

As we noted earlier, activation of a single excitatory synapse on a brain neuron will not cause it to "fire," or develop an action potential. Enough synapses have to be activated together and exert their influence together at the initial segment (Figure 4-5a). They sum together, a phenomenon often called *spatial summation*. Synapses at different places on the neuron have effects that sum together. If a few synapses are activated once together, it may not be enough to make the cell fire. However, if they are activated repeatedly at a fast enough rate, they will sum over time and generate an EPSP large enough to make the cell fire, a phenomenon called *temporal summation* (Figure 4-5b). A normally functioning neuron is continuously summing information over space and time and "deciding" whether or not to fire. The decision point is the action potential threshold at the initial segment of the axon.

FAST SYNAPTIC INHIBITION

A neuron can do only two basic things to influence other cells: it can increase or decrease their activity. Synaptic excitation increases the excitability and activity of a neuron. Inhibition does the opposite: it decreases the excitability and activity of a neuron. Fast synaptic inhibition occurs when inhibitory synapses on a neuron are activated.

An example of inhibitory synaptic input to a neuron is shown in Figure 4-6. Up to the point where the neurotransmitter acts on the chemical receptor molecules on the postsynaptic membrane, inhibition works just like excitation. An action potential arrives at the presynaptic terminal, Ca^{2+} rushes in, and neurotransmitter is released and diffuses across the synaptic space to attach to chemical receptor molecules. It differs from excitation in that only certain ion channels are opened, in particular Cl^- or K^+ or both. The Na^+ channels remain closed during inhibition.

In most vertebrate brain neurons the concentration of Cl^- is such that the equilibrium potential for Cl^- predicted by the Nernst equation is somewhat more negative than the actual resting potential. If the actual resting potential is −70 millivolts, the calculated Cl^- equilibrium potential might be −75 millivolts. When Cl^- channels that are normally closed are briefly opened, Cl^- moves into the cell, making it still more negative inside (Figure 4-7). A recording electrode can be used to detect this *hyperpolarization* (increased negativity), which is termed the *inhibitory postsynaptic potential* (IPSP). An IPSP is a membrane potential of the axon initial segment farther away from

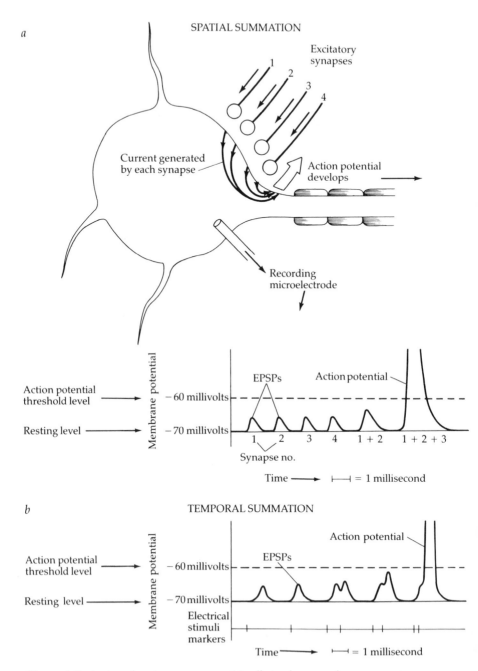

Figure 4-5 Action of excitatory synapses. Usually it takes several synapses acting together to cause the initial segment of the axon membrane to become depolarized to threshold. (*a*) The action of several synapses together at the same time is called spatial summation. (*b*) If one synapse is activated repeatedly over a short time, its actions can also add together to trigger the action potential; this is called temporal summation.

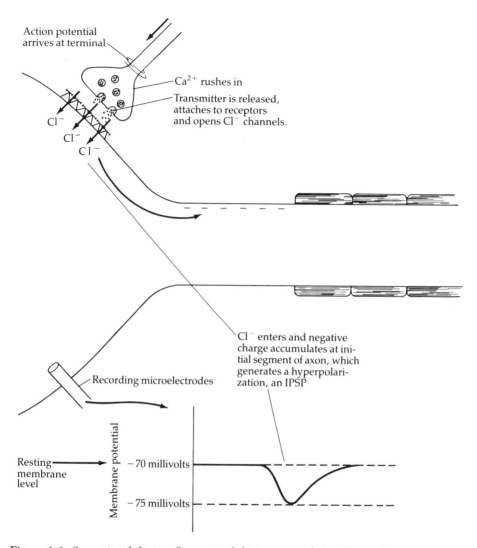

Figure 4-6 Synaptic inhibition. Synaptic inhibition proceeds just like excitation to the point where the inhibitory transmitter molecules attach to receptors on the postsynaptic membrane. Then only certain ion channels are opened, typically chloride or potassium ones. Here chloride channels open and negatively charged chloride ions move into the cell at the synapse, increasing the negative potential on the inside of the membrane even more than at rest and producing an inhibitory postsynaptic potential (IPSP), a hyperpolarization of the membrane.

the value of the spike threshold of the action potential than it is at rest; for example, −75 millivolts rather than −70 millivolts. IPSPs add together on the cell body and dendrites over space and time just as EPSPs do. When the cell

Figure 4-7 Interaction of excitation and inhibition. The inhibitory potential has a stronger action than the excitatory potential. When an inhibitory synapse is active, it acts as a shunt for the increased internal positive charge from the excitatory synapse to flow out, and the membrane at the initial segment is depolarized much less. This occurs even if the IPSP is depolarizing (bottom trace), which sometimes happens as a result of the concentrations of the inhibitory ion (chloride or potassium) inside and outside the neuron, that is, if the normally very low concentration of Cl^- inside the cell is higher, as happens in certain invertebrate neurons.

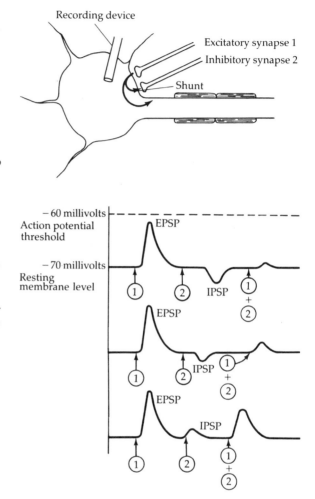

is being inhibited it has an IPSP; an excitatory synaptic action that normally would cause the cell to fire will not do so.

K$^+$ inhibition works in much the same way as Cl^- inhibition. As we saw in Chapter 3, the predicted K$^+$ equilibrium potential for neurons is typically a few millivolts more negative than the actual resting potential. If K$^+$ channels are opened at the synapse, the cell membrane potential becomes more negative than at rest, for example, −75 millivolts rather than −70 millivolts. The reason is that K$^+$ ions move out of the cell membrane, making it more negative inside.

Synaptic inhibition usually occurs as a hyperpolarization of the cell membrane potential in the mammalian central nervous system. The IPSP is characteristic of inhibition. In the case of Cl^--mediated inhibition, say of a motor neuron in the spinal cord, it is easy to show that the IPSP is due to Cl^- moving in through the briefly opened Cl^- channels. It moves in because the concentration of Cl^- is greater outside the cell than inside. If a microelectrode containing a solution with Cl^-, perhaps potassium chloride, is inserted into a neuron cell body and a small current is sent through the electrode to move Cl^- from the electrode into the cell, the concentration of Cl^- inside the cell will increase. As this happens, the IPSP will get smaller and eventually flip over and become a depolarizing potential. The same ion channels—the Cl^- channels—are opened each time, and Cl^- is crossing freely and shifting the membrane potential to the Cl^- equilibrium potential. However, the Cl^- equilibrium potential becomes less negative as the internal concentration of Cl^- increases. In each case, the membrane potential reached during the IPSP is correctly predicted by the Nernst equation applied to the inside and outside concentrations of Cl^-.

When IPSPs are being induced in a cell, synaptic excitation is less effective: the IPSP decreases the EPSP response of the cell. However, the relation is not a simple addition of positive and negative voltages, because inhibition turns out to be more powerful than one would predict from adding the IPSP and EPSP (Figure 4-7). Interestingly, in certain invertebrate neurons the IPSP is a depolarizing potential. The reason is simply that the Cl^- (or K^+) equilibrium potential for that neuron is less negative than the resting level. Yet these depolarizing IPSPs are still inhibitory. The equilibrium potential for Cl^- is determined by the internal and external concentrations of Cl^- and calculated with the Nernst equation (page 54). In most neurons, Cl^- has such a higher concentration outside that the calculated equilibrium potential is more negative (for example, -75 millivolts) than the normal resting membrane potential (for example, -70 millivolts). If the Cl^- concentration inside the cell were somewhat higher than its normal very low value, the Nernst equation would yield a somewhat less negative equilibrium potential, for example, -65 millivolts, for the IPSP. But it still can inhibit because the open chloride channels act as a shunt to leak off the increased internal positive charge (Na+ moving in) of EPSPs.

Inhibition is strong and can occur whether the IPSP is hyperpolarizing or depolarizing. The reason seems to be that during the peak of the inhibitory action, the IPSP, the ion gates of the Cl^- or K^+ channels or both are completely open. The cell membrane at the inhibitory synapse is completely freely permeable to Cl^- or K^+ or both. The cell membrane is held rather close to the equilibrium potential (for Cl^- or K^+) by the freely moving ions. They keep the membrane potential below the action potential threshold level.

Another reason inhibition generally tends to be stronger than excitation is that the inhibitory synapses tend to be on the cell body and to cluster near the initial segment of the axon. They are close to the place where the action potential is initiated and hence can exert a more powerful action on it than can excitatory synapses, which are mostly further away on the cell body and dendrites.

THE CHEMICAL RECEPTOR

The notion that chemical receptor molecules exist on neurons and are the mechanism by which transmitter chemicals exert their actions on neurons is perhaps the most important unifying concept in neuroscience. Receptor molecules exist in all cells and play critical roles in them, as in immune reactions. The reason a chemical transmitter such as ACh can function the way it does is because of the presence and properties of the ACh receptor molecules on the muscle or neuron membrane.

The receptor molecules for chemical neurotransmitters are large, complex protein molecules, and so their exact chemical structures have been difficult to determine. The receptors often are associated as we have seen with ion channels, functioning as chemically controlled gates on the channels. Receptors may also be separate from ion channels and can exert other kinds of influences on the neuron. Slow synaptic transmission seems to work through different receptors, as we shall see in Chapter 5. It is thought that particular receptors and transmitters are specific for each other because they are shaped in such a way that the transmitter molecule fits into the receptor like a hand fits into a glove (Figure 4-8a).

In the diagrams of synaptic transmission (particularly Figures 4-5 and 4-6), receptors were shown on the postsynaptic or target cell. Actually, neurotransmitter receptors are present on the presynaptic terminals as well and can regulate the activity of the terminals. In particular, if a given synaptic terminal releases ACh, it may also have ACh receptors on the terminal. These are termed *autoreceptors* and are believed to control the amount of release of ACh dependent upon the amount of ACh present in the synaptic space. Receptors for neurotransmitters other than the one released by the terminal may also be present on the terminal.

Chemical receptor molecules on neurons are not only on synapses and do not only handle synaptic transmitters. Hormone receptors are found in many neurons and in the cells of certain glands and other tissues. Hormones from the endocrine glands are released into the blood and circulate throughout the body, including the brain. Hormones act only on neurons and tissues that have chemical receptor molecules for the particular hormones.

For example, the pituitary gland releases certain opioids, substances like opium, that act only on certain neurons in the brain because only these neurons have the particular opioid receptor molecules (see Chapter 6).

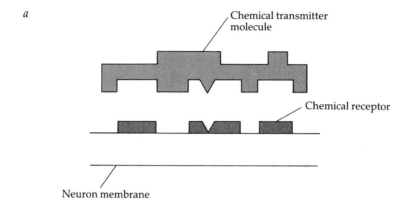

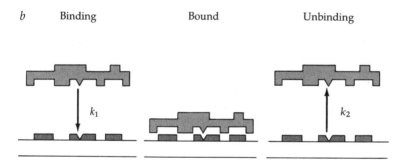

Figure 4-8 (*a*) The key-and-lock theory of how transmitter molecules fit into receptor molecules. (*b*) The transmitted molecule is shown binding (left), bound (center), and unbinding (right) from the receptor molecule. The rate of binding (k_1) is not necessarily the same as the rate of unbinding (k_2).

The acetylcholine (ACh) receptor molecule is the best characterized of all neurotransmitter receptor molecules. The reason is that ACh receptors are the sole receptors in the electric organ of some fishes and eels and hence a pure "culture" for study can be made with them. Because the receptors are protein molecules, *antibodies* can be manufactured against them. (Antibodies are specific proteins made by the body that attack foreign substances in the body or organisms invading it.) The antibodies can then be injected into an animal, where they will bind with the receptors wherever they are in the body. In the case of ACh, antibodies formed to receptors on cells from the electric organ of the torpedo fish can produce a condition in rabbits that appears identical to the human disease myasthenia gravis. This condition is characterized by increasing muscular weakness; the symptoms vary from mild to severe.

When ACh receptor antibodies from a torpedo fish are injected into a rabbit, they attach to and destroy ACh receptor molecules at neuromuscular junctions. This seems to be what happens in myasthenia gravis, but in the human disease, an *autoimmune reaction* destroys the receptors. For unknown reasons the afflicted individual develops antibodies to his or her own ACh receptors. The antibodies destroy varying numbers of the ACh receptors at the neuromuscular junctions, producing varying degrees of muscular weakness.

Cloning the ACh Receptor

Using the techniques of molecular biology, it is proving possible to identify the chemical structures of receptor molecules. This has been an extraordinary achievement. Receptor molecules are very large and complex proteins. Actually, most receptors are made up of several different subunits, each of which is a large protein molecule. All of these subunits together form the particular type of membrane channel (ion channel) characteristic of receptors that operate channels. The genes—the DNA sequences—that code for many of these receptor subunits are now known. Hence it is possible, using recombinant DNA methods, to make these receptor subunits.

Electron microscope photographs provide a very clear picture of the ACh receptor (look ahead at Figure 5-1 on page 114, the ACh receptors in the electric organ of the torpedo fish). Each receptor—there are hundreds in Figure 5-1—looks like a tiny sea anemone or a five-petaled flower. The little hole in the middle of each receptor is the ion channel; it is surrounded by five little blobs, each one a large protein molecule, that constitute the five subunits of the receptor. To analyze the structure of the receptor it must first be identified. As it happens, the poison of the cobra snake, cobratoxin, binds specifically to the ACh receptor and not to any other molecules in the cell membrane (this is part of the lethal action of the poison). Cobratoxin is tagged with a *radioactive label*, most often radioactive iodine, and infused onto the electric organ of the torpedo fish. The receptor can then be dissolved and purified, the concentration of radiolabel showing that it is a pure solution of ACh receptors.

The pure receptor is then injected into a rabbit; the rabbit makes specific antibodies against the receptor, as we noted earlier. From this antibody it is possible to prepare a DNA "library," and from the library one can obtain a DNA sequence that in turn defines the sequence of amino acids that form the protein. In this way the structure of each of the subunits of the ACh receptor was determined. The next step is cloning. The DNA (or RNA) that determines the structure of each receptor subunit is inserted into bacteria. The bacteria divide and multiply and produce large amounts of the receptor subunits for further study (see Appendix).

From this work, we now know that the ACh receptor is a very large protein with a molecular weight of 270,000 daltons (one dalton is equal to the mass of one hydrogen atom). It is composed of four types of subunits, termed α, β, γ and δ (alpha, beta, gamma, delta). The complete ACh ion channel has two alpha subunits and one each of the other types (Figure 4-9). Only the alpha subunits actually bind the ACh transmitter molecules, but all the subunits together form and control the ion channel. When the ACh transmitter molecules attach to the alpha subunits, the channel opens briefly and allows Na^+ ions to pass into the cell, causing depolarization— the EPSP.

Perhaps even more spectacular is the incorporation of the genetic codes for the receptor subunits into a vertebrate cell. The frog egg (oocyte) is the cell of choice because it has no ACh receptors of its own. The messenger RNA for the various receptor subtypes is microinjected into the frog egg. The RNA makes the receptor subunits and they are incorporated into the egg cell membrane. They can then be studied by the patch-clamp method (Figure 4-10). Using this procedure, it was found that the fully active Na^+ channel was formed only if all four types of subunits were present. Remember though, that only the alpha subunits are the receptors for ACh.

This discussion has concerned only the type of ACh receptor at the neuromuscular junction. There are actually two general types of ACh receptors, *nicotinic* and *muscarinic*, to be described in Chapter 5. The neuromuscular ACh receptor is of the nicotinic type (nicotine acts on it like ACh). But in the brain, as of this writing, nicotinic ACh receptors have only two subunits, alpha and beta, with the alpha occurring in at least three different forms and the beta in two. It seems likely that a number of different functional types of ACh receptors may be present in the mammalian brain.

Drugs and Receptors

Another extremely important aspect of chemical receptor molecules on neurons concerns the actions of drugs. Many drugs that have powerful effects on the brain and behavior do so because they act on chemical receptor molecules. Such drugs trick the receptor molecule into accepting them as it would the neurotransmitter, but once attached to the receptor, they may produce quite different actions. Curare is a deadly poison used by the South American Indians. In small amounts it produces immediate muscle paralysis and consequently death from respiratory failure: the chest and diaphragm muscles become paralyzed. Curare is known to attach to the ACh receptor molecules on the skeletal muscle cells in the body. It doesn't activate the receptor and consequently Na^+ channels; it just sits there. But it blocks the

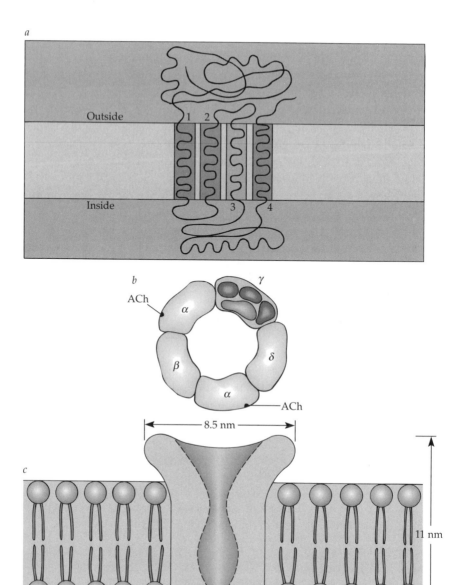

Figure 4-9 Acetylcholine (ACh) receptor and its associated ion channel. (*a*) How one of the subunits of an ACh channel fits into the membrane. The subunit, consisting of one polypeptide chain, traverses the membrane four times. (*b*) The five subunits that make up the channel are arranged in a circle to form an aqueous pore through which ions can move. Acetylcholine binds to the subunits. How the membrane-spanning regions are arranged in a subunit is indicated in the subunit. (*c*) Overall shape and structure of the ACh channel. It is 11 nm long and up to 8.5 nm wide on the extracellular side. The central pore is constricted at the level of the two phospholipid head groups of the membrane's bilayer.

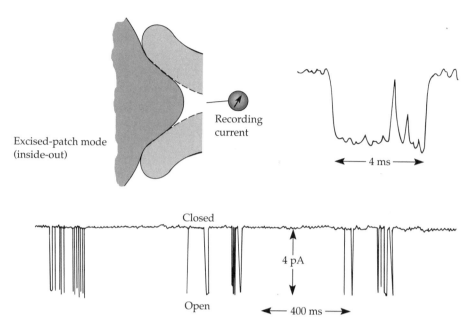

Figure 4-10 Actual patch-clamp recording of the actions of a single acetylcholine (ACh) receptor ion channel in the presence of applied ACh. Note that the channel shows frequent transitions between the open and closed states (Pa, picoamps, ms, milliseconds).

ACh molecules released by the motor nerve terminals from attaching to the receptor molecules and thereby produces total paralysis.

Drugs that act on chemical receptors on neurons and other cells have varying degrees of action on or attachment to a particular receptor. This is termed *affinity*. It might seem clear that the body's own neurotransmitters would have the highest affinity for their receptors, but that is not always the case. Some drugs have higher affinities than natural compounds for receptors and produce greater actions. Other drugs have a very high affinity for receptors but produce no action. Curare is an example of such drugs, which simply block the binding of the transmitter.

In general, when a neurotransmitter is released at a synaptic terminal, not all of the receptor molecules join to transmitter molecules. Binding occurs at different rates and to different degrees, and so does unbinding when transmitter molecules leave the receptors (Figure 4-8b). Neurotransmitters, drugs, and hormones—any substance that will bind to a chemical receptor—are all equally subject to these considerations. Any substance that binds to a receptor is termed a *ligand*.

A piece of neural tissue rich in a given type of receptor molecule can be prepared as a solution in a test tube in such a way that the receptors are still quite functional. When the appropriate transmitter molecules are tagged with a radioactive label and added to the receptor solution, the proportion of transmitter molecules that bind to the receptors can be determined, for example, by separating the receptors and the unbound transmitter molecules. This test is easy to do because receptors are large protein molecules and transmitters are small molecules. The transmitter molecules do not simply bind to receptors and stay there. They bind and release until a dynamic steady state is reached, which happens quite rapidly in a test tube.

Using this procedure we can determine the affinity of a transmitter or drug for a receptor. The general reaction is

$$L + R \underset{k_2}{\overset{k_1}{\rightleftharpoons}} LR$$

where L is the free ligand (the transmitter or drug), R is the free receptor, LR is the transmitter bound to the receptor, k_1 is the rate of binding and k_2 is the rate of unbinding. The affinity is the degree to which the ligand binds to the receptors or, more technically, the concentration of ligand necessary to bind to half the total number of receptor sites present. Note that the reaction goes both ways, between the free ligand and receptor on the left and the bound combination on the right. However, the rate of binding (k_1) and the rate of unbinding (k_2) are not necessarily the same.

The general point to remember is that neurotransmitter molecules do not all simply bind to their receptors. There is a *dynamic equilibrium*, or continuous process of binding and unbinding, between free and bound transmitter molecules and free and bound receptors. Each neurotransmitter-, drug-, or hormone-receptor combination has its own rates of binding and unbinding and hence achieves its own dynamic steady state.

To give a concrete example, opiate receptors in the brain bind both the drug morphine and the brain opioids released by neurons and the pituitary gland (endorphins and enkephalins). A drug called naloxone also binds to the opiate receptors and blocks both morphine and brain opiates from binding. Moreover, naloxone has a higher affinity for the receptor and will "knock off" and displace morphine and brain opioids. This effect of naloxone is so powerful and quick that a person dying from an overdose of heroin, which acts on opiate receptors, will be completely recovered just minutes after being given naloxone. These days, anyone brought into an emergency room comatose and without obvious injuries is routinely given naloxone. It has no known serious side effects and so is harmless to a person not under the influence of opiates. Naloxone will immediately revive people suffering from an overdose of a variety of opiate substances. (Opiates are treated in more detail in Chapter 6.)

AMINO ACIDS—THE FAST NEUROTRANSMITTERS IN THE BRAIN

Earlier we used ACh at the neuromuscular synapse as our prototypic example of fast excitatory synaptic transmission, in part because it is the best under-stood. Although ACh is also a neurotransmitter in several brain systems, it commonly acts more as a slow neuromodulator than as a fast neurotransmitter in the brain (see Chapter 5). Actually, several neurotransmitters in addition to ACh have both fast and slow synaptic actions. The actions a neurotrans-mitter has are determined by its receptors. Typically, slow synaptic actions are termed *neuromodulation*. The receptors activated by the transmitter do not directly control ion channels but rather interact indirectly via the intracel-lular biochemical machinery of the neuron. Fast synaptic actions occur with receptors that do directly open ion channels, as in the ACh neuromuscular junction. We will focus more on neuromodulation in Chapters 5 and 6.

Simple amino acids are believed to be the workhorse fast neurotransmit-ters in the brain. Amino acids are the building blocks of proteins; they are present in the foods we eat and are a normal part of cellular metabolism. Indeed, they are widely distributed throughout the tissues of the body and brain. This fact created difficulties in the study of amino acids as neuro-transmitters. How can one distinguish between an amino acid thought to be a neurotransmitter and the same amino acid present in all cells as a result of cellular metabolism? Part of the solution to this problem has come from iden-tification of the receptors on neurons for amino acid transmitters.

Glutamate

The evidence is now quite strong that *glutamate* is the primary fast excitatory transmitter in the brain (Figure 4-11). *Aspartate*, closely related to glutamate, is also thought to be an excitatory transmitter, but with less certainty. The evidence is also quite strong that GABA (gamma-amino butyric acid) and *glycine* are the primary fast inhibitory transmitters. GABA and glycine are also closely related chemically to glutamate (Fig. 4-11). Glycine appears to be the major inhibitory transmitter in the spinal cord and GABA in the brain. Here we focus on glutamate and GABA as the primary examples.

The glutamate synapse is schematized in Figure 4-12. Glutamate, derived from foods and from metabolism, is present in vesicles in the presynaptic terminal and is released at the synapse when the action potential in the axon arrives at the terminal and triggers Ca^{++} entry—the standard story. The re-leased glutamate acts on a particular receptor termed the *AMPA receptor*,

Figure 4-11 Glutamate molecule. The other amino acid transmitters can all be derived from this molecule. With one carboxyl group (– COO⁻) removed, the molecule becomes GABA; with one carbon group removed (– CH2⁻), the molecule is aspartate; with two carbon groups and the carboxyl group removed, the molecule is glycine.

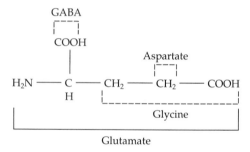

associated with sodium–potassium channels. The channels open briefly, sodium rushes in, and the EPSP develops. This glutamate–AMPA transmitter–receptor is the prototypic fast excitatory synapse in the brain. Glutamate rapidly disassociates from (leaves) the receptors and is inactivated by reuptake into the presynaptic terminal. Actually current evidences suggests that inactivation of the AMPA receptor is due more to a very rapid process of desensitization—the receptor stops responding while glutamate is still present. Part of the difficulty in analyzing the synaptic actions of glutamate is that until very recently there were no specific blockers, chemicals that could block the fast excitatory synaptic actions of glutamate. One such recently developed blocker, CNQX, is shown in Figure 4-12.

But there is much more to the glutamate story. It appears that glutamate and its associated receptors may prove to be the key system involved in memory storage in the brain. Two forms of long-lasting synaptic plasticity occur at glutamate synapses—*long-term potentiation* (LTP) and *long-term depression* (LTD). In both cases, particular patterns of synaptic activation can result in changes in the excitability of the synapses that last for hours or longer. Indeed, these two phenomena of synaptic plasticity are currently the most prominent candidates for mechanisms of memory storage in the mammalian brain.

Glutamate Synapses and Long-term Potentiation

In 1970 a Norwegian scientist, T. Lømo, and a British scientist, Tim Bliss, working in Per Andersen's laboratory in Oslo, were studying the synaptic responses of the hippocampus to electrical stimulation of its input pathways (Figure 4-13). They discovered that if a brief high-frequency train of stimuli was given to an input pathway (for example, at 100 Hz or 100 per second for only 1 second), the synaptic response of neurons in the hippocampus to single test-pulse stimuli to the same pathway had increased dramatically and remained so as long as it was tested. They termed this phenomenon long-term potentiation (LTP). Without going into detail, the increase in the synaptic

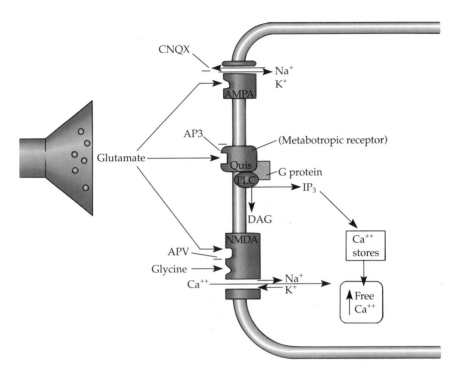

Figure 4-12 Glutamate receptor family. The AMPA receptor controls fast sodium and potassium channels; the NMDA receptor controls calcium channels; the quis-qualate or metabotropic receptor controls a second-messenger system via a G protein that acts on the intracellular machinery (IP3, ADAG) of the cell. The drug CNQX blocks the AMPA receptor, APV blocks the NMDA receptor, and AP3 is thought to block the quis receptor. Other receptor subtypes may also exist.

response occurred at the synapses on hippocampal neurons formed by the axon fibers stimulated—it was a *monosynaptic* (one synapse) *potentiation*. The remarkable aspect of this potentiation was that it lasted so long after such a brief period of stimulation. Subsequent work showed that LTP had many of the properties one would hope for in a mechanism of memory storage. Thus, it required stimulation of a certain minimum number of fibers to develop, a property termed *associativity*—activation of one or just a few synapses would not work. Although initially studied in the hippocampus, LTP has now been found in other brain structures as well, for example, the cerebral cortex and the amygdala. The possible role of LTP in memory storage will be examined in Chapter 11. Here we focus on the synaptic mechanism underlying LTP.

Synaptic pathways that exhibit LTP are believed to use glutamate as the primary neurotransmitter. The mechanism by which LTP is established, how-ever, does not seem to involve the AMPA receptors (Figure 4-12). But the

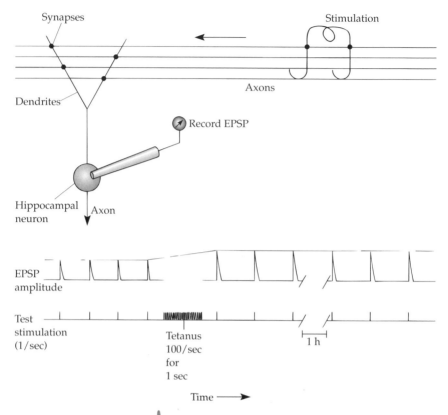

Figure 4-13 Long-term potentiation. Brief, high frequency stimulation of axons synapsing on hippocampal neurons causes a long-lasting increase in the responsiveness (excitability) of these synapses. LTP is initiated by sufficient activation of glutamate NMDA receptors and, according to some experts, is maintained by long-lasting increases in the responsiveness of AMPA receptors. (Glutamate is thought to be the neurotransmitter at these synapses.)

synaptic response that is potentiated is generated largely by the AMPA receptors. If this seems confusing, read on.

Another type of glutamate receptor, the *NMDA receptor*, plays the key role in the establishment of LTP (Figure 4-12). Although the NMDA receptor is a glutamate receptor, it is not activated by weak synaptic actions.

The primary ion channel associated with the NMDA receptor is a Ca^{++} channel. However this channel is normally blocked by magnesium (Mg^{++}) ions. When the cell membrane containing the NMDA channels is depolarized sufficiently, Mg^{++} leaves the channels and glutamate activation of the NMDA receptors opens the channels, allowing Ca^{++} to rush into the neuron. This is the critical event that results in the development of LTP. The conditions necessary to activate the NMDA receptors in hippocampal neurons are thus glutamate action together with sufficient depolarization of the neuron membrane potential to release the Mg^{++} block. This joint requirement explains the "associativity" property of LTP—a few active synapses release glutamate but are not enough to depolarize the neuron sufficiently.

Study of LTP was greatly facilitated with the development of a specific antagonist to the NMDA receptor—APV. This substance blocks the action of glutamate on the NMDA receptor. Consequently, it blocks the development of LTP. It has no effect on the normal fast synaptic excitatory action of glutamate that is mediated by the AMPA receptor. Under normal (that is non-LTP) circumstances the NMDA receptor does not play much of a role in fast excitatory transmission at glutamate synapses.

Our understanding of the complexity of the NMDA receptor is growing rapidly. There are now thought to be at least five different types of binding sites on the NMDA receptor that regulate actions on the calcium channel. These different binding sites are sites where different types of compounds are thought to act.

If activation of the NMDA receptor and associated influx of Ca^{++} produces LTP, how can it be that the increase in excitability of the synapses is seen at the glutamate–AMPA receptors? The reason seems to be that the NMDA receptors contribute relatively little to the fast excitatory response of the nerve cell membrane, as we noted. The persisting increase or potentiation of the synapses is due largely to a persisting increase in the response of the AMPA receptors to glutamate. This can occur in only two ways: a persisting increase in the amount of glutamate released by the presynaptic terminals or an increase of some kind in the responsiveness or affinity of the AMPA receptors to glutamate. At present some evidence supports both the presynaptic (increased glutamate release) hypothesis and the postsynaptic (increased AMPA receptor affinity) hypothesis.

But if LTP involves increased transmitter release from the presynaptic terminals, how could this be caused by activation of NMDA receptors in the postsynaptic membrane? The only way is if some chemical is released post-synaptically and diffuses back across the synaptic cleft to act on the pre-synaptic terminals. Two candidate substances at present are nitric oxide and arachadonic acid. On the other hand, convincing evidence now indicates that the postsynaptic AMPA receptors increase their affinity for glutamate when LTP develops. Perhaps both pre- and postsynaptic processes are normally involved in the maintenance of LTP.

Glutamate Synapses and Long-term Depression

The phenomenon of long-term depression (LTD) was discovered by Masao Ito and his colleagues working in Tokyo in 1981. They were studying responses of a type of neuron in the cerebellum called the *Purkinje cell*. The key relevant features of this type of neuron and its input pathways are indicated in Figure 4-14. The Purkinje neuron is the principal neuron in the cerebellar cortex, the only type of neuron that conveys information out from the cerebellar cortex to other brain structures. One type of input fiber to the Purkinje cell is the *climbing fiber*—there is one and only one to a Purkinje neuron and it is strongly excitatory—a fast synaptic action thought to use aspartate as the neurotransmitter. The other type of input, the *parallel fibers*, are extremely numerous, forming perhaps 200,000 synapses on each Purkinje neuron. They are also fast and excitatory and thought to use glutamate as their neurotransmitter. Ito discovered that if he gave a series of simultaneous stimulations to the climbing fiber and to a group of parallel fibers to the same Purkinje neuron, the sub-

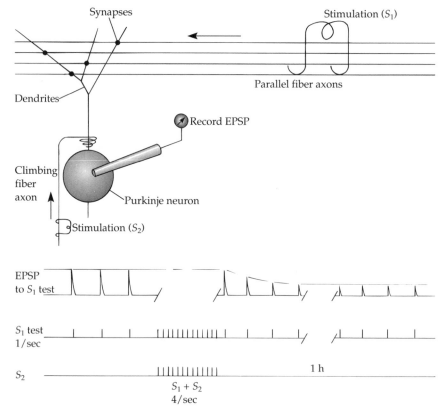

Figure 4-14 Long-term depression (LTD). In cerebellar cortex (see Chapter 9), if both parallel fiber axons (that synapse on Purkinje neuron dendrites) and climbing fibers (that also synapse on Purkinje neuron dendrites) are repeatedly stimulated simultaneously, the response of the Purkinje neuron to activation of the parallel fibers is markedly decreased for a period of hours. The mechanism appears to involve a long-lasting decrease in the responsiveness of the AMPA receptors activated by the parallel fibers.

sequent response of the Purkinje neuron to single test pulses to the parallel fibers was much reduced; this depression lasted for at least an hour.

Purkinje neurons do not have NMDA receptors but they do have AMPA receptors, which are thought to mediate the excitatory synaptic response to the parallel fiber synapses. However, activation of the Purkinje neuron by a climbing fiber results in a marked influx of Ca^{++}, analogous to activation of the NMDA receptors in hippocampal neurons. Current evidence indicates that another type of glutamate receptor, the *metabotropic receptor* (Figure 4-12), also plays a key role in the establishment of LTD. In sum, to establish LTD in Purkinje neurons, three things must happen more or less together: glutamate activation of AMPA receptors (normally from parallel fibers), influx of Ca^{++} (normally from action of the climbing fiber), and glutamate activation of the metabotropic receptor (again by action of the parallel fibers). The net result is a persisting decrease in the response of the AMPA receptors of the Purkinje neuron to glutamate activation by the parallel fibers. The possible role of LTD in memory storage will be considered in Chapter 11.

Although the net outcomes of LTP and LTD are opposite, persisting increased versus decreased synaptic excitability, they share several common features. Both occur at glutamate synapses, both require Ca^{++} influx, and both involve changes in excitability that are mediated via AMPA receptors. Current evidence suggests that the metabotropic glutamate receptor may also play a role in LTP. This metabotropic receptor, incidentally, would be classed as having a slow or modulatory action—it does not directly control ion channels. So glutamate, like ACh, has both fast and slow synaptic actions. It is surely significant that the two best known forms of long-lasting plasticity at synapses in the brain both involve the ubiquitous and very ancient excitatory neurotransmitter glutamate.

To complicate matters, as of this writing there are thought to be at least five different types of glutamate receptors. Molecular biologists have complicated the picture further. Although only one subunit of the NMDA receptor has yet been cloned, more than ten different subunits of the other subtypes of glutamate receptors have now been identified and cloned.

GABA

GABA stands for gamma-aminobutyric acid, a simple amino acid that is synthesized from glutamate in one simple step (Figure 4-15). When an action potential arrives at the terminal, the calcium channels open, Ca^{2+} rushes in, and the GABA vesicles release their contents into the synapse. The postsynaptic membrane has GABA receptors, onto which the GABA molecules attach. When these receptor molecules are activated, they open only Cl^-

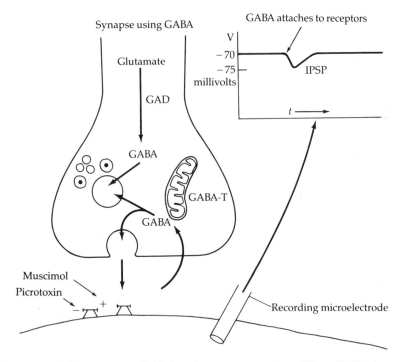

Figure 4-15 Synapse using GABA as the neurotransmitter. When GABA is released and attaches to its receptors, chloride channels open in the postsynaptic membrane and produce synaptic inhibition (IPSPs). The drug muscimol is an agonist (it acts like GABA) and picrotoxin is an antagonist (it blocks the GABA receptor). GABA is an example of a neurotransmitter that causes fast synaptic inhibition and is thought to be inactivated by being taken back up by the terminal. The receptor shown here is the GABA$_A$ receptor.

channels. As we saw earlier, if only Cl$^-$ channels open, the membrane will become more negatively charged inside than its normal level of –70 millivolts. More chloride ions are outside the membrane, and they tend to be kept out because some of their channels are normally closed. When Cl$^-$ rushes in, the inside of the membrane becomes more negative. This yields an inhibitory postsynaptic potential, the IPSP. Consequently, GABA produces synaptic inhibition: it decreases the excitability of the target neuron.

Actually, it is the opening of the Cl$^-$ channels that produce inhibition, as we noted earlier. Opening the Cl$^-$ channels always causes the membrane to go toward its equilibrium potential for Cl$^-$ and tends to hold it there. Another way of stating it is that the open Cl$^-$ channels act as a shunt. When an excitatory synaptic action occurs, an EPSP, it cannot depolarize the cell as well because the associated current is shunted or leaked off by the open Cl^- channels.

One of the most important questions to be answered about chemical neurotransmitter systems in the brain is where they are. It is known that certain anatomical systems in the brain use a given chemical transmitter. Such a system, using one chemical transmitter, may have a particular function in the brain, possibly in relation to behavior.

In order to identify and trace a chemical circuit in the brain, we need some kind of label for the particular chemical involved. As we noted, it is difficult to localize neuronal GABA and other amino acids that function as neurotransmitters in the brain because they seem to be almost everywhere. Like glutamate, GABA is also manufactured in the ordinary course of metabolism of certain foods by cells in both the brain and the rest of the body. Metabolic GABA is not used as a neurotransmitter, although it is chemically the same as neurotransmitter GABA, and herein lies the problem.

Eugene Roberts, a neurochemist at City of Hope Hospital in southern California and the discoverer of GABA, developed with his colleagues a powerful method for localizing neurotransmitter GABA. GAD, the enzyme that makes the neurotransmitter GABA, is involved in making only neurotransmitter GABA, as we have said: it is not involved at all in the manufacture of metabolic GABA. Consequently, GAD is present only in the neurons that make GABA as a neurotransmitter. The technique of Roberts and his colleagues identifies and localizes GAD, relying on the principles of immunohistochemistry. Such techniques, in which the body's immune system is used to label the presence of a substance in the brain, are now widely applied in brain studies. In the case of GAD, a chemically pure sample of GAD molecule was obtained from brain tissues and injected into animals, in which it caused an immune reaction. GAD is a protein, and the injection of a foreign protein into an animal brings the immune system into action. The animal's immune system makes an antibody that is specific to the foreign GAD preparatory to eliminating it from the body. The antibody can then be extracted from the animal's blood serum and labeled, for example, with a radioactive isotope. It is now injected into another experimental animal, say a rat. The labeled antibody along with its radiolabel now binds to GAD molecules, and only GAD molecules, wherever they are in the brain of the rat. The presence of radiolabeled GAD can be detected when sections of the rat's brain are placed on x-ray film.

Use of the labeled-GAD technique has brought scientists to the point where they think they know the distribution of neurotransmitter GABA in the brain. It is present in high concentrations in the gray matter throughout the brain and is found mostly in local interneurons that are presumed to be inhibitory in their actions. There are, however, two long axon neuron systems that also use GABA and are inhibitory, Purkinje neurons in the cerebellum and a class of neurons in the basal ganglia.

When an action potential causes the release of GABA, it diffuses across the synaptic cleft and combines with GABA receptors, which open Cl⁻ channels. Like glutamate, there is no enzyme in the synapse to break down or inactivate GABA. Instead, after its release from the receptor much of it diffuses back across the synaptic cleft and is taken up again by the presynaptic terminal, where it is stored in vesicles and used again. GABA is thought to be taken back up through *pinocytosis*, the same process used for the reuptake of glutamate. The terminal membrane folds around GABA molecules and incorporates them into the terminal. Some GABA is also taken up by the postsynaptic membrane. There is an enzyme inside the target cell that then metabolizes this GABA. However, the enzyme does not appear to be present in the synaptic cleft and does not play a direct role in the synaptic action of GABA. Apparently the only way GABA released at a synaptic terminal can be inactivated is by the receptors releasing it and the presynaptic terminal taking it up again.

Most readers are probably familiar with the disease epilepsy. Symptoms may range from momentary blackouts to massive general body convulsions. One type of epilepsy appears to be caused by damage to a region of the brain that then periodically develops seizure activity: runaway discharging of neurons. Seizure activity can spread to other regions of the brain. This kind of epilepsy can be produced experimentally in monkeys by implanting a small amount of an irritating substance such as alumina cream on the cerebral cortex. After the monkey recovers from the operation, it will gradually develop epilepsy, or an epileptic focus in the brain.

Roberts and his associates at City of Hope examined the GABA content of the brain region having the epileptic focus in such monkeys. They did it by measuring the presence of GAD using the labeled GAD technique described earlier. They found a marked reduction of GAD, and therefore of GABA, in the region of the epileptic focus, which makes good sense. The easiest way to produce runaway excitation of neurons is to remove the inhibitory effects of the neurons that normally keep the excitatory neurons under control, and this is what the effect of decreasing the amount of GABA, an inhibitor, would be.

The effect of removing the inhibitory controls of the GABA neurons can also be shown very clearly with drugs. To take one example, a drug called bicuculline is a rather specific antagonist to GABA. It causes convulsions and death in animals if it is injected into the brain even in very small amounts. The convulsions develop because the inhibitory GABA neurons no longer function to hold down the activity of the nervous system, and the excitatory neurons in the brain go into runaway excitation.

GABA and Anxiety Neurosis

It is commonly thought that the neuroses are basically learned disorders, fears and anxieties that develop as a result of life experience, whereas the major psychoses, such as schizophrenia and depression, result from fundamentally biological disorders of the brain. (We discuss the major psychoses in Chapter 5). However, recent evidence raises the possibility that one major form of neurosis, anxiety neurosis, may also be due to an underlying brain disorder.

Two major forms of anxiety neurosis are panic attacks and generalized anxiety. In the panic disorder, the person suffers sudden and terrifying attacks of fear that are episodic and occur unpredictably. The symptoms of a panic attack are dilated pupils, flushed face, perspiring skin, rapid heartbeat, feelings of nausea, desire to urinate, choking, dizziness, and sense of impending death. The activity of the sympathetic nervous system and pituitary-adrenal hormonal system increases and cortisol, the stress hormone, is released. The generalized anxiety disorder is a persisting feeling of fear and anxiety that is not associated with any particular event or stimulus.

Recent evidence suggests that both panic attacks and generalized anxiety have a significant genetic factor. Interviews of relatives of anxious patients in clinical studies indicated that up to 40 percent of the relatives also had anxiety neurosis. It is tempting to postulate that anxiety neurosis is learned: a person who grows up in a neurotic family seems likely to resemble the rest of the family in mental disposition. However, studies of twins show that if one identical twin has anxiety neurosis, the chances are greater than 30 percent that the other will too, whereas the chances of both twins having the disorder are only about 5 percent if they are not identical. Isolated cases in which one identical twin was adopted away from the family and the twins were raised separately show the same general result.

The discovery of Librium and other minor tranquilizing drugs opened up an intriguing new approach to understanding the anxiety neuroses. These drugs are all chemically closely related and are a class of compounds called the benzodiazepines. The benzodiazepines are remarkably effective in treating the symptoms of panic attack and anxiety.

In the mid-1930s dye compounds attracted the attention of chemists at the pharmaceutical company Hoffmann-La Roche. These chemists were attempting to make a particular group of dye compounds biologically active. They added a basic side chain that had often before imparted biological activity to compounds, without success.

The compounds were put aside, as were others. By 1957, the laboratory benches had become so crowded that a cleanup had to be instituted. As the chemists were throwing out various drugs and other compounds, one drug was submitted for pharmacological tests. It had extraordinary calming and muscle relaxant effects in animals. When the chemists analyzed the structure of the drug, it turned out to be a rather different compound than they thought they had made. It was, in fact, the benzodiazepine derivative that came to be known as Librium. The benzodiazepines all have a seven-membered ring (diazepine ring) attached to a standard six-membered benzene ring.

The benzodiazepines are now the drug treatment of choice for panic attack and anxiety. In proper therapeutic doses they are relatively safe, have few side effects, and are not particularly addicting. In higher doses they are addicting, both in terms of the tolerance that is built up to them (increasingly high doses are required to produce the same effect) and the variety of symptoms that follow withdrawal, including anxiety and emotional distress, nausea and headaches, and even death. The benzodiazepines have become drugs of abuse.

The benzodiazepines rather specifically ease anxiety and panic attack. There is a close correlation between the time courses of the mild withdrawal symptoms when drug treatment is stopped and the return of symptoms in individuals with anxiety neuroses. Benzodiazepines are of little help to schizophrenia, even for treating the anxiety symptoms associated with the disease, and they may even make depression worse. Interestingly, benzodiazepines are not particularly helpful in the treatment of specific phobias.

Study of the benzodiazepines sprang to prominence in neuroscience in 1977 with the discovery of specific receptors for these substances in the mammalian brain. The benzodiazepine receptors are distributed widely in the brain, with strong concentrations in such areas as the cerebral cortex, hippocampus and cerebellum (Figure 4-16).

Meanwhile, a growing body of evidence indicated that the benzodiazepines potentiate the effects of the inhibitory transmitter GABA. It soon became clear that the benzodiazepines were not merely analogues of GABA that acted just like it. Although regions of high concentrations of benzodiazepines also have high concentrations of GABA receptors, the converse is not true; some brain regions that have high concentrations of GABA receptors do not have high concentrations of the benzodiazepine receptor.

In sum, the benzodiazepine receptor seems to exist together with the GABA receptor but is not identical with it. The current model of the GABA and benzodiazepine receptors is that they are coupled at GABA synapses (Figure 4-17). In this model, activation of the benzodiazepine receptor by a benzodiazepine acts via an intermediary molecule, "gabamodulin," to increase either the binding of GABA molecules to the GABA receptor, or the coupling between the GABA receptor and the chloride channel, or both. The result is an increase in the inhibitory effects of GABA. GABA synaptic inhibition in the brain seems a good way to reduce at least the symptoms of anxiety, if not the causes.

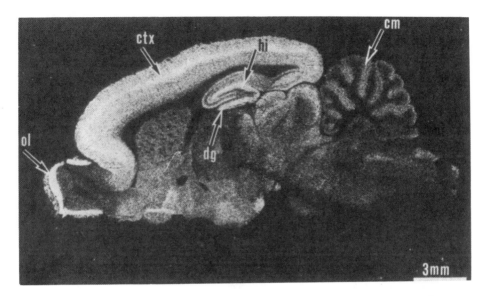

Figure 4-16 Distribution of benzodiazepine (BDZ) receptors in the rat brain. A radiolabeled substance that binds to the BDZ receptors was administered, and then images of the brain sections were developed on x-ray film. A sagittal, or longitudinal, section made near the midline of the brain is shown. The white areas are locations of BDZ receptors. They are particularly dense in the cerebral cortex, the hippocampus, the cerebellum, and the olfactory bulb.

The fact that a specific receptor exists in high concentrations in the brain for the benzodiazepines suggests that the brain or body may produce its own antianxiety substances. If this is so, perhaps either through inheritance or accident the brain of a person suffering from anxiety neurosis has too little of its own antianxiety substances. Many laboratories are currently hot on the trail after natural brain antianxiety compounds and have been since the late 1970s. Although several candidates have been proposed, as of this writing none has been proved to be a brain antianxiety compound.

As with other neurotransmitter receptors, studies show the GABA receptor to be more complex every year. There are now thought to be two types of GABA receptors, GABA$_A$ and GABA$_B$. Our discussion has focused on GABA$_A$, which is much better understood than GABA$_B$. At least seven different types of sites are now associated with the GABA$_A$ receptor. In addition to the GABA and benzodiazepine sites is a site specific for barbiturates and a site specific for steroid hormones. Molecular biologists have complicated the picture even more: at last count at least 20 different subunits of the GABA receptors have been cloned. It seems in-

Figure 4-17 Hypothetical scheme of the BDZ receptor as a complex with the GABA receptor at GABA synapses. The BDZ receptor appears to act to facilitate the opening of chloride channels by the GABA receptor, thus enhancing synaptic inhibition.

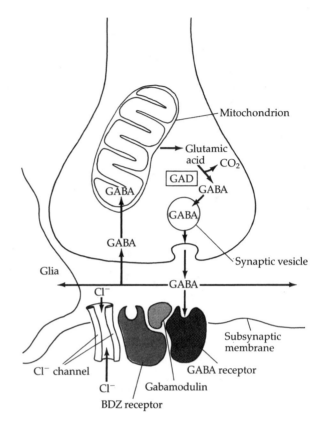

creasingly clear that neurotransmitter *receptors* hold the keys to the functioning of neurons and the brain.

ELECTRICAL SYNAPTIC TRANSMISSION

It was unclear whether synaptic transmission in the vertebrate central nervous system was chemical or electrical in nature until the 1940s, when John Eccles, then at Canberra, and others found the initial evidence pointing to chemical transmission. Eccles received the Nobel prize for this work. Synaptic transmission at neuromuscular junctions and at other peripheral synapses, such as the heart and autonomic nervous system, had been known much earlier to be chemical (specifically, to utilize ACh).

The great majority of synapses in the mammalian (and human) brain are chemical. But very recently, evidence has accumulated suggesting that there are some electrical synapses in the mammalian brain, even in higher structures such as the cerebral cortex. The difference between electrical and chemical synapses is an important one. A chemical synapse is by nature plastic; it can be altered in many ways and at many different steps to increase or decrease its activity. Electrical synapses are rigid and unchanging. What goes in always determines what goes out, and it cannot be altered short of major structural or chemical change. Learning and memory could not develop in a nervous system that had only electrical synapses.

An electrical synapse works much like an electrical transformer. The pre- and postsynaptic membranes are connected in "gap junction" synapses by a specialized structure. When an action potential arrives at the terminal of an electrical synapse, it induces an electric field in the postsynaptic neuron. If the field is large enough, the postsynaptic membrane reaches the action potential threshold, the voltage-gated sodium channels open, and an action potential develops. No transmitter chemical action need be involved.

The effectiveness of an electrical synapse depends very much on the size and geometry of the pre- and postsynaptic elements. In order to work reliably, the presynaptic terminal must be close to the size of the postsynaptic element. If the presynaptic element were too small, the electric field built up in the postsynaptic neuron would also be too small. You might wonder if there is any electric field effect like this in a typical chemical synapse (Figure 4-2). There is, but because of the existence of the synaptic cleft and the tiny size of the presynaptic element relative to that of the postsynaptic element, it is very small and has no significant influence on the postsynaptic membrane potential.

Simpler invertebrate animals have both chemical and electrical synapses. It seems likely that the first synapses to appear in evolution were electrical. Indeed, in such primitive animals as the sea urchin, when a fertilized egg begins to divide and develop, electrical synapses develop between the first cells to form. At the stage when the animal consists of only four or eight cells, two adjacent cells dissected out will be found to have functional gap-junction electrical synapses between them. It may be that electrical synapses play a critical role in the growth and development of the embryo.

Electrical synapses are much simpler than chemical synapses. Why did evolution go to all the trouble of developing chemical synapses? Further, why did chemical synapses win out in evolution? Why are most (but not all) synapses in the mammalian brain chemical? I noted earlier that there are many more possibilities for change and plasticity at chemical synapses. However, chemical synapses are present in animals that are very primitive and cannot learn anything except habituation. The sea anemone, a representative of the lowest phylum of animals to have a nervous system, has both chemical and electrical synapses and can show habituation. If touched, it contracts, if touched over and over, it contracts less and less: it habituates.

There is another and perhaps more important reason why the chemical synapse has been favored in evolution. The chemical synapse is typically very tiny, and so a great many chemical synapses can be packed into a small space. Not so with the electrical synapse. As we have seen, the presynaptic element must be almost as large as the postsynaptic element for an electrical excitatory synapse to work well. This limits the number of synapses to only a very few per neuron. The complexity of even the simpler invertebrate nervous systems could not have developed without the smaller chemical synapses.

One other major difference between chemical and electrical synapses has to do with synaptic delay. In the electrical synapse, the postsynaptic response develops at essentially the exact time that the presynaptic action potential does. In the chemical synapse there is a delay: the time required for the neurotransmitter to be released and diffuse across the synaptic space. This delay increases the ability of the cell to integrate information over time, as in temporal summation (Figure 4-5b).

Electrical synapses in the mammalian brain tend to exist between the cell bodies of immediately adjacent neurons that have the same function. Adjacent motor neurons in a motor nucleus tend to fire together to activate muscle fibers that are close to each other. Electrical synapses between them would increase their synchrony of action, so that when one motor neuron fired, the other would also fire at about the same time and vice versa. However, the vast preponderance of synapses in the mammalian and human brain are chemical. We are what we are because our brains are basically chemical machines rather than electrical ones.

SUMMARY

The key to understanding how the brain works is the process of synaptic transmission: how neurons transmit information to other neurons or muscle or gland cells. In overview, the process is straightforward. When an action potential arrives at an axon terminal (the presynaptic part of the synapse), it opens voltage-gated calcium (Ca^{2+}) channels in the terminal membrane that are normally closed. Calcium rushes in and triggers the release of a neurotransmitter chemical that diffuses across the synaptic cleft to act on receptors in the postsynaptic cell membrane of the synapse and hence trigger reactions in the postsynaptic neuron (or muscle or gland cell).

When calcium rushes into the presynaptic terminal, it causes the terminal to release neurotransmitter chemical by a process of exocytosis. The neurotransmitter is present in the presynaptic terminal in little spheres, or vesicles. When calcium rushes in, some of these vesicles fuse with the terminal membrane and dump their chemical content into the synaptic cleft. In the case of acetylcholine (ACh), the transmitter chemical at the neuromuscular junction, one vesicle contains about 10,000 molecules of ACh. This is termed one quantum of transmitter chemical. The action potential and subsequent calcium influx triggers the release of about 100 vesicles, or 100 quanta of transmitter. There is also a random spontaneous release of vesicles in the absence of the action potential, usually one or two or three at a time, causing miniature potentials that are thought to be simply "noise" in an imperfect system.

The neurotransmitter chemical attaches to chemical receptor molecules (proteins) in the postsynaptic membrane. These receptors then act to produce changes in the postsynaptic cell. In "fast" (less than a millisecond) synaptic transmission, these receptors directly control ion channels. This is yet another type of ion channel; it is not voltage-gated (opened) but rather can be opened only when the chemical transmitter attaches to the receptor that controls the channel (these are termed ligand-gated channels).

In fast excitatory synaptic transmission the receptors open sodium channels and sodium ions rush in, causing some depolarization (the local membrane potential becomes less negative). This excitatory response (EPSP: excitatory postsynaptic potential) is graded depending on how many receptors—Na^+ channels—are activated. If enough receptors are activated, the membrane potential at the initial part of the axon where it leaves the cell body (initial segment) is depolarized to reach the action potential threshold for the voltage-gated sodium channels there, and the action potential develops and travels down the axon. In fast inhibitory synaptic transmission, the receptors control normally closed chloride (Cl^-) channels. They open, Cl^- rushes into the cell, and the cell membrane becomes hyperpolarized (more negative than the resting potential); the cell is inhibited from generating an action potential (IPSP: inhibitory postsynaptic potential).

In recent years, molecular biology has provided the knowledge and tools to characterize neurotransmitter receptors (all of which are complex protein molecules). It is becoming increasingly clear that the "message" in synaptic transmission is in the receptor rather than simply in the chemical used as the transmitter. Thus, ACh can be an excitatory transmitter or an inhibitory transmitter, depending on the type of receptor it acts on. One type of ACh receptor (the receptor at the neuromuscular junction, which is excitatory) has a molecular weight of 270,000 daltons and is made up of four types of subunits. The reason so many drugs have such powerful effects on the brain is that they "fool" specific chemical receptors on neurons into thinking that they are neurotransmitters. That is, because of their chemical structure they attach to the receptor and either trigger it (agonist drugs) or block the normal transmitter chemical from attaching to the receptor (antagonist drugs).

Glutamate, an amino acid present in food and in all cells, is the workhorse fast excitatory neurotransmitter chemical in the brain. It also seems to play a key role in memory storage. An example is long-term potentiation (LTP). If a pathway using glutamate as a transmitter (in the hippocampus, for example) is stimulated rapidly, it can cause a persisting increase in excitability of the activated synapses. This potentiation is initiated by activation of one type of glutamate receptor, the NMDA receptor. The persistence of increased excitability seems to involve another type of glutamate receptor, the AMPA receptor, which mediates fast excitatory transmission (opening

Na$^+$ channels). Changes in the presynaptic terminals may also occur. Another process of synaptic plasticity, long-term depression (LTD), can also occur at glutamate synapses (for example, in the cerebellum) and involves a long-lasting decrease in the excitability of glutamate AMPA receptors.

GABA (gamma amino butyric acid) is the workhorse fast inhibitory neurotransmitter in the brain. Its receptors control chloride (Cl$^-$) channels in neurons. The tranquilizers (benzodiazepines) act on the GABA receptors to increase their actions and hence to increase inhibition. They are effective in treating certain types of anxiety.

SUGGESTED READINGS AND REFERENCES

Books

Baudry, M., & Davis, J. L. (1991). *Long-term potentiation: A debate of current issues.* Cambridge, MA: MIT Press.

Eccles, J. C. (1964). *The physiology of synapses.* Berlin: Springer-Verlag.

Edelman, G. M., Gall, W. E., and Cowan, W. M. (1987). *Synaptic function.* New York: John Wiley & Sons.

Kandel, E. R., Schwartz, J. H., and Jessell, T. M. (1991). *Principles of neural science* (3rd ed.). New York: Elsevier.

Kuffler, S. W., Nicholls, J. G., and Martin, A. R. (1984). *From neuron to brain: A cellular approach to the function of the nervous system* (2nd ed.). Sunderland, MA: Sinauer Associates.

Shepherd, G. M. (1988). *Neurobiology* (2nd ed.). New York: Oxford University Press.

U. S. Congress, Office of Technology Assessment (1992). *The biology of mental disorders.* Washington, D. C.: U. S. Government Printing Office.

Articles

Bliss, T. V. P., and Lømo, T. (1973). Long-lasting potentiation of synaptic transmission in the dentate area of the anesthetized rabbit following stimulation of the perforant path. *Journal of Physiology, 232,* 331–356.

Cotman, C. W., Monaghan, D. T., and Ganong, A. H. (1988). Excitatory amino acid neurotransmission: NMDA receptors and Hebb-type synaptic plasticity. *Annual Review of Neuroscience, 11,* 61–80.

Ito, M. (1989). Long-term depression. *Annual Review of Neuroscience, 11,* 85–102.

Madison, D. V., Malenka, R. C., and Nicoll, R. A. (1991) Mechanisms underlying long-term potentiation of synaptic transmission. *Annual Review of Neuroscience, 14,* 379–397.

Nicoll, R. A. (1988). The coupling of neurotransmitters to ion channels in the brain. *Science, 241*, 545–553.

Sakmann, B. (1992). Elementary steps in synaptic transmission revealed by currents through single ion channels. *Science, 256*, 503–512.

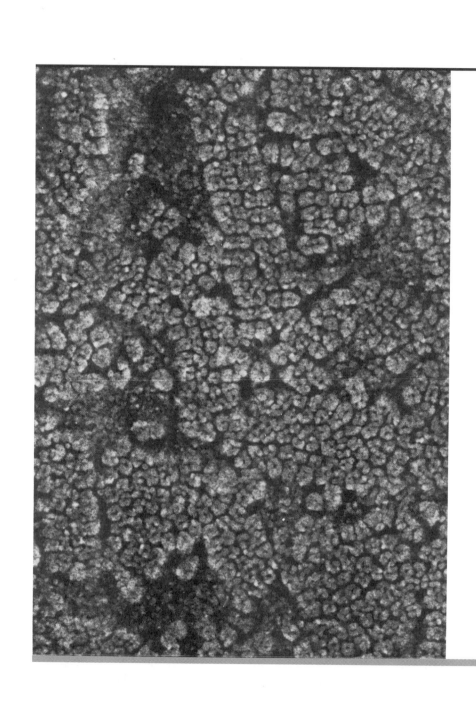

5

Neurotransmitters and Chemical Circuits in the Brain

Investigations of the chemistry of synaptic transmission in the brain—the communication among its neurons—holds promise for the solution of such fundamental questions about the brain and behavior as how the brain stores memories, why sex is such a powerful motivation, and the biological basis of mental illness. Sorting out the connections of the circuits chemical synapses form is a difficult task, but here, too, progress has been made, for example, in detecting the circuits that may be at fault in Alzheimer's and Parkinson's diseases. The study of chemical transmitter substances and circuits in the brain and drug actions on these circuits and neurons began only a few years ago but has greatly expanded to become the largest field of neuroscience.

Before we look at particular neurochemical transmitters, a few general points that apply to all of them are worth noting. We have already seen how the action potential triggers the release of neurotransmitters at the axon ter-

Figure 5-1 ACh receptors and ion channels in the electric organ of the torpedo fish. This electron photomicrograph shows them as molecular structures consisting of five subunits surrounding an ion channel.

minal by causing Ca^{2+} to rush through the membrane and the way the transmitter acts on its receptors on the postsynaptic cell membrane by altering the excitability of the cell (Figure 5-1). From a chemical point of view, other steps in the process of synaptic transmission are equally important.

The chemical transmitter must first be synthesized. All synaptic transmitters identified so far are rather simple chemicals that are available either as the products of normal metabolism or from common foods. Indeed, some transmitters are simply amino acids like glutamate and GABA, parts of the proteins in food. Once the transmitters have been synthesized or eaten, they must be transported to the axon terminal (unless they are synthesized there) and stored in vesicles ready for release. The amount of any neurotransmitter available for use in the brain is always limited, in order not to flood the brain. Usually one critical step or factor in the synthesis and storage of the transmitter limits the amount available; this is the *rate-limiting factor*. Determination of rate-limiting factors is important, because many brain disorders, such as major depression, may result from too little or too much of a neurotransmitter. If the rate-limiting factor is known, the possibility exists of treating the disorder by increasing or decreasing the amount of neurotransmitter in the brain.

Another critical aspect of synaptic transmitter actions is *inactivation*. If a transmitter stayed on its receptors and continued to act, the brain would go out of control. Once the transmitter has attached to the receptors and exerted its action, it must be inactivated. This can occur in several ways. An enzyme may break down the neurotransmitter at the receptor, or the transmitter may attach only briefly to the receptor and then be released and taken away by some other process. Inactivation always takes place, as we noted in our discussion of receptor kinetics in Chapter 4; however, the rate at which it occurs can vary widely. After the transmitter has been inactivated it must be dealt with in some way. In general, transmitter chemicals or critical parts of them are taken back up by the terminals and reused (pinocytosis).

One might think that if a transmitter is taken back up and reused, then there would always be enough. Although the reuse of transmitters is a remarkable example of economy of function in neurons, it is far from perfect. Some transmitter is lost and ultimately metabolized and excreted from the body. If no new transmitters were made, the stores would gradually be depleted. The rate-limiting factor is critically important in the synthesis of transmitter. It may take a long time for a change in a rate-limiting factor to become apparent, but eventually it will. For example, drugs given to treat such severe mental illnesses as schizophrenia and depression often do not begin to change the rate-limiting factor or show their effects for a week or more.

ACETYLCHOLINE

Acetylcholine (ACh) is the transmitter at the neuromuscular junction, as we saw in Chapter 4, and at certain other peripheral synapses of the autonomic nervous system (such as in the heart). It is the most thoroughly studied transmitter and perhaps the most familiar. In 1924 Otto Loewi, in one of the classic experiments in the field of neuroscience, discovered ACh and settled the argument about whether synaptic transmission from the vagus nerve to the heart muscle (and other synapses) was electrical or chemical.

Loewi's experiment, a model of simplicity, is well worth describing here. The vagus nerve is one of the major nerves that controls the heart. In a frog the vagus nerve and the heart can be removed and kept alive in a dish of Ringer's solution. (Ringer's solution resembles blood in its salt constituents.) Electrical stimulation of the vagus nerve, both in the live animal and in a dish, slows the heart rate.

Loewi stimulated the vagus nerve of a heart in a solution of Ringer's many times, which caused repeated slowing of the heart rate. He then removed some of the solution from the dish containing the stimulated heart and applied it to another frog's heart in another dish. This heart also slowed. This simple experiment proved that synaptic transmission is chemical. Loewi named the unidentified substance "Vagusstoff"; it was soon shown to be ACh.

Fast Transmitter Actions in the Periphery

The synthesis of ACh is shown in Figure 5-2. It is made in one step from acetyl coenzyme A (acetyl CoA) and choline. *Acetyl CoA* is present in large amounts in the mitochondria of all cells. It is involved in the citric acid cycle, which makes biological energy in the form of ATP by metabolizing glucose and takes place in part in the mitochondria.

There is one important peculiarity about energy metabolism in the brain. Whereas other tissues and organs in the body can make biological energy by metabolizing substances other than glucose, such as proteins and carbohydrates, neurons, so far as we know, can make biological energy, or ATP, only from the metabolism of glucose. Hence, the brain is totally dependent on the glucose supplied by the blood in order to function, and as we have seen, its demands are great: although the human brain is only about 2 percent of body weight, it gets 15 percent of the blood supply. The brain also requires great amounts of oxygen, which is necessary for the metabolism of glucose. Glucose and oxygen are used to make ATP, and in the process a number of products such as acetyl CoA and acetate are formed. The final outcome of the metabo-

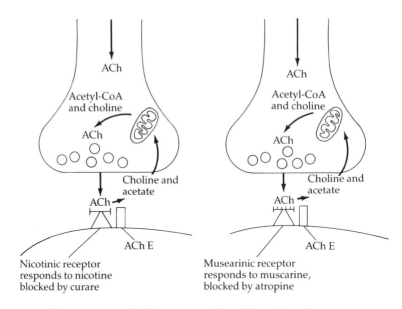

Figure 5-2   The two types of ACh synapses. They differ only in their receptors, which causes them to be acted on differently by drugs. The nicotinic receptor is activated by nicotine and blocked by curare, whereas the muscarinic receptor is activated by muscarine and blocked by atropine.

lism of glucose is water and carbon dioxide; the latter passes back to the blood and is exhaled from the lungs.

Choline, which combined with acetyl CoA forms acetylcholine, is not manufactured by the body and must be obtained from foods. Egg yolks are a rich source of choline, as are many vegetables. After digestion of choline-containing foods, choline passes into the blood and is taken up by neurons. As it happens, the amount of choline available to neurons is the rate-limiting factor in the synthesis of ACh. Acetyl CoA and choline acetyltransferase, the enzyme that facilitates the synthesis of ACh from acetyl CoA and choline, are always present in ample amounts in cells. Consequently, if a person is suffering from a disorder thought to be brought on by insufficient amounts of ACh, one safe and simple treatment might be more choline-containing foods in the person's diet. As we shall see, this simple treatment may in fact be helpful for some elderly people who are just beginning to exhibit the distressing early signs of senility.

The inactivation of ACh at the receptors is accomplished very rapidly by the enzyme *acetylcholinesterase* (AChE). This enzyme is present in close association with the ACh receptor molecules and breaks ACh down into acetate and choline in a matter of microseconds, freeing the receptor to respond to new ACh. Much of the choline is then taken up by the axon terminal to be made into ACh and reused. The acetate is used by all cells in the citric acid cycle.

Acetylcholine is either formed at the axon terminals or synthesized in the cell body of the neuron and transported down the axon to the terminals (Figure 5-2). This process of *axoplasmic transport* takes hours to days in a long axon. When an action potential arrives at the terminal, Ca^{2+} rushes in and the vesicles release their contents of ACh into the synapse. As we noted earlier, one action potential causes the release of about 100 vesicles, each containing about 10,000 molecules of ACh. The ACh molecules diffuse across the synapse and attach to the ACh receptors, which, on skeletal muscles, open Na^+ channels, causing the muscle cell to develop an action potential and contract. Almost immediately after the ACh binds to the receptors, AChE breaks it down into acetate and choline, which are reused.

Drugs could act at many places to interfere with the ACh synapse. They could block the synthesis of ACh, its transport down the axon, its formation into vesicles, its release into the synapse, its attachment to the receptor, its breakdown by AChE, and so on. Early on in the history of pharmacology it was hoped that drugs producing the same effect on people would turn out to have a common chemical structure. A glance at the many places drugs could act on the ACh synapse shows that for the most part this was a case of wishful thinking. For example, curare and botulin, a poison found in improperly canned foods, both cause paralysis, but are quite different chemicals. Curare, as we saw earlier, blocks the ACh receptors and so prevents ACh from acting. Botulin, however, blocks the release of ACh from the presynaptic terminals. Hence these two chemically unrelated drugs have a common effect, blockage of the ACh synapse, but they do it in very different ways.

An earlier point may have been puzzling. In describing Otto Loewi's experiment on the vagus nerve of the frog, I stated that stimulation of the vagus nerve releases ACh, which causes the heartbeat to slow. ACh inhibits the activity of cardiac muscle cells, yet it excites the activity of skeletal muscle cells. It has opposite actions, excitatory and inhibitory, on two different types of muscle cells. As it happens, different drugs can block these two synapses. Curare blocks the ACh synapses of skeletal muscle cells but has no effect on the ACh synapses of heart cells; atropine, on the other hand, blocks the ACh synapses of heart cells but has no effect on the ACh synapses of skeletal muscle cells. The ACh that normally acts at both kinds of muscle synapses is identical in chemical composition, and so the receptors must be different (Figure 5-2). This is a good illustration of the fact that the kind of effect produced by a neurotransmitter depends not only on the nature of the transmitter but also on that of the receptor. Studies of ACh synapses of muscle and peripheral tissues in the autonomic system in pure culture showed many years ago that there must be two types of ACh receptors. Some drugs activate only one or the other receptor. Nicotine, the active ingredient in tobacco, acts like ACh on ACh synapses of skeletal muscle cells but has no effect on the ACh receptors on heart muscle cells. The skeletal-muscle-type ACh receptor is therefore called the *nicotinic receptor*.

Another drug, a poison called muscarine, acts just like ACh on the ACh synapses of heart muscle cells and on most of the ACh synapses in the autonomic nervous system. However, muscarine has no effect on the ACh receptors of skeletal muscle cells. The ACh receptors activated by muscarine are called *muscarinic receptors*.

Muscarine, incidently, is an extract of a poisonous mushroom called *Amanita muscaria*, or fly agaric. (Muscarine does not kill flies outright but makes them groggy so that they can be more easily killed.) This substance is a hallucinogen and was favored in its mushroom form by the early dwellers of Siberia. It is not inactivated in the body, which led, according to the pharmacologist Robert Julian, to the custom among the Siberians of drinking the urine of those who had eaten the mushrooms. According to report, the effect lasted to the fourth or fifth person.

As of this writing there appear to be several different types of nicotinic receptors in neurons in the brain (combinations of two different alpha and three different beta subunits) and five types of muscarinic receptors.

The actions of many different *cholinergic drugs* (drugs that act on acetylcholine neurons) can be understood in terms of how the ACh synapse works. Drugs that act specifically on the nicotinic or muscarinic receptors will clearly have different effects on the nervous system and body. Curare acts on the nicotinic receptor (for example, at neuromuscular junctions on skeletal muscles) and causes total paralysis, whereas atropine acts on the muscarinic receptors and interferes with certain aspects of the autonomic nervous system.

Drugs such as botulin that block the release of ACh work with equal effect on both nicotinic and muscarinic synapses. Similarly, drugs that block AChE, leading to prolonged ACh action and hence to convulsions and sometimes death, act on both kinds of receptor systems. Physostigmine, the first AChE blocker discovered, is an extract of the Calabar bean. According to Julian, the Nigerians called the Calabar bean the ordeal bean and used it as a test of guilt. The suspect was forced to eat the bean. If he lived, he was innocent; if he died, he was guilty. The insecticide malathion, of recent fame in the battle against the Mediterranean fruit fly in California, also acts to block AChE, as do some of the most deadly nerve gases developed for warfare.

Acetylcholine Circuits in the Brain

Surprisingly, much less is known about ACh neurons and circuits in the brain than about several other neurotransmitters. The identification of ACh-containing neurons and receptors in the brain has proved difficult. The ease with which ACh can be studied in pure culture in such peripheral synapses as the neuromuscular junction is why so much has been learned about the neuromuscular ACh synapse.

In a few places in the spinal cord and brain stem ACh has been proved to be a fast transmitter for nicotinic receptors. Motor neurons of the spinal cord and cranial nerve nuclei have their cell bodies in the spinal cord and brain stem and send their axons out to synapse with skeletal muscle cells. They all use ACh, and the muscle receptors are nicotinic. These motor neurons typically give off collateral axon fibers that synapse on smaller interneurons near the motor neurons. ACh is the synaptic transmitter at these synapses as well, and the receptors on the interneurons seem to be of the nicotinic type. Cranial nerve ACh synapses in the brain are fast excitatory ones. The interneurons activated in this way typically act back on the motor neurons to inhibit them, a case of *negative feedback* (Figure 5-3). Judging by the widespread distribution of nicotinic receptors in the brain, it seems very likely that there are ACh-nicotinic receptor systems in many places in the brain in addition to actions of motor neuron collaterals.

It may come as a surprise that ACh synapses between the motor neuron axon collaterals and interneurons are the only synapses in the mammalian central nervous system where we are *certain* what the neurotransmitter is— and that it is ACh. The evidence implicating other neurochemicals as neurotransmitters ranges from very strong to weak at this point because of the extraordinary experimental difficulties involved in proving that a substance is a synaptic transmitter in the brain. It is impossible to make a pure culture of one type of synapse in the brain, as has been done to study the neuromuscular junction. We shall provisionally assume, as do most neuroscientists, that certain chemicals are very likely to be neurotransmitters. It should be remembered, though, that some degree of doubt remains.

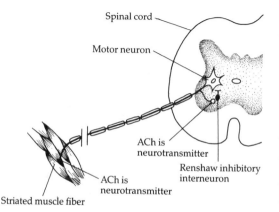

Spinal cord

Motor neuron

ACh is neurotransmitter

ACh is neurotransmitter

Renshaw inhibitory interneuron

Striated muscle fiber

Figure 5-3 A synapse in the spinal cord in which it is certain that the transmitter is ACh. The synapse is a terminal formed by a small branch of the motor neuron axon that acts on a small inhibitory interneuron (Renshaw cell), which in turn acts to inhibit the motor neuron. This is an example of a negative feedback loop.

The major ACh neuron systems in the brain are sketched in Figure 5-4. Brain systems that appear to use ACh as their neurotransmitter seem not to be fast synapses but rather to use the slower, *second-messenger type of synaptic action* (except for the motor neuron axon collateral synapses noted earlier). The cell bodies of the neurons lie in the brain stem in two principal regions, the *septal nuclei* (often called the nuclei of the diagonal band) and the *nucleus basalis*. Some anatomists feel that these two nuclei actually form a continuous band of ACh neurons, so that there is really only one ACh nucleus in the forebrain, the nucleus basalis. This structure lies in the lower or basal part of the forebrain (Figure 5-4). The axons project to forebrain regions, particularly the hippocampus and cerebral cortex. Both types of ACh receptors are present, although the muscarinic ones tend to predominate in the higher regions. (The presence of nicotinic receptors in the brain may be part of the reason that smoking tobacco is so addictive).

Little is known about the functions of the brain ACh systems. However, very recent discoveries suggest that they may be critical for normal intellectual functions. It has been known for some time that the performance of animals on learning and memory tasks can be altered by drugs that act on the ACh system.

A recent increase in our understanding of Alzheimer's disease came in part from work by Joseph Coyle and his associates at the Johns Hopkins School of Medicine. They examined the brains of a number of patients who

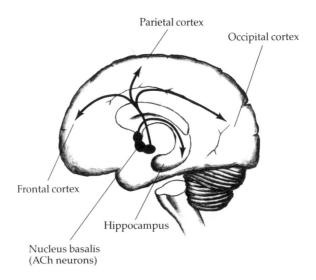

Figure 5-4 The brain ACh system. The ACh cell bodies are in a nucleus at the base of the brain, the nucleus basalis, and project widely to the cerebral cortex and hippocampus.

had died from Alzheimer's disease, a severe form of senility, and found in all cases a massive loss of cells in the nucleus basalis, which contains the ACh neurons that project to the cerebral cortex. In addition the levels of chemicals associated with the ACh system are lower in Alzheimer individuals. We shall consider these new findings further in Chapter 10.

SLOW SYNAPTIC ACTION: THE SECOND-MESSENGER SYSTEMS

To this point we have discussed in detail only fast synaptic transmitter actions, transmission that occurs in less than a millisecond. Synaptic transmitter actions of another major class occur more slowly, taking anywhere from a few milliseconds to seconds or even minutes to be completed. This type of synaptic transmission has been recognized only in the past few years. Actually, the mechanism of action was first determined for hormones and then for neurotransmitters. These slower chemical actions work by way of what are called second-messenger systems.

Like fast synaptic neurotransmitters, the slower-acting hormones and neurotransmitters first attach to specific protein receptor molecules on the surface of or in the neuron (and often in the case of hormones on other target cells). For a slow synaptic transmitter, the events of synaptic transmission are the same as for fast transmitters up to the attachment to the receptor molecule: an action potential arrives at the terminal, Ca^{2+} rushes in, and transmitter chemical is released, diffuses across the synapse, and attaches to the receptor molecule. From this point on the story differs.

In second-messenger synapses the protein receptor molecule is not directly associated with an ion channel. Instead, it triggers a sequence of chemical events within the cell membrane. The outcome of these chemical reactions may ultimately be an action on ion channels so that the cell becomes excited or inhibited, with associated changes in membrane potential, but the action on the channels is indirect. It might in the end affect the metabolic ion pump, which would change the concentration of certain ions inside the cell. A change in Na^+ concentration could change the excitability of the cell without influencing the membrane potential of the cell. Thus if the Na^+ concentration inside the cell increased, it would have no effect on the resting membrane potential, which is determined by K^+ concentrations, but when EPSPs opened Na^+ gates, less Na^+ would rush in and the EPSP would be smaller. Other second-messenger chemical actions involve the DNA in the nucleus of the cell, influencing it to make more or less of certain substances or to make different substances. The latter type of action could result in profound and even permanent changes in the neuron.

An example of the initial step in the activation of a second-messenger system is shown in Figure 5-5. ATP, the chemical source of biological energy in cells, is, as we have seen, formed by the metabolism of glucose. It has a high-energy phosphate bond that can easily be used as a source of energy for chemical and biological activities. Remember that the metabolic ion pump that pumps Na^+ out and K^+ into neurons uses ATP as its source of energy.

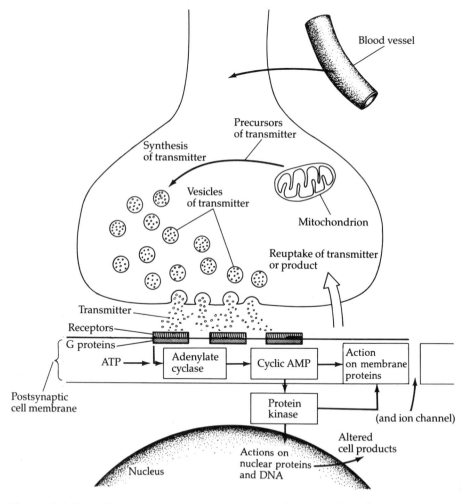

Figure 5-5 Second-messenger synaptic action. Up to the point where the transmitter molecules attach to the postsynaptic receptors, synapses utilizing second messengers work like the fast excitatory and inhibitory synapses. But after the receptor is activated and acts on the G protein, it triggers a set of chemical reactions in the cell membrane in which ATP is converted into AMP. Cyclic AMP can exert a variety of influences on the cell, ranging from changes in the membrane to changes in the activity of the DNA in the nucleus.

ATP is present throughout the cell. When the receptor molecule is activated by its chemical messenger or transmitter (the *first-messenger system*), it causes ATP to undergo a chemical reaction that produces another chemical, *cyclic adenosine monophosphate* (cAMP). The enzyme that catalyzes this reaction is called *adenyl cyclase* (Figure 5-5). CyclicAMP can initiate actions that result in changes in ion channels, the ion pump, DNA and so on. Because cAMP is the substance that initiates these actions, it also acts like a transmitter or messenger, but within the cell, rather than from one neuron to another: it is a second messenger. There are other second messengers as well. These compounds are called second messengers because they act after the first messenger, the transmitter chemical, has crossed the synaptic cleft and attached to receptors.

In general terms, the neurotransmitter chemical systems that act via the slower second-messenger system rather than via the fast first-messenger route can be thought of as modulators of the activity of neurons and systems in the brain. When you touch something hot, you jerk your hand away. Information must cross two or three sets of synaptic junctions in the spinal cord and one set at the neuromuscular junctions of your arm and shoulder muscles to initiate withdrawal of your arm. These are fast synaptic actions, as indeed they must be if we are to survive and avoid injury in this uncertain world. At the same time, the pain from the burn may cause the release of brain opioids (endorphins) from the pituitary, which could modulate the pain somewhat so that it is not too incapacitating. The modulatory opioid action is by way of the second-messenger system.

An important point to keep in mind about neurotransmitter systems is that the actions produced by a neurotransmitter on a neuron and ultimately on you are determined by the receptor molecules and how they act. The same neurotransmitter can have a fast excitatory effect at some synapses and a fast inhibitory effect at others, depending on the ion channels the receptor molecule opens. It can also act more slowly via second-messenger systems. The nicotinic ACh receptors are thought to be fast, first-messenger systems and all the muscarinic ACh receptors involve slow second-messenger systems. The message is in the receptor molecule and its actions as well as in the neurotransmitter.

Current research on receptors gives us a very nice categorization of the fast and slow receptors. As noted, fast neurotransmitter receptor systems (e.g., nicotinic ACh, AMPA–glutamate, $GABA_A$) are directly coupled to ion channels and act in less than one millisecond. The slow transmitter-receptor systems (e.g., muscarinic ACh and most systems discussed in this chapter) all involve second-messenger systems and have much slower actions: they take hundreds of milliseconds. Some of these slow systems are coupled to ion channels and others are not, but in all cases their actions are modulatory; they either enhance or dampen the fast neurotransmitter–receptor systems. Some slow systems also act to regulate other aspects of the biochemical machinery of the cell, including changes in gene expression.

It turns out that all the slow systems have one element in common, the G *proteins* (guanine nucleotide-binding proteins). All the different slow receptors are coupled to G proteins (Figure 5-5). When the receptor is activated by its transmitter, its action is always to activate a G protein. This in turn results in activation of a second-messenger system. The adenylyl cyclase system involving conversion of ATP to cAMP is an example of a second-messenger system. Two other major second-messenger systems have now been characterized, one involving guanyl cyclase and one involving phospholipid hydrolysis (Figure 5-6). Although these three different systems involve different biochemical reactions or "cascades," they all can result in diverse actions on the machinery of the cell, including modulatory actions on ion channels in the cell membrane.

CATECHOLAMINES: DOPAMINE AND NOREPINEPHRINE

The catecholamines constitute a group of chemical substances that are widely present in both the brain and the peripheral nervous system. Only two catecholamines need concern us here: dopamine (DA) and norepinephrine (NE).

The synthetic pathway for these transmitters is shown in Figure 5-7. They are known as catecholamines, incidentally, because they all have what is called a catechol nucleus (a benzene ring with two hydroxyl groups) and an amino group. The pathway is quite simple. Tyrosine naturally occurs as an amino acid in protein foods. In a series of steps tyrosine is converted into L-Dopa, then into dopamine, then norepinephrine, and finally epinephrine. Each of these steps requires an enzyme. Neurons that use dopamine as a transmitter have the first and second enzymes but not the third, and so tyrosine is converted as far as dopamine. Neurons that use norepinephrine as a transmitter have the first, second, and third enzymes, and so tyrosine is converted all the way into norepinephrine.

Epinephrine (sometimes called adrenaline) is not commonly used as a neurotransmitter by neurons in the brain. It is, of course, a major substance secreted by the adrenal gland in states of emotion or stress. Cells in the adrenal gland that secrete epinephrine possess the enzymes for all four steps, so tyrosine is converted all the way into epinephrine, which remains in the adrenal glands for release.

The enzyme that converts tyrosine into L-Dopa, called tyrosine hydroxylase, is the rate-limiting step for the formation of these substances; consequently, how much tyrosine hydroxylase is present in a neuron determines how much dopamine or norepinephrine will be synthesized. Whether a neuron contains dopamine or norepinephrine depends on whether it has only the first two enzymes or all three. So far as we know, all neurons that use dopamine or norepinephrine as transmitters have ample amounts of the en-

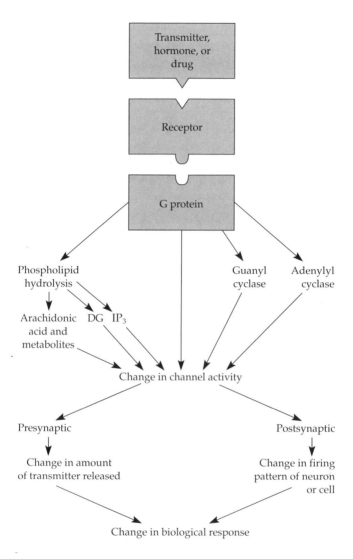

Figure 5-6 Major pathways involving second-messenger systems in synaptic transmission. In all cases, the transmitter or hormone acts on a receptor that acts on a G protein. The G protein can then act on one of several different sets of biochemical machinery inside the cell. These systems may then alter cell excitability by acting on ion channels in the neuron membrane but may in addition or instead have other actions on the cell, including altered gene expression. DG = diacylglycerol; IP = inositoltriphosphate.

zyme that converts L-Dopa into dopamine, so they never store L-Dopa, only dopamine or norepinephrine.

The problem of identifying neurons in the brain that contain dopamine or norepinephrine was solved when a group of scientists working in Sweden made a dramatic discovery. They found a chemical procedure that makes these

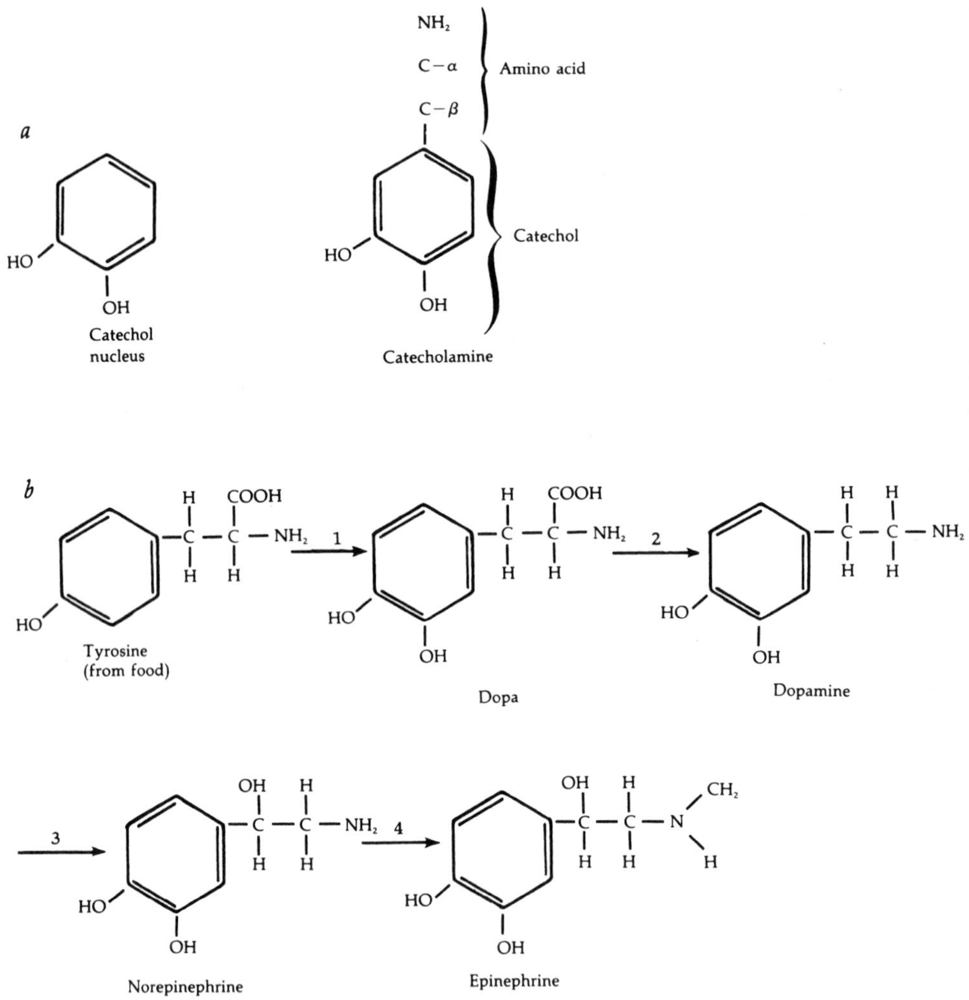

Enzymes that make the reactions go:
1 Tyrosine hydroxylase
2 Aromatic amino acid decarboxylase
3 Dopamine-β-oxidase
4 Phenylethanolamine-*N*-methyl transferase

Figure 5-7 (*a*) General structure of the catecholamines. They all share the catechol nucleus, a benzene ring with two adjacent hydroxyl (OH) groups. (*b*) Structures and synthesis of the catecholamines. Tyrosine, an amino acid found in foods, is converted into Dopa, then into dopamine, next into norepinephrine and finally into epinephrine, depending on which enzymes (1–4) are present in the cell.

neurons fluoresce, or give off colored light, when an appropriate light source is shined on them. When so treated, both dopamine- and norepinephrine-containing neurons will shine with a greenish light. Unfortunately, they both give off the same color. They can, with some difficulty, be distinguished, since dopamine shines after a shorter treatment than epinephrine.

Norepinephrine can be clearly identified as a neurotransmitter in parts of the peripheral nervous system, in particular in the sympathetic portion of the autonomic system. The *sympathetic nervous system* consists of a series of ganglia, or collections of neuron cell bodies lying just outside the spinal cord. The ganglia send fibers to the heart, blood vessels, viscera, sex organs, skin, and other places in the body, but not to the skeletal muscles (see Chapter 1). A simplified diagram of the sympathetic nerve connections to the heart is shown in Figure 5-8. The sympathetic system tends to excite its target organs, for example, the heart. When an individual is aroused and angry or afraid, it

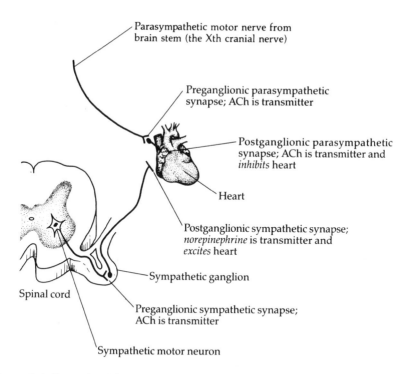

Figure 5-8 Example of the dual innervation of organs by the sympathetic and parasympathetic parts of the autonomic nervous system and the transmitters they use. The preganglionic fibers are motor neurons from the brain stem and spinal cord. These fibers all use ACh, and the receptors are nicotinic. The postganglionic parasympathetic fibers also use ACh, but the receptors are muscarinic. The postganglionic sympathetic fibers use norepinephrine as their neurotransmitter.

becomes active. The nerves that connect from the sympathetic nervous system to such organs as the heart use norepinephrine (NE) as neurotransmitter. When they are active, they cause the heartbeat to increase. NE is an excitatory transmitter of the heart, in contrast to ACh, which inhibits it. Part of the reason so much is known about NE is that it is an identified synaptic transmitter at places such as the heart.

Schematic diagrams of DA and NE synapses in the brain are shown in Figures 5-9 and 5-10. Tyrosine is transported down the axon to the terminal, where it is converted into dopamine (and in some terminals into norepinephrine) and stored in vesicles. Two types of vesicles appear to contain DA or NE. Under the electron microscope one type of vesicle looks clear; these vesicles are thought to hold and release the transmitter at the synapses. The clear vesicles are the standard synaptic vesicles, present in all the axon terminals of all chemical synapses. The other type is larger and has a dense or dark-staining core. It is thought that the dense-core vesicles hold reserves of synaptic terminals containing DA or NE. However, only the smaller, clear vesicles are immediately involved in synaptic transmission.

When an action potential arrives at the terminal, Ca^{2+} flows into the terminal and the clear vesicles of NE or DA release their contents into the synaptic space. The molecules of NE or DA diffuse across the synaptic space and attach to their receptors, which causes changes in the postsynaptic membrane. Then the receptors release the NE or DA, and some of it diffuses back and is taken up by the presynaptic terminal. So far, the story is much like that for glutamate and GABA synapses.

An important enzyme in both DA and NE synaptic systems (and in other cells of the body) is monoamine oxidase (MAO). The enzyme is present both in the presynaptic terminal and in the postsynaptic cell, where it breaks down excess amounts of DA or NE. The products of the breakdown are then further metabolized and ultimately excreted by the body. The other inactivating enzyme present in the postsynaptic cells of DA and NE synapses is catechol methyltransferase (COMT). However, MAO and COMT in the postsynaptic cell do not seem to participate in the inactivation of DA or NE that is being used in synaptic transmission. The transmitter molecules are inactivated by being released from the chemical receptors in the postsynaptic membrane and taken up again by the terminals, just as was the case for GABA.

When DA or NE molecules attach to postsynaptic receptors, they cause changes in the membrane of the target cell. It is here that the story diverges from that of ACh at the neuromuscular junction and that of glutamate and GABA in fast synaptic transmission and resembles that of the brain ACh system. The receptor molecules for DA and NE do not directly open ion channels in the postsynaptic membrane; instead, they activate second-messenger systems.

Synapse using dopamine

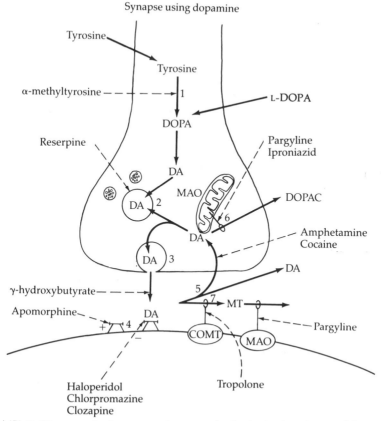

Figure 5-9 Diagram of a dopaminergic neuron in the brain showing possible sites of drug action. Numbers refer to steps in the process of synaptic transmission.

1. Synthesis of DA. Certain drugs (for example, α-methyltyrosine) can inhibit the synthetic enzyme.

2. Storage of DA. Reserpine interferes with the uptake–storage mechanism. The depletion of dopamine produced by reserpine is long lasting.

3. Release of DA. The drug γ-hydroxybutyrate blocks release of dopamine by blocking action potentials in dopaminergic neurons.

4. Receptor effects. Apomorphine stimulates dopamine receptors. Chlorpromazine, clozapine and haloperidol are dopamine receptor-blocking drugs.

5. Reuptake of DA by the terminal. Dopamine has its action terminated by being taken up into the presynaptic terminal. Amphetamine and cocaine are potent inhibitors of the reuptake process.

6. Enzyme actions: Monoamine oxidase (MAO). Dopamine present in a free state within the presynaptic terminal can be degraded by the enzyme MAO. Dihydroxyphenylacetic acid (DOPAC) is a product of the action of MAO on dopamine. Pargyline is an effective inhibitor of MAO, as is iproniazid. Some MAO is also present outside the dopaminergic neuron.

7. Enzyme actions: Catechol-o-methyl transferase (COMT). Dopamine can be inactivated by the enzyme COMT, which is believed to be localized outside the presynaptic neuron. Tropolone is an inhibitor of COMT. MAO further degrades the product and is inhibited by pargyline.

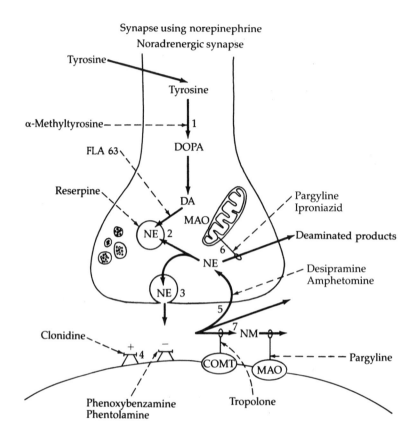

Figure 5-10 Diagram of an NE neuron in the brain showing possible sites of drug action. Numbers indicate steps in transmission.

1. Enzymatic synthesis of NE. The step from tyrosine to Dopa is blocked by α-methyltyrosine, and the step from Dopa to NE is blocked by Fla-63.

2. Storage of NE. Reserpine and tetrabenazine interfere with the uptake–storage mechanism of NE, as with DA in Figure 5-9.

3. Release of NE.

4. Receptor effects. Clonidine appears to be a potent receptor-stimulating drug. Phenoxybenzamine and phentolamine are effective blocking agents for one type of NE receptor (alpha type).

5. Reuptake of NE by the terminal. Norepinephrine has its action terminated by being taken up into the presynaptic terminal. The tricyclic drug desipramine is a potent inhibitor of this uptake mechanism, as is amphetamine.

6. Enzyme actions: Monoamine oxidase (MAO). Effects are the same as for DA (Figure 5-9). Norepinephrine present in a free state within the presynaptic terminal can be degraded by the enzyme MAO. Pargyline and iproniazid are effective inhibitors of MAO.

Dopamine Circuits in the Brain

Three major dopamine circuits have been discovered in the brain. (For some reason, dopamine-containing cells also occur in the retina of the eye, which need not concern us here.) All three of the dopamine circuits consist of one-neuron pathways. The neuron cell bodies of the dopamine-containing neurons are in the brain stem, and they send their axons to other brain regions.

One of the circuits is very simple. The neuron cell bodies are in a region of the hypothalamus, and they send their axons just a short distance into the pituitary gland (Figure 5-11). This dopamine system is believed to function like other parts of the hypothalamus–pituitary system, the endocrine-gland master control system. The hypothalamus either manufactures hormones and

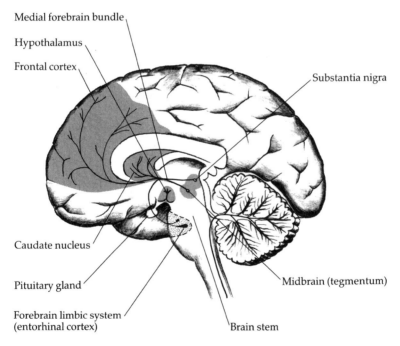

Medial forebrain bundle

Hypothalamus

Frontal cortex

Substantia nigra

Caudate nucleus

Pituitary gland

Midbrain (tegmentum)

Forebrain limbic system (entorhinal cortex)

Brain stem

Figure 5-11 The three dopamine systems in the brain. One is a local circuit in the hypothalamus; another is the pathway from the substantia nigra to the caudate nucleus of the basal ganglia, which is involved in motor functions and Parkinson's disease; the third consists of cell bodies in the brain stem and midbrain (tegmentum) that project widely to the cerebral cortex and forebrain limbic system (entorhinal cortex). The third DA system is thought to be involved in schizophrenia.

holds them in its nerve terminals in the pituitary gland for release or triggers the release of hormones held in cells in the pituitary gland. These hormones are released directly into the bloodstream (Chapter 6).

The second dopamine system is the best understood. There is a very unique structure in the lower midbrain, the *substantia nigra* (dark substance), so called because the cell bodies in it contain a dark-colored pigment. Many cell bodies in the substantia nigra contain dopamine as well. The dopamine-containing substantia nigra cells project to the basal ganglia. As we saw in Chapter 1, the basal ganglia are large masses of neurons situated in the depths of the cerebrum (forebrain). They are below the cerebral cortex and surrounded by the white matter, the masses of fibers going to and from the cortex (see Chapter 9). The dopamine-containing cells of the substantia nigra project directly to the basal ganglia.

The majority of dopamine-containing neurons, holding roughly three-quarters of all the dopamine in the brain, are in this substantia-nigra-to-basal-ganglia system. This dopamine system plays a major role in the regulation of movement. It is the system that is deficient in Parkinson's disease (see Chapter 9). For unknown reasons, the dopamine-containing neurons in the substantia nigra gradually die and disappear as the disease progresses. This produces the symptoms of Parkinson's disease: tremors and repetitive movements of the hands, "pill-rolling" movements of the fingers, and increasing difficulty in standing and initiating general body movements such as walking. When this system was discovered to be at the root of Parkinson's disease a few years ago, a very helpful treatment was developed, the administration of L-Dopa. Remember that L-Dopa is the substance from which dopamine is made in the neurons in the brain (Figure 5-7b).

The third dopamine system is thought to be involved in some major way in schizophrenia, the most severe mental disorder. The functions of this dopamine system are actually not well understood, although the pathway itself has been well characterized (Figure 5-11). The dopamine-containing cell bodies lie in the midbrain just next to the substantia nigra. They project to higher brain regions, the cerebral cortex and limbic system. In particular, they project to the frontal lobes of the cerebral cortex, to the septal areas, and to a region of limbic cortex called the entorhinal cortex. The entorhinal cortex is the major source of neurons projecting to the hippocampus.

Schizophrenia: The Dopamine Hypothesis

Given the great complexities of the human mind and its disorders, psychiatry, psychology, and neuroscience have made surprising progress in understanding such disorders over the past 50 years. A broad distinction is commonly made between neurosis and psychosis. Neurotic conditions can be severely incapaciting, as in extreme anxiety, but the person does not lose contact with reality (see Chapter 4). The major psychoses, schizophrenia and depression, are far more serious and debilitating than the neuroses. People suffering from these disorders can lose contact with reality to varying degrees. The dopamine neurotransmitter system appears to be critically involved in schizophrenia; depression, on the other hand, appears to involve the norepinephrine and serotonin neurotransmitter systems. I discuss depression later in the chapter after describing the serotonin system.

Persons suffering from schizophrenia lose contact with reality. They have false beliefs and disordered thought processes. They often have hallucinations, for example, hearing sounds that do not exist, in particular voices addressing them and instructing them to do things. It is not uncommon to see such an individual in the downtown area of a large city. The person will be carrying on a loud and lively conversation with the empty air. Actually, there are two categories of symptoms characteristic of schizophrenia, positive and negative. The symptoms I have just described are the *positive symptoms* and are easily recognized. The *negative symptoms* are more subtle. They include the absence of normal emotional reactions and expressions, termed flat or flattened affect, loss of motivation, general loss of interest and social withdrawal. A final point to keep in mind is that in some people suffering from the disorder, the positive symptoms can wax and wane. At times these people are relatively normal and at other times they become severely disturbed.

Schizophrenia afflicts about 1 percent of the world's population, independent of race, culture, and, apparently, life experiences. Schizophrenia has a genetic basis and therefore runs in families. A person with an identical twin who is schizophrenic has a 50-50 chance of becoming so; a person with a schizophrenic brother or sister has one chance in eight of becoming schizophrenic. If none of a person's close relatives is schizophrenic, the base rate chance of developing the condition is about one in 100. These figures show a clear genetic factor in schizophrenia and also that schizophrenia is not due to a simple genetic cause, such as a single recessive gene. If it were, a person whose identical twin developed the condition would invariably also develop it. Perhaps experience plays a key role; a genetic predisposition may not by itself always be sufficient to cause the disease. On the other hand, perhaps there are several genes involved and the degree to which they are expressed depends on developmental factors rather than on experience as such. Much is still not known.

It would be satisfying if one could say that basic research in neuroscience led to a clear understanding of schizophrenia, which in turn led to the development of helpful treatments for the disorder, but that is not the way it happened. Instead, the first drug of great benefit in treating schizophrenia was discovered quite by accident. This led to the current view that because a drug has proved effective in treating schizophrenia, the condition is due in part to chemical disorders in the brain. The wonder drug was originally a product of the nineteenth-century German dye industry, which had manufactured a number of new dyes in the search for better ways to color cloth. One chemical group of these dyes is called phenothiazines. Previously it had been found that some dyes help malaria, and so the phenothiazines were tried out on people with malaria, but without success.

Physicians, apparently convinced that the new dyes had to be good for something in medicine, tried them on several disorders. A French surgeon noted in 1949 that the phenothiazine dyes had a marked calming effect on some surgical patients. Soon after, one of these drugs, *chlorpromazine* (see Figure 5-9), was found to have remarkably beneficial effects on schizophrenics. By 1954 chlorpromazine was approved in the United States as a treatment for schizophrenia, and it is from this date that the remarkable decline in patients in mental hospitals began in the United States.

Until the introduction of chlorpromazine, many of the over 2 million schizophrenics in the United States had to be hospitalized because little else could be done for them. Chlorpromazine does not cure schizophrenia, but it is often effective in treating the more severe positive symptoms. Many patients become calmer and more rational and are then able to live on their own outside the hospital.

The extraordinary success of chlorpromazine led to the hope that schizophrenia might be understood at the chemical level by understanding the chemistry of chlorpromazine. However, other drugs were discovered that were also helpful in treating the symptoms of schizophrenia. For example, *haloperidol* is equally helpful in treating schizophrenia, but it has a chemical structure quite different from that of chlorpromazine (Figure 5-9). This kind of puzzle is common in neuroscience. Different drugs having very different chemical structures can have the same effect on the brain and behavior.

When faced with a puzzle like this, it is helpful to simplify the situation as much as possible. The chemical activity of the human schizophrenic brain cannot, of course, be studied directly, but the effects of drugs on particular neurotransmitter systems of the brain can be examined in a test tube. All mammals have essentially the same neurotransmitter systems in the brain, and so the relevant brain tissue can be removed from an animal and its chemical reactions studied in the laboratory.

From these experiments it was learned that chlorpromazine, haloperidol, and all the other antipsychotic drugs that help in the treatment of schizophrenia interfere with the neurotransmitter dopamine in the brain of the rat and other laboratory animals by binding to dopamine receptors. In fact, haloperidol binds even better to the dopamine receptors than dopamine, the real transmitter. The effectiveness of all of the antipsychotic drugs used in treating schizophrenia can be predicted rather accurately by measuring how well they can displace haloperidol from the dopamine receptors.

When dopamine is released at synapses and binds to dopamine receptors, it activates the dopamine-receiving neurons. Activation takes place through a second-messenger system, which can effect changes in the cell membrane, chemical reactions within the cell and even the genetic material, the DNA, in the nucleus of the cell, as described earlier in the chapter. When the antipsychotic drugs bind to dopamine receptors, they do not activate the dopamine-receiving neurons. They apparently are inactive, other than binding to the receptors. The reason they have such powerful effects is because they block dopamine from attaching to the receptors, just as naloxone blocks opiate receptors. They are antagonists. The extraordinary fact that all of the drugs effective in treating schizophrenia block the dopamine receptor and are effective in proportion to how much they block it seems to imply that schizophrenia is caused by too much dopamine. This is the "dopamine theory" of schizophrenia. Basically, the theory postulates that the third dopamine system projecting from the brain stem to the cerebral cortex and limbic system is overactivated. It is only a theory, however, and much is still not known. For example, the actions of the antipsychotic drugs on dopamine receptors were determined in a test tube and on brain tissue from animals, but as far as we know, animals do not develop schizophrenia.

In several studies the brain levels of dopamine have been measured in schizophrenic patients who died. The results are negative: the brain level of dopamine appears to be normal. Some very recent work indicates that schizophrenic individuals do have a significant increase in the number of dopamine receptors in the brain. If this is verified, it would fit with the results from the chemical studies. The schizophrenic brain would be much more sensitive to dopamine than the normal brain because it has more dopamine receptors in target neurons. It is not that there is too much dopamine in the schizophrenic brain, but rather that the normal amount of dopamine has too powerful an action. By blocking dopamine receptors with antipsychotic drugs, the system can be brought back toward a normal level of sensitivity and function.

Recent work has provided additional evidence in support of the dopamine hypothesis of schizophrenia. So far I have focused on the positive symptoms; chlorpromazine and other dopamine antagonists treat the positive symptoms. On the other hand, the same drugs can make the negative symptoms, flattened affect and social withdrawal, worse. Hence the current dopamine hypothesis proposes that *too much* dopamine action in the third dopamine system yields the positive symptoms and that *too little* action yields the negative symptoms. Thus, one might wonder whether Parkinson's disease, resulting from too little dopamine, and schizophrenia, possibly due to too much dopamine, are somehow related. No actual relation is thought to exist, because Parkinson's disease involves the second dopamine circuit, from the substantia nigra to the basal ganglia, and schizophrenia appears to involve the third dopamine system, from the midbrain to the cerebral cortex and limbic system.

Unfortunately, however, there is a relation in terms of drug effects. The dopamine neurons and synapses appear to work in the same way in both systems. Thus a drug cannot be given that will act on one system but not on the other. When L-Dopa is given to a Parkinson's patient, it should also increase dopamine levels in the "schizophrenic" circuit, and, in fact, a significant number of Parkinson's individuals initially develop schizophrenialike symptoms when they are treated with L-Dopa.

Drugs used to treat schizophrenia reduce the dopamine content of dopamine neurons in the brain. Consequently, individuals given these drugs ought to develop the symptoms of Parkinson's disease, and indeed many do. These symptoms can be helped with other drugs. There is, however, a much more serious consequence of the use of the schizophrenia drugs. This effect has only recently been appreciated because it appears to develop after a long course of repeated treatment with the antipsychotic drugs, a course as long as years. A significant number of individuals treated with antipsychotic drugs develop a disorder called *tardive dyskinesia*. The symptoms are repeated and bizarre movements of the face and mouth, which the person cannot control. This disorder is thought to be the mirror image of Parkinson's disease: an abnormality of movement control by the basal ganglia due to too much dopamine in the substantia-nigra-to-basal-ganglia system. Tardive dyskinesia is a tragic example of an "iatrogenic" illness, an illness that is caused by a medical treatment.

Why is tardive dyskinesia thought to result from too much dopamine? Drugs used to treat schizophrenia reduce dopamine content, not increase it. The following general principle, however, appears to operate for all chemical synapses and in fact for all chemical receptors on neurons. If the normal functioning of a given transmitter or receptor system is somehow interfered with so that less of the normal transmitter is available, the neurons and receptors try to compensate. The neurons make more transmitter and the chemical receptors increase in number or affinity (up regulation), apparently in an attempt to maintain normal function. This mechanism is sometimes called *disuse supersensitivity*. In the case of schizophrenia drugs, the second dopamine circuit, that involved in Parkinson's disease, is thought to be initially normal but reduced in function by the drugs. The system slowly compensates by making more and more dopamine and more receptors. At some point it overcompensates and makes far more than enough to overcome the drug effects. The result is tardive dyskinesia. The same mechanism of compensating for drug effects is believed to underlie the development of withdrawal symptoms in drug addiction (see Chapter 6).

A further problem with drugs that act primarily to block the brain dopamine systems is that they are effective in helping the symptoms of schizophrenia in only about 40 percent of patients. More recently, a drug called *clozapine* (trade name Clozaril) has been used with greater success. This drug seems to help a much larger percentage of schizophrenic patients. Further, it appears to treat both positive and negative symptoms of the disease. From this fact you might conclude that the drug does not act on the brain dopamine systems. You would be partly correct. It blocks both dopamine and serotonin actions (see Figures 5.9 and 5.14) but has a relatively greater action on serotonin synapses. This would seem to raise further problems for the dopamine theory of schizophrenia.

Like other drug treatments, clozapine has drawbacks. In 1 to 2 percent of cases it causes destruction of the immune system, leading eventually to death. Fortunately, this side effect can be monitored by weekly blood tests and the drug treatment can be stopped before permanent damage occurs to the immune system. But it means weekly medical visits, resulting in an annual cost of several thousand dollars. (But the annual cost to the United States of schizophrenia is about 129 billion dollars.) Clozapine has produced remarkable recovery in many schizophrenic patients, which makes the relatively rare development of the immune disorder all the more tragic. Phil, age 36, had been severely schizophrenic for 13 years and did not respond to dopamine-blocking drugs. He was "awakened" by clozapine and recovered to the extent that he could work part time and begin to lead a social life. Then the immune disorder began to develop and he had to be taken off the drug. "He has his voices and moods again," his father said sadly. "We'll just have to wait for something else to come along."

Norepinephrine Circuits in the Brain

The NE circuits in the brain are rather unusual in that a few small collections of cell bodies in the brain stem containing NE send their fibers to almost all the structures and regions in the brain (Figure 5-12). These fibers make direct connections from the brain stem to the cerebellum, hypothalamus, thalamus, cerebral cortex, hippocampus, septum, basal ganglia, amygdala, and on and on. The NE fibers go almost everywhere, yet they come from relatively few cell bodies. In terms of the neurotransmitter content of the brain, NE accounts for only about 1 percent. What could be the function of such a sparse, diffuse, yet widespread chemical circuit? The simplest answer is that the brain NE system must serve some kind of very general and nonspecific function, perhaps basic level of excitability or arousal.

Many of the NE cell bodies are situated in a small nucleus in the brain stem called the *locus ceruleus*. These cells are pigmented and have a bluish color. They give rise to a pathway called the *dorsal bundle*, which projects to most of the higher brain regions noted as being connected in the NE brain

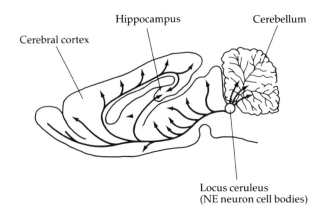

Figure 5-12   NE projection system in the brain of the rat. The cell bodies are in the locus ceruleus and adjacent regions of the brain stem and project widely to the forebrain and cerebellum and to the brain stem and spinal cord.

circuit (Figure 5-12). The rest of the NE cells in the brain stem are situated near the locus ceruleus in several cell groups. Their axons form the *ventral bundle*, which projects more deeply in the brain to the reticular formation and hypothalamus.

A parallel of sorts can be drawn between the adrenal gland and the brain NE circuit. Both systems release NE, the adrenal gland into the bloodstream and the NE pathway via axon terminals. Both systems yield an overall increase in the amount of NE present throughout the brain. It is known that the adrenal gland secretes NE (and epinephrine) in response to stress- or arousal-producing events in the environment. Although we do not yet know the conditions that lead to increased activity of the brain NE system, we might speculate that it is also related to arousal. One small problem with this idea is that NE appears to be more inhibitory than excitatory in its actions on brain cells, at least when it is directly applied to them.

One rather prosaic hypothesis is that the brain NE system actually innervates (connects to) only blood vessels in the brain, not neurons. In times of arousal or stress it could then increase blood flow in the brain. This is, in fact, the kind of action the sympathetic part of the peripheral autonomic system exerts on blood vessels in the body. It also uses NE as the chemical neuromuscular transmitter in synapses with the smooth muscle fibers of the blood vessels. For this reason, the brain NE system is sometimes called the sympathetic nervous system of the brain.

Current evidence, however, argues strongly that the more important circuits in the brain NE system do connect to neurons. One of the major reasons the brain NE system is believed to be involved in behavioral arousal is because of the effects of certain drugs. Amphetamine is a potent brain stimulant and acts on the NE (and DA) systems, as does cocaine. Certain antidepressant drugs that are used to treat people who are seriously depressed appear to act primarily on the NE system.

There is evidence that NE in the brain and in the rest of the body may play an important modulatory role in the processes of learning and memory retrieval. The levels of NE in the brain and body are related to how well an animal or human learns or remembers. To take a simple example, people tend to remember events that were associated with strong emotions such as anger, fear, or grief. These emotional states typically involve increased blood levels of NE released from the adrenal gland and probably in the NE brain circuits as well. We consider this at greater length in Chapter 11.

A diagram of an NE axon forming synapses in the cerebral cortex is shown in Figure 5-13. The axon does not form a terminal; instead it has a number of swellings. Each of these swellings is an NE synapse. The NE is presumably released from all of the swellings when an action potential travels out the axon. The released NE probably acts on immediately adjacent neurons but may also diffuse to nearby neurons.

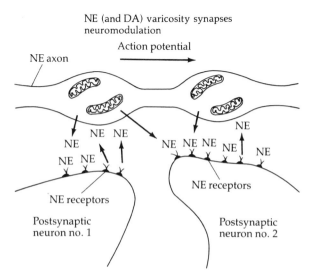

NE (and DA) varicosity synapses
neuromodulation

Action potential

NE axon

NE NE
NE
NE NE

NE receptors

Postsynaptic
neuron no. 1

NE NE NE NE
NE
NE

NE receptors

NE

Postsynaptic
neuron no. 2

Figure 5-13 NE is thought to function more as a neuromodulator or local hormone than as a cause of discrete synaptic actions that would convey specific information. The NE axons have many varicosities along their length that release NE when activated, which acts on nearby neurons. There are also NE synaptic terminals that form discrete synapses (not shown).

The NE and DA synaptic actions are quite slow, involving second-messenger systems, and take up to seconds or even minutes to be completed as opposed to less than one millisecond for fast synaptic transmitters. Also, NE and DA are not rapidly broken down by enzymes but must be reabsorbed by the axon swellings to become inactivated. Perhaps the NE and DA synaptic systems are best considered as existing in an "equilibrium." Under normal basal, or resting, conditions, steady-state actions would be exerted by some level of NE or DA present at neurons in the vicinity of the NE or DA axon swellings. This basal level would be maintained by ongoing release and reuptake. When the systems are activated, then the amount of NE or DA would increase for a time, fluctuating with the activity of the NE or DA neurons. Rather than a fast all-or-none action, the amount of NE or DA present would change gradually. The amount present would then correspondingly modulate the activity of the neurons that are influenced by NE or DA. In this sense, the catecholamine systems in the brain, the DA- and NE-containing neurons, may actually function more like suppliers of local hormones than like traditional synapses.

SEROTONIN

Serotonin, the last neurotransmitter we shall discuss in detail, was initially thought to be involved in high blood pressure. This was because it is present in blood serum and induces a very powerful contraction of smooth muscles, for example in the intestines and blood vessels. Later, when serotonin was found in brain tissue, it became the favored substance to explain various forms of mental illness. Although many of these views are no longer held, serotonin remains of interest as a neurotransmitter because of its apparent involvement in depression, sleep, and the regulation of body temperature. Also, the actions of LSD on the brain seem to involve serotonin.

Serotonin has a somewhat more complicated molecular structure than the transmitters we have discussed so far. It is manufactured in two steps in certain brain cells from the naturally occurring amino acid tryptophan. (Bananas are loaded with tryptophan.) Tryptophan is converted into an intermediate product, called 5-HTP, which is then converted into serotonin (5-hydroxytryptamine, 5-HT). The first step, from tryptophan to 5-HTP, is brought about by the enzyme tryptophan hydroxylase and is thought to be the rate-limiting step. Although serotonin does not have a catechol group, as do NE and DA, it does have an amino group like NE and DA. Hence, NE, DA, and 5-HT are all termed *monoamines* (one amino group).

A serotonin synapse is shown in Figure 5-14. Tryptophan is transported down the axon to the terminal, where it is converted into serotonin and

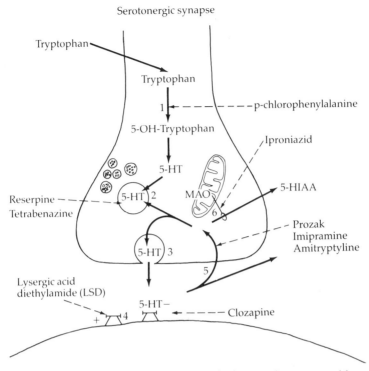

Figure 5-14   Diagram of serotonergic neuron in the brain indicating possible sites of drug action. Numbers refer to steps in synaptic transmission.

1. Enzymatic synthesis of 5-HT. Tryptophan is taken up into the serotonin-containing neuron and converted to 5-OH-tryptophan (5-HT) by the enzyme tryptophan hydroxylase. This enzyme can be inhibited by *p*-chlorophenylalanine.

2. Storage of 5-HT. Reserpine and tentrabenazine interfere with the uptake–storage mechanism, causing a marked depletion of serotonin.

3. Release of 5-HT. As of this writing, no drug is known that acts specifically to block release.

4. Receptor effects. Lysergic acid diethylamide (LSD) acts as a partial agonist (that is, it acts like 5-HT) at serotonergic synapses in the CNS. Clozapine blocks the receptors (it is an antagonist).

5. Reuptake of 5-HT by the terminal. Tricyclic drugs such as imipramine and amitriptyline appear to be inhibitors of this uptake mechanism, as does prozak.

6. As with DA and NE, serotonin that is inactivated by reuptake in the presynaptic terminal is broken down by MAO, a process that is inhibited by iproniazid.

stored in vesicles. Both small, clear vesicles and larger, dense-core vesicles seem to be present in serotonin terminals, as in catecholamine terminals. When an action potential arrives at the serotonin terminal, serotonin molecules are released into the synaptic cleft and act on serotonin receptors on the surface of the postsynaptic neuron. The serotonin is then released from the receptors and taken back up the terminals. As is the case for GABA and the catecholamines, there is no specific enzyme at the receptors to break down serotonin. In common with the catecholamines, excess serotonin is metabolized by the enzyme MAO, which acts primarily within the presynaptic terminals. As of this writing, seven different subtypes of serotonin receptors have been identified. Some are thought to be fast, e.g., controlling ion channels, particularly Cl^-, and others activate second-messenger systems.

The cell bodies of serotonin-containing neurons in the brain are situated in a narrow band of nuclei (collections of cell bodies) that runs along the brain stem from the medulla to the midbrain. These nuclei are collectively called the *raphe* (seam) *nuclei*. As in the NE system, the serotonin neurons send their axons to many higher regions of the brain (Figure 5-15). However, the distribution of serotonin terminals is not so widespread. For example, the serotonin fibers that project to the hypothalamus go primarily to one nucleus, the suprachiasmatic nucleus, which is thought to be involved in the control of basic biological rhythms such as sleep and waking. Serotonin fibers also project to the septum, the hippocampus, the cerebral cortex, the basal ganglia, and the amygdala.

Surprisingly, the structure in the brain that has the highest concentration of serotonin is the *pineal gland* (see Figure 1-4). This remarkable little gland is not actually a part of the brain, because although it is physically within the brain the blood–brain barrier separates it from the brain. The pineal gland receives nerve fibers not from the brain but from the sympathetic part of the

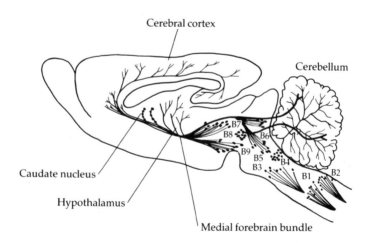

Figure 5-15 Serotonin circuit in the brain of a rat. The serotonin-containing neurons are in a number of nuclei in the brain stem called the raphe (seam) nuclei (labeled B1–B9). They project to rather localized regions of the hypothalamus, cerebral cortex, and other structures.

peripheral autonomic nervous system. These fibers, incidentally, use NE as their transmitter. Serotonin in the pineal gland is converted into a pigment called melatonin, which acts on skin pigmentation and influences the activity of the female gonads. Both serotonin and melatonin in the pineal are under the control of the day–night cycle. The light–dark cycle exerts its influence on the pineal via the sympathetic nerve fibers. This system exerts powerful control over the female reproductive cycle in many species of animals and may also play a key role in sleep and waking.

Current behavioral interest in the brain serotonin system centers around three topics, sleep, LSD, and depression. If the raphe nuclei are destroyed, the behavioral result tends to be an animal that is insomniac, or does not sleep much. A similar effect is produced by drugs that deplete brain stores of serotonin. The serotonin system, then, has something to do with sleep, but it is not yet clear just what. Sleep patterns eventually become relatively normal in serotonin-deprived animals.

LSD is one of the most potent psychoactive drugs; minute amounts produce hallucinations. LSD is a powerful inhibitor of serotonin-sensitive tissue responses, perhaps because the structure of the LSD molecule is quite similar to that of serotonin.

Serotonin is present not only in the brain and pineal gland but also in certain body tissues, particularly smooth muscle, and in one of the types of blood cells, the blood platelets. If a drug that acts on serotonin is given systemically (that is, injected into the bloodstream), it will act on all serotonin, not just on the serotonin in the brain circuits. Consequently one must be very careful in drawing conclusions from such drug effects about the actions of serotonin in the brain, as a given drug might affect primarily non-brain serotonin targets and only at second hand the brain.

DEPRESSION: THE MONOAMINE HYPOTHESIS

Depression is a condition everyone has experienced. We all feel sad, blue, or down in the dumps on occasion. Normal people become sad and depressed for good reasons: loss of a loved one, a financial setback, and so on. However, psychotic depression occurs for no good reason, at least none that is apparent to anyone except the depressed person. The symptoms of psychotic depression are the same as those of normal depression, only more so. The depressed individual typically just sits there and feels miserable. Unlike schizophrenia, thought processes are normal, except for unreasonable feelings of worthlessness.

There are actually two different forms of depression: the condition just described, which is often called *major depression*, and a condition now called *bipolar depression*. The older term for bipolar depression is manic–depressive

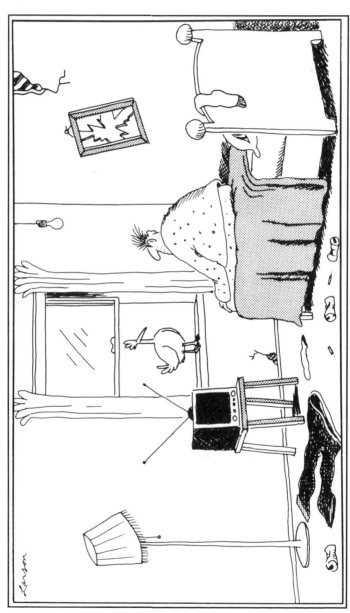

The Bluebird of Happiness long absent from his life, Ned is visited by the Chicken of Depression.

psychosis. Individuals classified as bipolar depressives have had at least one episode of mania: wild and unreasonable euphoria and feelings of intense joy and power, resulting in bizarre, manic behavior. Manic episodes are quite rare in the condition; the depressed phase is much commoner. Although major depression and the depressed phase of bipolar depression seem basically to be the same, the most effective treatments for the two conditions differ.

Major depression is a most serious and common condition: 20 percent of women and 10 percent of men have at least one episode in their lives. Many people have repeated episodes throughout life. Successful suicide, the tenth leading cause of death in the United States, is usually the result of psychotic depression. Bipolar depression is much less common than major depression; only about 1 percent of the population in this country suffer from it.

Both types of depression show a strong genetic predisposition, particularly the bipolar disorder. If one identical twin has the disorder, the chances are 72 percent that the other will develop it, whether they have been raised together or apart.

In recent years Seymour S. Kety, then at Harvard University, developed a large-scale approach to determining whether or not major psychoses have a strong genetic component. The studies were done mostly in European countries, particularly Denmark, primarily because the public-health records are superior to those in the United States but also because the courts permit scientists access to medical records for legitimate research purposes.

A major study on bipolar depression was done in Belgium. All children who had been diagnosed as bipolar depressive and who had been adopted by nonbiological relatives as infants were identified. The biological parents and parents of an equivalent sample of normal children were interviewed and diagnosed. The results were striking: 18 percent of the biological parents were also bipolar depressives, whereas only 1 to 4 percent of the parents of the normal group of children were so affected.

Some evidence indicates that at least one of the genes responsible for the bipolar disorder is on the X sex chromosome. In several studies the inheritance of the bipolar gene was tracked by the use of marker genes. The gene for colorblindness is situated on the X chromosome. It could be shown that the relatives of people who are both colorblind and develop the bipolar disorder tend to have the two traits together more often than would be expected on the basis of chance. This does not mean that colorblind people are predisposed to the bipolar disorder! The two abnormal genes just happen to be situated on the same X chromosome in some people, and the colorblindness trait can be used to indicate that the X chromosome, and moreover the particular piece of it on which the colorblindness gene is situated, is transmitted when the bipolar-disorder gene is transmitted. Genes that are close together on a chromosome show linkage: during the process of cell division, chromosomes break and swap pieces, but they do not break into such small pieces that genes close together are ordinarily separated. The colorblindness gene and the bipolar gene seem to be linked. However, the bipolar-disorder gene is also linked to Xga; the gene for another disorder called ocular albinism. The locus, or location, of the bipolar gene on the X chromosome may be between the color-blindness gene and the Xga gene.

Chromosome marker studies of depression are recent and few and must be viewed with caution. It is important to remember that a person who has the bipolar or depression "gene" does not necessarily develop or have the disorders. Even in identical twins, who have identical genes, the concordance, or agreement, rate of the bipolar disorder is 72 percent, not 100 percent.

Major depression or the bipolar disorder can strike adults of any age, but they rarely develop in children. Stress and other experiences in life do not seem to be immediate causes of the disorders. Drug treatments have proved extraordinarily successful with these disorders. With drug treatment, the symptoms of depression and the bipolar disorder often disappear, and the patient becomes normal again. Some people recover fully. They are not necessarily "cured." Many must remain on drug treatment, but so long as they do, they are their former mentally healthy selves.

The most effective treatments for depression and the bipolar disorder are quite different. Drugs that seem to potentiate, or increase, the action of mono-amine synapses, particularly those utilizing the monoamine transmitters norepinephrine and serotonin, work for depression, and the element lithium, in the form of a simple lithium salt, works for the bipolar disorder.

Reserpine, a drug first used to treat high blood pressure, was later found to be helpful in treating schizophrenics. Early on in the use of reserpine for high blood pressure it was noted that some patients being treated with the drug developed depression. The major action of reserpine is to make the catechol-amines dopamine and norepinephrine less available for synaptic transmission (Figures 5-9 and 5-10). Normally, these neurotransmitters are present in vesicles in the presynaptic terminals. When the terminal is activated by an action potential, some vesicles release their transmitter into the synaptic cleft. Reserpine causes dopamine and norepinephrine to leak out of the vesicles into the intracellular medium of the terminals, where it is less available for release at the synapse and where much of it is eventually destroyed by the breakdown enzyme monoamine oxidase (MAO). Reserpine is no longer used because newer drugs are more effective in treating schizophrenia, as we noted earlier.

Meanwhile, a drug called iproniazid was being used to treat tuberculosis (see Figures 5-9, 5-10, and 5-14). It was noted that iproniazid often markedly improved the depressed mood of tubercular patients. The drug was then found to be an effective treatment for depression. The primary action of iproniazid on neurons is to inhibit MAO. The neurotransmitters norepinephrine, dopamine, and serotonin are all monoamines. The most important point here is that MAO is a normal mechanism for breaking down and inactivating norepinephrine, dopamine, and serotonin. If a drug is given that inhibits MAO, more of these neurotransmitters will be available for incorporation into vesicles and for release at the synaptic terminals. Inhibition of MAO increases the activity of the monoamine neurotransmitter systems.

Another class of drugs was discovered to be effective in the treatment of depression. Imipramine, the first of these to be used, also increases the activity of monoamine synapses but in a different way than does iproniazid. Remember that the primary way neurotransmitters are inactivated at monoamine synapses is by reuptake into the presynaptic terminal; this is true for dopamine, norepinephrine, and serotonin (Figures 5-9, 5-10, and 5-14). Unlike ACh, which is broken down at the synapse by the enzyme AChE, the breakdown enzyme for monoamines, MAO, is present only inside cells and cell terminals. The only way to eliminate monoamines after they have been released at synapses is reuptake into the terminal. Imipramine blocks this process.

Imipramine is an example of the class of drugs called the tricyclics, so named because of their common core chemical structure. All of these drugs that are effective in the treatment of depression block the reuptake of monoamines, but they are somewhat selective. Imipramine blocks the reuptake of norepinephrine and serotonin but not the reuptake of dopamine. Another tricyclic, amitriptyline, blocks the reuptake of serotonin, and another, desipramine, has its greatest effect on the reuptake of norepinephrine. Remember that blocking reuptake means that more of the transmitter is active at the synapse. Recently, a drug that selectively blocks only reputake of serotonin, Prozac, has become popular in the treatment of depression.

The fact that these tricyclic drugs, all effective in the treatment of depression, act to increase the amount of norepinephrine and serotonin present and active at synapses leads to a straightforward biological explanation of depression: depression is brought on by too little norepinephrine and serotonin (Figures 5-10 and 5-14). This seems to be a case, however, where the treatment, which came first, is more effective than the theory. There are many problems with the too-little-norepinephrine-and-serotonin hypothesis of depression. For one thing, increasing the level of either transmitter at the synapse seems to work. Yet norepinephrine and serotonin are neurotransmitters in rather different circuits in the brain. Another difficulty with this theory is the lack of completely convincing evidence that depressed individuals have lower than normal levels of norepinephrine and serotonin in the brain. Metabolic breakdown products of both transmitters can be measured in the urine. Some depressed people have low levels of the norepinephrine product, some have low levels of the serotonin product, and some have low levels of both; but not all have low levels of either one. Further, the degree to which the urinary products reflect brain metabolism of monoamines is not really known.

Another problem with characterizing depression simply as a shortage of norepinephrine and serotonin concerns the time course of the action of the tricyclics. The tricyclics act on norepinephrine and serotonin synapses within minutes after their administration, yet their beneficial effects on depression take one to two weeks to develop. This problem is similar to that encountered in the dopamine theory of schizophrenia; antipsychotics act rapidly on dopamine receptors but require days to produce their antipsychotic effects. The long time course of the therapeutic actions of both kinds of drugs implies that processes of neuronal plasticity have a long time course, perhaps involving major changes in receptor sensitivity, an increase or a decrease in the number of receptors on postsynaptic cells, or even alterations in the physical structure of the synapse.

The antidepressant drugs are not as helpful in the treatment of the bipolar disorder, which, as we have seen, is periods of depression with at least one episode of mania. Fortunately, lithium carbonate, a salt of the element lithium, is enormously effective in treating bipolar depression.

Lithium is a very dangerous substance, literally a poison, and overdoses can kill. The level of safe dosage varies from person to person and as a function of repeated use. If blood levels are regularly monitored, it can be taken with relative safety. A manic individual given Lithium is calmed, and it prevents subsequent depression. Lithium is helpful to about 80 percent of individuals with the bipolar disorder. It is much less helpful in the treatment of major depression.

The reasons for Lithium's effectiveness are still largely obscure. It appears to act on both norepinephrine and serotonin synapses. Its actions are complex, involving both increases and decreases in transmitter availability at the synapses. Lithium also inhibits a second-messenger system, the synthesis of cyclic AMP, that is normally activated by norepinephrine. As is the case for tricyclics and the antipsychotics used to treat schizophrenia, the synaptic actions of Lithium are immediate, but its therapeutic effects on mania require one to two weeks to develop.

COMMENT

The most is known about the least common transmitters in the brain—the catecholamines DA and NE. These transmitters and the neurons that contain them can be identified, localized, and studied in a variety of ways. Yet they account for only a few percent of the total amount of neurotransmitter in the brain. There are about 10,000 NE neurons and 35,000 DA neurons in the rat brain and perhaps four times as many in the human brain—relatively speaking a very small number of neurons. The bulk of neurotransmitters consists of the workhorse amino acids. A growing number of peptides and hormones are also thought to function as neurotransmitters or neuromodulators in the brain; the brain opioids are examples (see Chapter 6).

Although it is tempting to associate behavioral functions with transmitters, for example, sleep with serotonin or general arousal with NE, it really cannot yet be done with any certainty. The message or meaning is not in the molecule. For example, ACh is the neurotransmitter at the neuromuscular junction. The "function" of ACh is not movement. The reason it produces movement is that it happens to be the transmitter between motor neuron axons and muscle fibers. Further, a given transmitter, like ACh or glutamate, can have both fast actions on ion channels and slow actions on second-messenger systems, depending on the receptors. It is the wiring diagrams, the ways neurons in the brain and body are interconnected, that determine particular behaviors. To understand the brain, both the neurotransmitter receptors and the wiring diagrams must be taken into account. A phenomenon as complex as consciousness presumably has as its basis the immensely complex circuitry of the cerebral cortex. To know whether glutamic acid or aspartic acid is an excitatory transmitter at certain neurons in the cortex is not enough to unravel the problem of consciousness or other brain functions. We must also know the patterns of interconnections among the neurons. Although some recent substantial advances have been made in this area, we are only beginning to understand the functional circuitry of the brain.

SUMMARY

Acetylcholine (ACh) is perhaps the best understood of the chemical neurotransmitters because it acts at neuromuscular junctions and can be studied in "pure culture." There are two major types of ACh receptors, those on skeletal muscles that are excitatory (nicotinic receptors) and those that act on the heart muscle, for example, and are inhibitory (muscarinic receptors). Much less is known about ACh circuits in the brain. The major ACh brain circuit has its cell bodies in the nucleus basalis (projecting widely to the cerebral cortex) and the septal nuclei (projecting to the hippocampus).

ACh in brain circuits appears to exert not fast synaptic actions (as it does on muscles) but rather slow or modulatory synaptic actions via second-messenger systems. In slow synaptic transmission the steps up to and including attachment of the transmitter to receptor molecules in the post synaptic membrane are the same as in fast synaptic transmission, but from this point the story differs. These slow-acting receptors are not directly coupled to ion channels. Instead they activate G proteins that in turn activate second-messenger systems. An example of such a system is the conversion (by the G protein) of ATP into cAMP, which in turn can act through complex biochemical processes within the cell to alter its excitability or even to change pattern of gene expression in the DNA of the cell.

Two well-characterized neurotransmitters in the brain are dopamine (DA) and norepinephrine (NE), both catecholamines. They are made in cells from tyrosine, an amino acid common in foods. Tyrosine is converted to L-dopa, then into dopamine, then to norepinephrine (and finally epinephrine). The final product, dopamine or norepinephrine, depends on what enzymes are present in the cell.

There are three major dopamine neuron circuits in the brain, one in the hypothalamus, one projecting from the substantia nigra to the basal ganglia, and one projecting from the brain stem to the cerebral cortex and other forebrain structures. In Parkinson's disease, the dopamine-containing neurons in the substantia nigra degenerate. The symptoms of the disease are brought on by the consequent decrease of dopamine transmission in the basal ganglia. Treating patients with injections of L-dopa (which converts to dopamine in the brain) has proved helpful. The dopamine system that projects to the forebrain appears to be involved in the severe mental illness schizophrenia. In general, drugs that help to treat the symptoms of schizophrenia block dopamine synapses in the brain. Hence a widespread theory of the cause of schizophrenia is that the forebrain-projecting dopamine system becomes overactive.

The norepinephrine (NE) circuits in the brain all arise from a small collection of neurons in the brain stem (in the locus ceruleus) and project to virtually all forebrain structures. In general, this NE system is thought to modulate level of arousal and may be involved in the consolidation of memory.

Serotonin is another neurotransmitter manufactured in cells from an amino acid present in foods, tryptophan (bananas are loaded with tryptophan). Its chemical structure is similar to those of DA and NE (they are all monoamines). The cell bodies of the brain serotonin circuit lie mostly in the raphe nuclei in the brain stem and project to the hypothalamus and forebrain structures.

Severe depression seems to involve the norepinephrine and serotonin circuits in the brain. There are two types of depression, one that is consistently severe depression and one that involves severe depression with at least one episode of mania (now termed bipolar depression, it used to be called manic–depressive disorder). In general, drugs that potentiate or increase the actions of the norepinephrine and serotonin circuits in the brain are helpful in the treatment of sever depression. They are not particularly helpful in treating bipolar disorder, but another substance, Lithium, in the form of a lithium salt, does seem to help those suffering from bipolar disorder.

All these neurotransmitter systems in the brain that seem critical for mental health and illness appear to act primarily via second-messenger systems. Interestingly, they account for only a few percent of the total neurotransmitters in the brain. The fast transmitters such as glutamate and GABA are much more common and widespread.

SUGGESTED READINGS AND REFERENCES

Books

Cooper, J. R., Bloom, F. E., and Roth, R. H. (1991). *The biochemical basis of neuropharmacology* (6th ed.). New York: Oxford University Press.

Gottesman, I. I. (1991). *Schizophrenia genesis: The origins of madness.* New York: W. H. Freeman.

Julien, R. M. (1992). *A primer of drug action: A concise, nontechnical guide to the actions, uses, and side effects of psychoactive drugs* (6th ed.). New York: W. H. Freeman.

Kaplan, H. I., and Sadock, B. J. (1988). *Comprehensive textbook of psychiatry* (5th ed.). Baltimore, MD: Williams & Wilkins.

Lickey, M. E., and Gordon, B. (1983). *Drugs for mental illness: A revolution in psychiatry.* New York: W. H. Freeman.

Snyder, S. H. (1986). *Drugs and the brain.* New York: W. H Freeman.

U. S. Congress, Office of Technology Assessment (1992). *The biology of mental disorders.* Washington, D. C.: U. S. Government Printing Office.

Articles

Bloom, F. E. (1988). Neurotransmitters: Past, present and future directions. *Federation of American Societies for Experimental Biology Journal, 2,* 32–41.

Depue, R. A., and Iacono, W. G. (1989). Neurobehavioral aspects of affective disorders. *Annual Review of Psychology, 40,* 457–492.

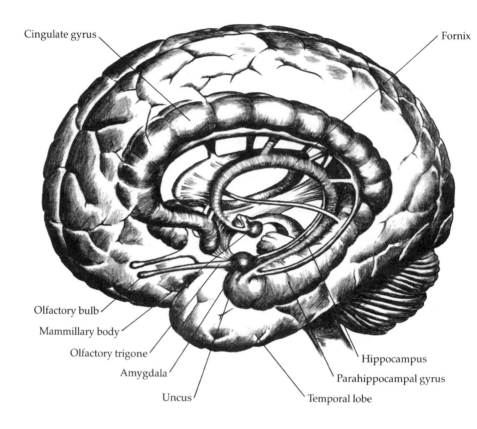

Cingulate gyrus

Fornix

Olfactory bulb

Mammillary body

Olfactory trigone

Amygdala

Uncus

Hippocampus

Parahippocampal gyrus

Temporal lobe

6

Peptides, Hormones, and the Brain

The recently discovered brain opioids are examples of a number of peptide substances that have been discovered in the brain in the past few years. *Opioids* are substances present in the pituitary gland and brain that act like opium (Figure 6-1). Many of the newly discovered peptides are *hormones* produced either by the pituitary gland or body tissues and organs, but some are produced in neurons. (A *peptide*, incidentally, is simply a relatively short chain of amino acids connected together. Proteins are much larger and more complex combinations of amino acids.) Progress has been rapid in elucidating the mechanism of action of the opioids because so much is known about the pharmacology of morphine and related opiates.

Opium, an extract of the opium poppy, has been used since ancient times for both pain relief and pleasure. *Morphine* and *codeine* are the two active ingredients in opium. Morphine was purified in the early nineteenth century and became widely used soon afterward; patent medicines later in the nine-

Figure 6-1 Opiate receptors are present in high concentration in many of the limbic structures of the brain. Certain of these regions (for example, the cingulate gyrus, hippocampus, amygdala, and mammillary body) appear to be particularly involved in experiences of pleasure and pain and the emotions.

teenth century were loaded with it (Figure 6-2). Today more addicts use intra-venous injections of heroin than of morphine. *Heroin* is synthesized from morphine and has a more potent and much more rapid action, primarily because it crosses the blood–brain barrier faster. It appears that heroin is converted into morphine in the brain and that the primary action is of mor-phine.

Morphine is among the best understood of all the drugs that act on the brain. In large part this is because similar chemical molecules can be syn-thesized that have very specific antagonistic actions to morphine. *Naloxone* is

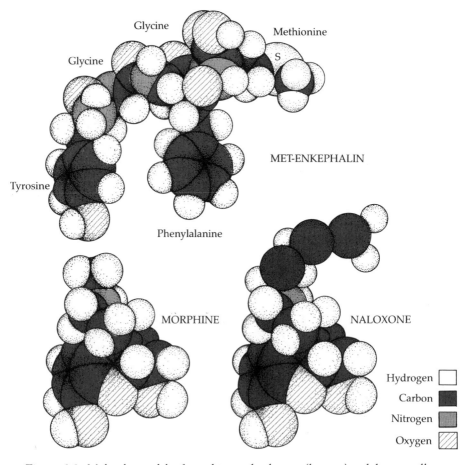

Figure 6-2 Molecular models of morphine and naloxone (bottom) and the naturally occurring brain opioid peptide met-enkephalin (top). Note that the bottom left part of each molecule is very similar. It is thought that morphine can "fool" the met-enkephalin receptors in the brain. Naloxone has a side group that resembles the phenylalanine group of met-enkephalin. Naloxone attaches to the opioid receptors in the body and brain more powerfully than morphine does and hence blocks the action of morphine.

an example of such a chemical (Figure 6-2). Naloxone has no obvious effect at all when it is given to a normal animal or human, but it very rapidly and completely reverses the effects of morphine, as we saw earlier.

OPIATE RECEPTOR AND BRAIN OPIOIDS

The fact that naloxone, a drug very similar in chemical structure to morphine, is a specific antagonist to morphine suggested that there might be a specific receptor molecule on neurons for morphine. The first evidence that such a receptor existed in the brain was developed by Avram Goldstein at Stanford University; the definitive work was done by Solomon Snyder and a graduate student, Candice Pert, at the Johns Hopkins University in 1974. Snyder and Pert used radioactively labeled naloxone and showed that it bound very specifically to receptors on neurons in several regions of the brain, specifically throughout the slow pain system.

This finding immediately raised a most puzzling question. Why on earth had the brain developed an elaborate receptor system for an extract of a poppy plant? Opium was not even available to humans until about 5000 years ago, when it was first extracted from the poppy. Yet the opiate receptor system exists in the brains of all higher vertebrates. Only one answer seemed possible: the brain must make or use chemical substances very similar to opium. This was actually proposed by Goldstein in 1967. The search was on after the receptor was found in 1974. John Hughes and Hans Kosterlitz at the University of Aberdeen in Scotland isolated a substance from the brains of pigs in 1975 that had the same actions as morphine and named it *enkephalin* (in the head). Chemically, enkephalin is composed of two similar and relatively simple substances, each containing five amino acid units. Although at first glance enkephalin does not seem to resemble morphine in chemical structure, it turns out that one part of the molecule does (Figure 6-2).

Subsequently, other brain opioids have been discovered. The group as a whole is termed either *endorphins* (endogenous morphine) or *brain opioids*. *Beta-endorphin* is a much larger molecule than the enkephalins and is found almost entirely in the pituitary gland rather than in the brain proper. It is derived from a larger precursor molecule in the pituitary called proopiomelanocortin, from which ACTH, beta-endorphin, and other hormones are made (Figure 6-3). At the moment, beta-endorphin is properly considered a hormone that is released from the pituitary gland. It is an opioid that has actions similar to those of morphine. The smaller enkephalin molecules are present in nerve terminals in a number of brain regions, particularly in the slow pain system (discussed later). At this point they are believed by some to act as neurotransmitters, but still with much uncertainty.

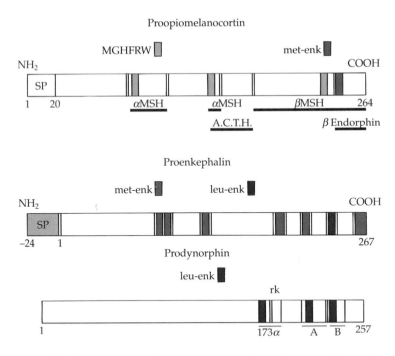

Figure 6-3 The "superhormones" or prohormones, from which opioid peptides and several hormones are made. Shown are the structural relationships among the prohormones, precursor forms of the three major branches of the opioid peptides, depicted as a bar diagram, whose length in amino acid residues is indicated by the smaller number at the corresponding C-termini. The location of the repeating peptide sequences are indicated.

Still other brain opioids have been discovered. At Stanford, Goldstein isolated a substance called dynorphin that is more than 200 times more potent than morphine. He and coworkers at the California Institute of Technology determined its chemical structure and synthesized it.

Current work in molecular biology has clarified the story of the manufacture of brain opioids. There are three "superfamilies" of proteins or peptides expressed by genes in neurons. The first is the *proopiomelanocortin family* noted earlier (Figure 6-3). This family is expressed primarily in the pituitary gland but also in a group of neurons in the hypothalamus, and it is a long chain of 264 amino acids (peptide or protein). Beta-endorphin is cleaved from this chain and is only 31 amino acids long. Another hormone, melanin-stimulating hormone (MSH, discussed later), is also cleaved from the large peptide, as is adrencorticotrophin hormone (ACTH). The second family of brain opioids, *met-* and *leu-enkephalin*, are formed in different neurons from a quite different super peptide called proenkephalin, a chain of 267 amino acids. Met-

and leu-enkephalin are only 5 amino acids in length. Neurons expressing the enkephalins are distributed widely through the brain, as are neurons expressing the third type of opioids, the *dynorphins*. The dynorphins arise from a quite different gene that expresses prodynorphine, a chain of 257 amino acids. Four different, much smaller peptide dynorphins are formed from this peptide. All of these brain opioids act on opiate receptors to varying degrees and all show *cross-tolerance* to morphine (if an animal is made tolerant—addicted—to morphine, it will also show tolerance to all the opioids).

To complicate the picture further, there are currently thought to be four different types of opioid receptors, labeled mu, delta, epsilon, and kappa. There is some degree of selectivity of action of the various brain opioids in the different receptors. Thus, dynorphins act primarily on the kappa receptors. Naloxone, the opiate antagonist that reverses the effects of morphine, antagonizes all the receptors but has its most potent actions on mu and delta receptors. At this point little is really known about the possible differential functions of the different brain opioids and the different opioid receptors.

Why do we and other vertebrates have these substances in our brains? What roles do they play in brain function and behavior? The answers are not yet entirely clear, but there are some tantalizing hints. The most obvious possibility is that these substances are released by the pituitary gland and neurons in the brain in times of stress to minimize pain and enhance adaptive behavior. For example, a minor injury received during athletic activity or another vigorous activity is sometimes not even noticed until later.

The other side of the coin is that release of these substances in the brain can produce a feeling of euphoria and well-being. A common example is the "high" experienced by most serious joggers. They report that if they jog regularly and go sufficiently long distances, they develop a genuine high: a strong feeling of joy or euphoria. It could be that jogging is a sufficient stress to induce the release of the brain opioids that act on the pleasure system in the brain. This of course is speculation. Morphine counters pain and produces a strong feeling of joy or pleasure. It is this pleasurable effect of morphine that appears to be responsible for its having become a seriously abused substance. Heroin addicts may first start using the drug because it gives them an intense high, often called a "rush." With repeated use, the high becomes more elusive and the more sinister aspects of morphine addiction, such as withdrawal symptoms if the individual attempts to stop using it, take over.

PAIN PATHWAYS IN THE BRAIN

Certain brain opioids or their chemical receptors or both are found in close association with pain pathways in the brain. There are two pain systems in the brain: the *fast pain system* and the *slow pain system*. Correspondingly, two classes of nerve fibers carry pain information from the skin and body tissues: fast and slow nerve fibers. The *fast nerve fibers* are relatively small and myelinated and conduct at about 5 to 30 meters per second. The *slow nerve fibers* are tiny, unmyelinated C fibers that conduct at about 0.5 to 2 meters per second. Slow fibers conducting from the foot could take as long as 2 seconds to signal pain to the brain. The fast pain fibers and their nerve-ending receptors service only the skin and mucous membranes, but the C fibers service all of the skin and all body tissue except the nervous tissue of the brain itself, which is insensitive to pain.

There is now evidence that the C fibers contain a particular peptide called *substance P*. It was discovered in 1931 in the dried acetone powder of an extract of neural tissue. P stands for powder but has come to mean pain, at least for C fibers. The chemical structure of substance P has been worked out and has been synthesized.

Substance P is present in C fibers, in the pain pathways of the spinal cord, and in a number of brain regions, including the basal ganglia and cerebral cortex. Although the evidence is clear that C fibers contain substance P, it is still not proved that substance P is the neurotransmitter at the synapses the C fibers make in the spinal cord. These fibers also contain glutamate, the workhorse fast excitatory neurotransmitter.

Although many details of the pain pathways in the spinal cord and brain remain to be worked out, the broad outlines are clear. Both the fast and the slow pain fibers synapse with neurons in a dorsal region of the spinal cord called the *substantia gelatinosa* (from its gelatinous texture). The majority of these neurons cross to the other side of the body to ascend to the brain, but some ascend on the same side. The fast pain pathway travels in close association with the primary somatic sensory system that mediates touch, pressure, and joint and limb movement senses (Figure 6-4). However, it forms relays through the reticular formation and terminates in two thalamic nuclei: the *ventrobasal complex* (the same thalamic nucleus that relays touch and pressure sensations) and the *posterior nucleus*. Both of these nuclei relay to the cerebral cortex.

The slow pain system takes a more tortuous route. In the brain stem it forms relays through the reticular formation and through a region called the *periacqueductal gray* (PAG), so named because it is a region of cell bodies (gray matter) surrounding the upward continuation of the spinal canal (aqueduct) in the brain stem and midbrain. This region is extremely important in pain sensation and the control of pain and may even be critically involved in learned fear and anxiety. From the periaqueductal gray the slow pain pathway projects to the hypothalamus, to a portion of the thalamus called the *in-*

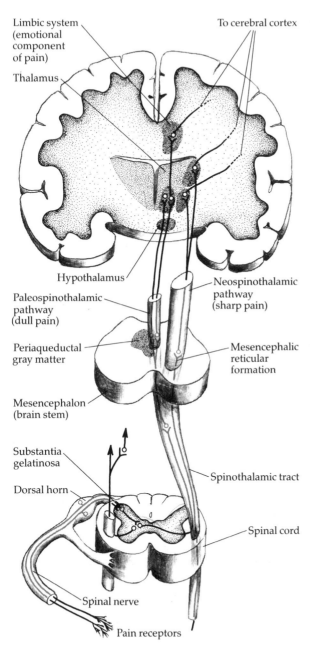

Limbic system
(emotional
component
of pain)

Thalamus

To cerebral cortex

Hypothalamus

Paleospinothalamic
pathway
(dull pain)

Periaqueductal
gray matter

Mesencephalon
(brain stem)

Substantia
gelatinosa

Dorsal horn

Neospinothalamic
pathway
(sharp pain)

Mesencephalic
reticular
formation

Spinothalamic tract

Spinal cord

Spinal nerve

Pain receptors

Figure 6-4 Pain systems in the spinal cord and brain. The slow or dull pain system mediates aching and burning pain, has high concentrations of opiate receptors, and is acted on powerfully by morphine. The fast and sharp pain system conveys sharp pricking pain rapidly to the cerebral cortex, does not have opiate receptors, and is not acted on by morphine.

tralaminar nuclei and to portions of the limbic system, such as the amygdala. The organization and activities of these higher regions of the slow pain system are not well understood. It is generally believed that they are involved in emotional and motivational aspects of pain, the subjective experience of pain.

The fast pain system and the slow pain system are functionally quite different. The fast pain system, which conveys information about painful stimuli to the cerebral cortex, is thought to be a more recent evolutionary development. The older slow pain system is present in more primitive vertebrates that have little or no cerebral cortex. Interestingly, morphine and other opiates have little or no effect on the fast pain system but a very powerful blocking action on the slow pain system.

The distribution of opiate receptors in the central nervous system is shown in Figure 6-1. They are present in the substantia gelatinosa of the spinal cord, the reticular formation, the periaqueductal gray, the hypothalamus, the intralaminar thalamic nuclei, the amygdala, and other regions of the limbic system. In short, they are distributed throughout the slow pain (and "pleasure") system in the brain.

Enkephalin-containing neurons are found in close association with the lower levels of the slow pain system. An example at the level of the spinal cord is shown in Figure 6-5. The function of this class of neurons is thought to be to control or gate how much of the slow pain information received from body tissues is relayed up the spinal cord to the brain.

The enkephalin interneuron appears to act synaptically on the incoming slow pain fibers that use substance P and/or glutamate as neurotransmitters. The enkephalin interneuron appears to inhibit transmission from the substance P fiber terminal to its target neuron, which sends pain information to the brain. The enkephalin interneurons could in turn be activated by local circuits in the spinal cord and by descending pathways from the brain. One of these pathways is believed to excite the enkephalin interneuron, which would inhibit incoming pain information in the substance P fibers. Interestingly, this descending pathway is believed to use serotonin as its neurotransmitter. The existence of these descending pain control pathways provides a means for the brain to control the amount of pain input it receives from the spinal cord.

Recent evidence from the laboratory of William Willis at the Marine Biomedical Institute at Galveston, Texas, has shed further light on this pain input system. He used injections of capsaicin in the skin of anesthetized animals (capsaicin is the active ingredient in pepper). This causes activation of the neurons in the substantia gelatinosa and also a process of sensitization—the neurons become increasingly more responsive over time. This sensitization could account for the persisting and severe pain following some types of injury—for example, burns—where chemicals released by the injury, for example, histamine, could act like capsaicin. He found that infusion in this region of the spinal cord of an antagonist to the AMPA-type glutamate recep-

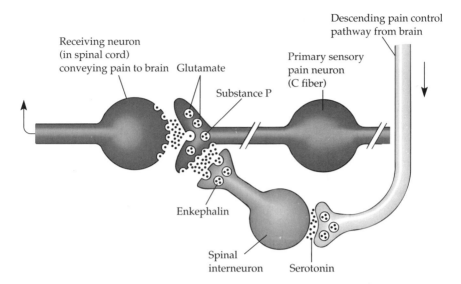

Figure 6-5 Certain interneurons in the spinal cord appear to use enkephalin as their neurotransmitter. They act directly on the terminals of the incoming sensory fibers conveying slow pain information to the spinal cord from the body and apparently inhibit this pain input from being relayed to the brain. The slow pain fiber terminals contain substance P and glutamate. Glutamate appears to be the fast transmitter, and substance P acts to modulate its actions. A descending pain control pathway from the brain is thought to act on the enkephalin interneurons; it appears to use serotonin as its transmitter.

tor blocked the responses of the neurons to the afferent input. However, an antagonist to the NMDA-type glutamate receptor did not block activation but completely prevented the sensitization process. So the critical synaptic processes appear to be glutamate–AMPA receptors for fast transmission and glutamate-NMDA receptors for sensitization, a result somewhat analogous to the glutamate receptor processes in hippocampal LTP (see Chapter 4).

ADDICTION AND THE OPIATE RECEPTOR

Drug addiction is one of the most devastating problems in our society. Alcohol is perhaps the most serious drug of abuse; there are about 10 million alcoholics in the United States. Although there are many fewer heroin addicts, heroin has received more publicity than alcohol, and it is indeed a serious and dangerous drug of abuse. Barbiturates and amphetamines, joined recently by cocaine, are also much abused and dangerous addicting drugs. Contrary to popular opinion, cocaine can be among the most addicting of substances.

From a medical point of view, nicotine obtained from the smoking of tobacco is the most serious drug of abuse because of the much increased incidence of emphysema, lung cancer, other forms of cancer, and heart disease in smokers. Heavy smoking of marijuana carries all of these dangers and may have other serious consequences as well. Another common substance of abuse is caffeine, present in substantial amounts in coffee and some soft drinks, which is at least as widely abused as nicotine. It may come as a surprise that food is a serious substance of abuse. Several million Americans have developed severe medical problems because they are addicted to eating too much food and have become obese or extremely overweight.

There are three related phenomena in substance abuse (abuse of food is a possible exception): addiction, tolerance, and withdrawal. *Addiction* is really a behavioral term; it means that the user seeks out and takes the substance with increasing frequency. *Tolerance* means that increasing amounts of the substance must be used to produce the same effect. The heroin user has to keep increasing the dose to get the same sense of euphoria, the same "rush." *Withdrawal* refers to the symptoms and feelings that develop when the user stops taking the substance.

Essentially all drugs of abuse give rise to marked tolerance. All addicting drugs do. However, some drugs to which tolerance is built up do not appear to be very addicting. For example, great tolerance is built up to LSD, but the drug does not appear to be addicting. Marijuana use also results in tolerance and the substance may be addicting, but much less so than heroin.

The severity of withdrawal symptoms varies enormously with the drug of abuse. Heroin withdrawal, despite the attention it has received, almost never directly causes death. Withdrawal from barbiturates, however, can cause death, and so can withdrawal from alcohol. In this sense, they are more dangerous than heroin. The nicotine withdrawal symptoms experienced by a heavy smoker who is trying to kick the habit are much less obvious and do not seem to be severe. They are subtle and persistent, often described as the inability to think clearly and increased tension and irritability.

Most of the symptoms of withdrawal from a drug of abuse can be predicted quite accurately from the direct effect of the drug itself. In every case they are the opposite of the drug's effects. Heroin slows down stomach contractions, and withdrawal brings on stomach cramps. Nicotine (from tobacco smoking) causes an increased heartbeat rate, and withdrawal causes a slowing of the heart. Amphetamine causes a sense of almost manic well-being, or euphoria. Withdrawal causes severe depression.

The striking opposite effects of the actions of drugs and withdrawal from them led to the general theory of withdrawal and addiction termed the *hypersensitivity theory*, which simply states that the body and brain attempt to counteract the effects of the drug. The body ordinarily tries to maintain a constant optimal state. When this state is altered by a drug, the body tries to compensate. For example, suppose that a drug causes an increase in heart rate, as nicotine does. The brain and nervous system might increase the activity of the vagus nerve, which causes a slowing of the heart rate. With repeated use of the drug, the increased compensatory activity of the vagus nerve could become long lasting and relatively permanent. When the drug is withdrawn, the vagus nerve would continue to be more active for some period of time. The heart rate will then be slower than normal for the same period of time.

The severity of withdrawal symptoms is closely related to the time course of action of the drug itself. Heroin is a fast-acting drug, and withdrawal is correspondingly rapid and severe. Methadone, a synthetic relative of heroin, produces the same effects as heroin but has a much slower time course of action. Withdrawal symptoms for methadone are much slower to develop and less severe, although more prolonged. This has led to the methadone maintenance treatment program for heroin addicts. Since methadone and heroin (and morphine) are very similar drugs, they show marked cross-tolerance. If tolerance has developed for one, it will be present for the other, just as the brain opioids show cross-tolerance to morphine, as we noted earlier.

There is no clear relationship between the severity of physical withdrawal symptoms and the addiction potency of drugs. The withdrawal symptoms from cocaine addiction are much less obvious than those from morphine, yet cocaine appears to be more addicting. Remember that addiction is primarily a behavioral phenomenon; it refers to repeated use of a drug. Many psychological as well as biological-chemical factors are involved.

Withdrawal symptoms are perhaps the most important reason such drugs as heroin, barbiturates, and alcohol are so severely addicting. The heroin user begins to use heroin because of the intense pleasurable feelings it produces and in many cases because of peer-group influences. When all of the other people in a group use heroin, someone wishing to be a part of the group will feel considerable pressure to join in. Once heroin is tried, biology often takes over. Humans and monkeys can become regular users after a few experiences with it. Initially, it is used for pleasure, but as use continues, tolerance develops and more and more of the drug must be used to get the same "kick." Eventually, the kick is hard to get, even with massive doses. A severely addicted person, incidentally, can tolerate a dose of heroin that would be fatal to a nonuser. The greater the tolerance, the more severe and unpleasant the withdrawal symptoms will be if use of the drug is stopped. Soon the addict takes heroin primarily to stave off the pain and suffering of withdrawal. What begins as a pleasure-seeking activity ends up as a pain-avoiding one.

The discovery of the opiate receptor led to the development of a straightforward theory of opiate addiction at the level of the chemical receptor. It is simply an extension of the supersensitivity theory of withdrawal symptoms.

Opiate receptors are believed to exert their action by way of a second-messenger system. In brief, neurotransmitter molecules attach to the receptors on the neuron membrane and, according to the theory, trigger a decrease in the synthesis of cyclic AMP. The decrease can act on the protein synthesis machinery of the cell to cause long-lasting changes in cell function. The opiate receptor is best thought of as a hormone receptor. The endorphins, remember, are present largely in the pituitary gland and are probably released normally at some rate into the bloodstream. In times of chronic pain or stress, their release is believed to increase. The increased blood levels of these brain opioids would then act on opiate receptors on neurons in the slow pain and pleasure systems of the brain to protect against the pain or stress.

Suppose that the brain opioids' primary action via the receptors is to reduce the formation of cyclic AMP in the target neurons. When artificial opiates such as heroin are administered, they act on the opiate receptors. Suppose that their action is also to decrease the synthesis of cyclic AMP. The cell now counteracts this effect by manufacturing more cyclic AMP. With repeated use of heroin, the cell develops a long-lasting increase in the manufacture of cyclic AMP to counter the depressing action of heroin. If the heroin is now withdrawn, the cell continues to make too much cyclic AMP and produces the symptoms of withdrawal.

The opiate receptor model of addiction has been adopted by some workers in the field as the basic model for all forms of addiction. This is not to say that all addictions involve the opiate receptor. In particular, barbiturate, amphetamine, cocaine, nicotine, and alcohol addiction do not have to do with the opiate receptor. Many of these drugs do act via certain neurotransmitter–receptor systems in the brain; for example, nicotine acts on nicotinic ACh receptors and amphetamine and cocaine are thought to act on the catecholamine receptors and the synapses for norepinephrine and dopamine. Barbiturates presumably act on the barbiturate site on the $GABA_A$ receptors, as well as having other actions. The addictive process could follow the same course of receptor adaptation in these systems as occurs in the opiate receptor system. So far as is known, however, alcohol does not have specific receptor actions.

Recent work on the "pleasure" system in the brain may offer an explanation for the initially pleasurable feelings caused by addicting drugs. As we noted, most addicts begin using these substances for the pleasurable sensations they cause, which can be intense with drugs like heroin and cocaine. It appears that there is a "reward" or "pleasure" system in the brain. As we will see in Chapter 7, the final target of this pleasure system appears to be a nucleus in the forebrain called the *nucleus accumbens* (Figure 7-3), and it is activated by an ascending pathway that uses dopamine as the neurotransmitter. A wide range of addicting drugs seem to influence this system.

Brain and body chemistry seem to be the most powerful determinants of addictive behavior, but behavioral and psychological factors can also be very important. One of the most interesting aspects of morphine addiction is that tolerance of morphine can to some degree be conditioned or learned. Rats given repeated injections of morphine in the same surroundings develop marked tolerance to the drug and can survive a dose of morphine that would kill them if it were given to them in different surroundings. This phenomenon of learned tolerance may account for some of the deaths from overdose among heroin addicts, for example, if they take the high dose to which they have become tolerant in a different and unusual environment.

HORMONES AND THE BRAIN

The brain opioids are chemically parts of much larger molecules from which some hormones are made in the hypothalamus–pituitary gland, as noted earlier. Indeed, beta-endorphin is released from the pituitary gland and is almost by definition an endocrine hormone. The fact that it does not easily cross the blood–brain barrier complicates our understanding of its possible functions.

Endocrine System

The *endocrine system* is the second great communication system of the body, the first being the nervous system. The endocrine system communicates by way of the blood. The master gland, the *pituitary*, and its hypothalamic connection secrete control hormones into the circulating blood. These hormones activate specific receptors in target organs, which release other hormones into the blood that act on other tissues and also back on the pituitary gland and the brain. The endocrine system is critically important for the activation and control of such basic behavioral functions as sex, emotion, and response to stress and in the regulation of basic bodily functions such as growth, energy use, and metabolism.

The key to the specific effects of hormones is the *hormone receptor molecule*. Hormone receptors are closely analogous in function to neurotransmitter receptors. A given hormone receptor will be activated only by its particular hormone (and by compounds that are chemically closely related, such as synthetic hormone analogues). The only cells in the body that respond to a particular hormone are those that have receptor molecules for that hormone. Oxytocin acts only on tissues in the breast and uterus of the female because only these tissues have oxytocin receptors. It does not cause contractions of other muscle tissues because they have no oxytocin receptors.

Some of the major *endocrine glands* are the gonads (ovaries and testes), the adrenal gland, the thyroid gland, the pancreas, the thymus, the pineal gland, and of course the pituitary gland (Figure 6-6). The kidneys and gastrointes-

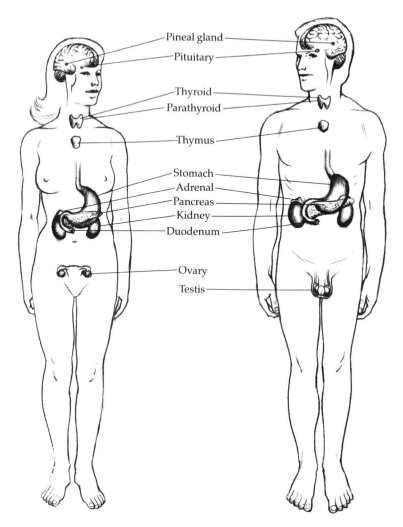

Pineal gland
Pituitary
Thyroid
Parathyroid
Thymus
Stomach
Adrenal
Pancreas
Kidney
Duodenum
Ovary
Testis

Figure 6-6 Locations of the major endocrine glands.

tinal tract also function as endocrine glands. The word endocrine means within; endocrine glands secrete within the body into the bloodstream (Table 6-1). *Exocrine glands* secrete substances outside the body. Examples are the sweat glands, tear glands, and salivary glands.

The activity of all the endocrine glands is under the direct control of the pituitary gland, situated at the base of the brain immediately next to the hypothalamus (Figures 6-6 and 6-7). The pituitary gland in turn is under the direct control of the *hypothalamus*, a small structure at the base of the brain composed of a number of different groups of neurons. The hypothalamus is

TABLE 6-1 Summary of the major endocrine hormones released into the general circulation

Gland	Hormone	Major function is control of:
Anterior pituitary	Growth hormone (GRH)	Growth; organic metabolism
	Thyroid-stimulating hormone (TRH)	Thyroid gland; metabolism
	Adrenocorticotropic hormone (ACTH)	Adrenal cortex
	Prolactin	Breasts (milk synthesis)
	Gonadotropic hormones:	Gonads (gamete production and
	Follicle-stimulating hormone (FSH)	sex hormone synthesis)
	Luteinizing hormone (LH)	
Posterior pituitary (hypothalamus)	Oxytocin	Milk secretion; uterine motility
	Antidiuretic hormone (ADH, vasopressin)	Water excretion
Adrenal cortex	Cortisol	Organic metabolism; response to stress
	Androgens	Growth and, in women, sexual activity
	Aldosterone	Sodium and potassium excretion
Adrenal medulla	Epinephrine	Organic metabolism; cardiovascular
	Norepinephrine	function; response to stress
	Opioids	
Thyroid	Thyroxine	Energy metabolism; growth
	Triiodothyronine	
	Calcitonin	Plasma calcium
Parathyroids	Parathyroid hormone (parathormone, PTH, PH)	Plasma calcium and phosphate
Gonads		
Female: ovaries	Estrogens	Reproductive system; growth and development
	Progesterone	
Male: testes	Testosterone	Reproductive system; growth and development
Pancreas	Insulin	Organic metabolism; plasma glucose
	Glucagon	
	Somatostatin	
Kidneys	Renin	Adrenal cortex; blood pressure
	Erythropoietin (ESF)	Erythrocyte production
	1,25-Dihydroxy vitamin D_3	Calcium balance
Gastrointestinal tract	Gastrin	Gastrointestinal tract; liver; pancreas; gallbladder
	Secretin	
	Cholecystokinin	
	Gastric inhibitory peptide	
	Somatostatin	
Thymus	Thymus hormone (thymosin)	Lymphocyte development
Pineal	Melatonin	Sexual maturity(?)

Source: Modified from A. J. Vander, J. H. Sherman, and D. S. Luciano, *Human Physiology: The Mechanisms of Body Function*, 5 ed, McGraw-Hill, New York, 1991.

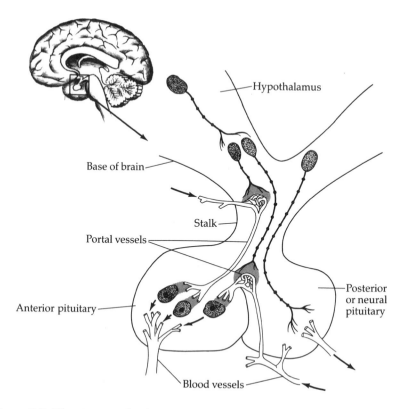

Figure 6-7 The pituitary gland extends from the base of the brain as an "out-growth" of the hypothalamus. The posterior pituitary is really just supporting tissue to hold the nerve terminals of nerve fibers from the hypothalamus that release hormones into the bloodstream. The anterior pituitary is a true gland, and its cells release hormones into the bloodstream when stimulated by hormones released from neurons in the hypothalamus. The hypothalamic hormones flow in the portal blood vessels directly from the hypothalamus to the anterior pituitary gland.

critically important in the regulation of basic bodily functions. It controls the autonomic nervous system and the functioning of the heart and blood vessels, temperature regulation, eating and drinking, sex, and pleasure. The hypothalamus acts through the brain and the rest of the nervous system and through the endocrine system by its control of the pituitary gland.

The pituitary gland is often referred to as the master gland of the endocrine system. Physically it is immediately next to and continuous with the hypothalamus. Actually, the hypothalamus is more properly considered as the master gland: it controls the activity of the pituitary gland directly and tightly. A clear understanding of the relation between the hypothalamus and the pituitary gland was developed only in recent years. The hypothalamus is made up of neurons and is of course not technically a gland at all, whereas a part of the pituitary is glandular tissue that has no neurons.

Let us take an example of how the system works. Under conditions of stress, the hypothalamus produces a hormone called corticotropin releasing hormone (CRH) that is transported through the portal blood supply directly to cells in the anterior pituitary, where it causes them to release adrenocorticotropic hormone (ACTH) into the general circulation (see Tables 6-1 and 6-2). ACTH acts directly on cells in the cortex of the adrenal gland, causing them to release cortisol into the bloodstream. Cortisol is the stress hormone and mobilizes the body to deal with stress (see Chapter 7).

This general sequence of events is true for all endocrine gland actions. There is one more very important step: *feedback control.* The increased blood level of cortisol acts back on the hypothalamus and pituitary gland to decrease their release of CRH and ACTH. This is an example of a negative feedback system, similar to the regulation of temperature by a thermostat. As the blood level of cortisol goes up, the "thermostats" in the hypothalamus and pituitary are turned off; as it goes down, they are turned on.

The pituitary gland is really two glands: the anterior pituitary and the posterior pituitary (Figure 6-7). Embryologically, the *posterior pituitary* is derived from the neural crest, which are the cells that form the nervous system; it is really just a part of the hypothalamus that sticks out from the brain and is not a gland in its own right. The posterior pituitary is simply a collection of cells that support and maintain the nerve terminals of neurons whose cell bodies lie in two regions of the hypothalamus. These nerve terminals are the only functional part of the posterior pituitary gland as far as the release of hormones is concerned. Hormones made by the neuron cell bodies in the hypothalamus are transported by axoplasmic flow to their terminals. They are then stored in the nerve terminals in the posterior pituitary. When these neurons are appropriately stimulated, their terminals release hormones directly into the bloodstream. The hypothalamic nerve terminals in the posterior pituitary are known to release only two hormones: *oxytocin* and *vasopressin.*

The *anterior pituitary* is a true gland. It contains no neurons from the hypothalamus. Yet its activities are tightly controlled by the hypothalamus. How this could be so was a puzzle for many years. The answer turned out to be surprising and simple. Several regions of the hypothalamus are heavily supplied with blood vessels, which go directly from the hypothalamus to the anterior pituitary gland, and they supply all of its gland cells. This vascular system is called the *portal system.* Regions of the hypothalamus connected with the portal system release hormones directly into it. The hormones are transported by the blood vessels directly to the endocrine cells of the anterior pituitary, stimulating them to release their hormones into the bloodstream and hence into the general circulation (Figure 6-8). Pituitary hormones are transported to all of the organs and tissues in the body. The major hypo-

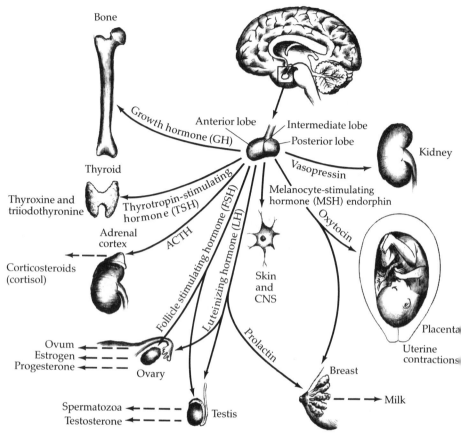

Figure 6-8 Target organs and actions of the anterior and posterior or pituitary hormones.

thalamic hormones that act on the anterior pituitary are summarized in Table 6-2.

All the hormones secreted by the neurons of the hypothalamus (except dopamine) are relatively small peptides, ranging in length from 3 amino acids for TRH to 34 for GnRH. All of the hormones released from secreting cells of the anterior pituitary are either peptides or peptides with attached carbohydrate groups, termed *glycoproteins*. Body hormones have several different types of structures, including peptides. Those concerned with sexual functions and stress are *steroid hormones*, derived ultimately from cholesterol, and are completely different from peptides in structure.

The chemical structures of all but one of the hypothalamic hormones (PRF) are now known, as are the structure of all the anterior pituitary hormones. The structures of most body hormones are also known. As you will no

TABLE 6-2 **Major hypothalamic releasing hormones and their effects on the anterior pituitary**

Hypothalamic releasing hormone*	Effect on anterior pituitary
Corticotropin-releasing hormone (CRH)	Stimulates secretion of ACTH (adrenocorticotropin)
Thyrotropin-releasing hormone (TRH)	Stimulates secretion of TSH (thyrotropin)
Growth-hormone-releasing hormone (GRH)	Stimulates secretion of GH (growth hormone)
Somatostatin (also known as growth-hormone-release-inhibiting hormone (GIH)	Inhibits secretion of GH (growth hormone)
Gonadotropin-releasing hormone (GnRH)	Stimulates secretion of LH and FSH
Prolactin-releasing hormone (PRH)	Stimulates secretion of prolactin
Prolactin-release inhibiting hormone (PIH)	Inhibits secretion of prolactin

*The structures of all the hypothalmic hormones (they are peptides) are known except for PRH. PIH is actually the neurotransmitter dopamine.
Source: Modified from Berne, R. M. and Levy, M. N. 1988. *Physiology.* 2nd Ed. St. Louis: C. V. Mosby Co .

doubt guess, all the brain hormones act on receptors in the cell membranes of cells in target organs in the body to activate second-messenger systems. They are all peptides (or peptides with some carbohydrate molecules) and function as blood-borne neurotransmitters. On the other hand the steroid hormones released by the gonads and adrenal gland have a quite different mode of action on target cells (Figure 6-9). They are transported intact across the cell membrane and attach to intracellular receptors that act directly on the DNA.

Another very important fact about the hypothalamic hormones only recently appreciated is the pattern of release: it is pulsatile. The hormones are released in pulses, little bursts of release, rather than continuously. This pulsatile release is necessary to trigger the appropriate secretions of the target hormones in the anterior pituitary. The necessity of pulsatile release confounded earlier studies on effects of hypothalamic hormones infused in the blood. Such hormones injected in the same concentration as the natural hormone had little effect because they were injected continuously or in one pulse. But when they are injected in the pulsatile pattern, they produce exactly the same effect as the natural hormones.

It is worth emphasizing again that hormone actions can be very specific. Oxytocin is released by the posterior pituitary (hypothalamic nerve terminals)

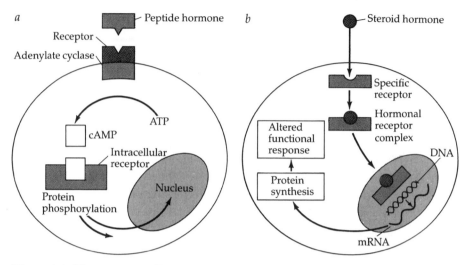

Figure 6-9 The two types of hormone actions on target cells. (*a*) Peptide hormones attach to receptors on the cell membrane and activate second-messenger systems. (*b*) Steroid hormones are instead transported intact across the cell membrane (translocated), attach to receptors inside the cell, and exert actions directly on the DNA-RNA in the nucleus, thus influencing the synthesis of proteins.

into the bloodstream and carried to all the tissues and cells in the body. Yet it acts on only two tissues, the breasts and the uterus in the female, and it acts only under certain conditions. Its action on breast tissue causes the ejection of milk, but only if the female has adequate milk production, that is, has recently given birth and is nursing. Oxytocin also causes uterine contractions at the end of pregnancy. The high degree of specificity is due to the presence of receptors on breast and uterus cells that are active only at the end of pregnancy and during nursing. The specific cells that are acted on by a hormone are called target cells.

For many neurotransmitter systems, the result of the second message is changes in the ion channels in the neuron membrane that cause increased or decreased activity, that is, action potentials. For most hormones, the second-messenger system does not cause changed ion permeability (except in muscle cells, as in the uterus) but does cause a number of other changes in the activity of the target cell. The hormone-receptor complex can act on the DNA, the genetic material in the nucleus, and the RNA (ribonucleic acid), which is involved in protein synthesis, in such a way that the cell manufactures new substances and otherwise alters its activities (Figure 6-9).

Colocalization of Peptides and Transmitters

When I was a student, Dale's law was absolute. It stated that a neuron uses one and the same chemical transmitter at all its synaptic terminals on other neurons or target cells. The transmitter or its precursor is made in the nucleus and transported to the terminals where it is readied for release. How could the axon branches send one transmitter down one branch and another transmitter down another branch? Posed in this way the answer is no way. It is perhaps possible that a common precursor of several transmitters could be sent down all branches and that different terminals could make it into different transmitters. As of this writing no instances of this occurrence have been observed. But the same neuron transmitter can of course have different action on different target neurons, depending on the postsynaptic receptors. Thus, a neuron releasing ACh could exert a fast excitatory action on one neuron (nicotinic receptor) and a slower inhibitory action on another (muscarinic receptor). And this does not violate Dale's law.

A very recent set of discoveries adds complications to Dale's law. Many neuron terminals contain more than just a neurotransmitter; they also contain peptides that could serve as transmitters. This colocalization of transmitters and peptides is widespread in the brain, as indicated in Table 6-3. Not a great deal is yet known about the functions of these colocalized peptides. A case in point is substance P in the C fiber terminals (Figure 6-5). These fibers also contain the fast excitatory transmitter glutamate. Both substance P and glutamate exert excitatory actions. Substance P may act to enhance and prolong the excitatory actions of glutamate at the C fiber terminal target neurons in the substantia gelatinesa. Indeed, current evidence favors glutamate as the actual neurotransmitter and AMPA receptors as mediating the fast excitatory transmission, as we noted earlier.

HORMONES AND SEX

Sexual behavior is extraordinary. It is of no importance for the survival of the individual yet the sex drive is extremely powerful. A mature male rat will freely cross an electrified grid that delivers an almost unbearable shock to reach a female rat in heat. The human literature is unfortunately replete with similar examples; witness the recent emergence of date rape as a serious problem on American campuses. Sexual behavior, as well as physical sexual characteristics, is under the control of the endocrine system. Neurons in certain regions of the brain have high concentrations of hormone receptors that are

TABLE 6-3　**Some examples of coexistence of classical neurotransmitters and peptide transmitters (after Hokfelt et al. 1986)**

Classical transmitter	Peptide	Brain region
Dopamine	CCK	Ventral mesencephalon
	Neurotensin	Ventral mesencephalon
		Hypothalamic arcuate nucleus
Norepinephrine	Enkephalin	Locus coeruleus
	NPY	Medulla oblongata
	Vasopressin	Locus coeruleus
Epinephrine	Neurotensin	Medulla oblongata
	NPY	Medulla oblongata
	Substance P	Medulla oblongata
	Neurotensin	Solitary tract nucleus
	CCK	Solitary tract nucleus
5-HT	Substance P	Medulla oblongata
	TRH	Medulla oblongata
	Substance P+TRH	Medulla oblongata
	CCK	Medulla oblongata
	Enkephalin	Medulla oblongata, pons
		Area postrema
Ach	Enkephalin	Superior olive
		Spinal cord
	Substance P	Pons
	VIP	Cortex
	Galanin	Basal forebrain
	CGRP	Medullary motor nuclei
GABA	Motilin(?)	Cerebellum
	Somatostatin	Thalamus
		Cortex, hippocampus
	CCK	Cortex
	NPY	Cortex
	Galanin	Hypothalamus
	Enkephalin	Retina
		Ventral pallidum
	Opioid peptide	Basal ganglia
Glycine	Neurotensin	Retina

From: Black, I. B. 1991. *Information in the brain: A molecular perspective.* Cambridge, MA: MIT Press. See Source and Cooper, Bloom and Roth, 1991, for more details.

specific for the products of the endocrine system. Moreover, sex hormones are now believed to exert direct control over the growth and development of one region of the brain itself. We examine this system as an example of how the brain and hormones interact.

Hormonal control of sexual development, of maintenance of physical sexual characteristics, and of sexual behavior is pervasive. Before we treat the development of male and female sexual characteristics it is necessary to know a little more about the sex hormones and the control systems that underlie them. The master control system is the hypothalamus and pituitary. It is currently thought that the hypothalamus releases one and only one hormone to activate the anterior pituitary gland to release sex hormones. This hypothalamic hormone is *gonadotropin-releasing hormone* (GnRH), which is secreted by neurons in the preoptic area of the hypothalamus. GnRH is transported directly to the anterior pituitary gland in the portal blood vessels and causes the release of two hormones from the anterior pituitary: *follicle-stimulating hormone* (FSH) and *luteinizing hormone* (LH). The names refer to the actions of the hormones on the female reproductive system. The *follicle* is the developing ovum (egg) cell and its surrounding tissues in the ovary. The *corpus luteum* is a structure in the ovary formed from the follicle. When FSH and LH were named it was believed that different pituitary hormones were involved in the male; subsequently it was shown they are identical in both sexes. In both males and females, the gonads are the only target organs for these anterior pituitary sex hormones. In the male, FSH and LH act only on the testes and in the female they act only on the ovaries (see Figure 6-10).

From this point on, the hormone story diverges sharply for the two sexes. In the mature male, LH causes cells in the testes to make and release *testosterone*, the male hormone, and FSH causes the development and growth of *sperm cells*. Testosterone in turn acts on many tissues to maintain the typical male sexual characteristics. It also decreases release of GnRH and pituitary FSH and LH, an example of a negative feedback system (Figure 6-10). In the mature female, at the beginning of a reproductive cycle FSH stimulates the maturation of the follicle in the ovary. FSH in combination with LH promotes rapid growth of the follicle and increased secretion of *estrogen* (estradiol) by the ovary. When blood estrogen levels approach a critical level, the pituitary reduces the output of FSH and GnRH, another example of a negative feedback system. A separate gonadal product, inhibin, feeds back to selectively inhibit FSH release (Figure 6-10). The high level of blood estrogen also causes an increase in pituitary LH secretion, which in turn produces *ovulation*. At this time the output of another pituitary hormone, *prolactin*, increases and facilitates corpus luteum formation.

The corpus luteum is a "temporary endocrine gland," formed in the ovary, and it secretes estrogen and progesterone. *Progesterone* acts on the reproductive system to prepare it for the implantation of a fertilized egg and to maintain gestation and lactation. In the absence of a fertilized ovum the corpus luteum degenerates, along with the hormones it produces, and the cycle repeats, with another corpus luteum forming. The recycling occurs because the

Figure 6-10 Regulation of LH and FSH secretion. The gonadal steroids estradiol in women and testosterone in men exert negative feedback (1) at the pituitary level by blocking GnRH stimulation of LH and FSH secretion and (2) at the hypothalamus level by inhibiting GnRH release. A separate gonadal product, in-hibin, feeds back to selectively suppress FSH release. Negative modulation by endorphins and dopamine and positive modula-tion by norepinephrine are also important in regulating LH and FSH secretion.

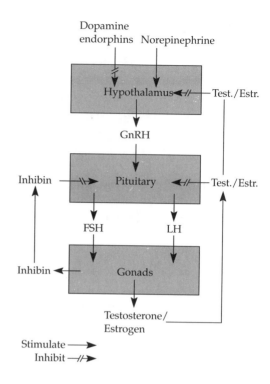

level of circulating estrogen inhibiting pituitary FSH production decreases with the demise of the corpus luteum.

The mechanism by which the corpus luteum is preserved after conception is not fully understood. Estrogen and progesterone are maintained by the corpus luteum at levels that prevent normal cyclic estrous activity. (Some birth control pills contain estrogen and progesterone.) During pregnancy several changes occur to ensure the maintenance of the fetus and adaptive responses on the part of the mother to the presence of this growing "foreign body." Another factor is the steady increase in prolactin secretion from cells in the anterior pituitary over the course of pregnancy, causing increased growth of breast tissues and, at the time of birth, synthesis of milk protein (casein). It also, blocks the synthesis of GnRH, which prevents the normal release of LH and thus prevents ovulation.

In our discussion to this point we have stressed the predominant sex hormone actions. But some cells in the ovaries release testosterone and some cells in the testes release estradiol, and these cells are thought to play roles in feedback regulation of the secretion of the brain sex hormones. Neurotransmitters also play key roles in the regulation of brain sex hormones (Figure 6-10). Note in Table 6-2 that dopamine is released as a hypothalamic hormone (PIH). Dopamine also markedly inhibits the release of prolactin from the anterior pituitary, and chemical analogues of dopamine successfully treat disorders resulting from too much prolactin release.

Sex hormones are also secreted by the adrenal gland. A part of the adrenal gland, the *adrenal cortex*, secretes hormones that have actions similar to testosterone (androgens) and hormones concerned with responses to stress and other functions. *Androgens* are secreted by the adrenal glands of both men and women. In women, the adrenal androgens are thought to play some role in sex drive. In males, testosterone appears to play a more critical role in sex drive. In both sexes the adrenal androgens play an important role in growth and development.

All of the hormones secreted by the adrenal cortex have very similar chemical structures, which are closely related to the structures of the sex hormones. They are all steroid compounds. A *steroid* is a type of lipid (fat) molecule having a characteristic arrangement of four carbon rings. Steroid compounds consist of the same steroid structure and differ only in a side chain.

All of the steroid hormones are derived from cholesterol. Cholesterol may not be good for you in excessive amounts, but clearly it is essential for a normal sex life. Not all of the chemical pathways involved in the manufacture of the various steroid hormones operate in any given target cell. Testosterone is predominantly made in the testes, estrogen and progesterone in the ovaries, and androgens and *cortisol* (the stress hormone) are made in the adrenal cortex. The reason is that only the specific enzymes necessary to make the compounds appropriate to a given target cell are present in the greatest amounts in the cell. Thus, the enzymes necessary to make cortisol are present only in the cells of the adrenal cortex.

Sex Hormone Receptors in the Brain

Receptors for estrogen and testosterone have been identified in the brain, using radiolabeled hormones. They are proteins, as are other neurochemical receptor molecules, but their exact structures are not known. The estrogen receptor is highly specific for estrogen and had previously been found only in tissues such as the uterus, on which estrogen acts. The brain estrogen receptors are primarily in the pituitary gland and hypothalamus but are also present in certain regions of the midbrain and in a structure of the limbic system, the amygdala.

The distribution of estrogen and testosterone receptors in the brain seems to agree well with the effective sites of action of these hormones. The sites are concentrated within certain nuclear regions of the hypothalamus, in agreement with the primary distribution of receptors noted earlier. The existence of sex hormone receptors in a limbic brain structure such as the amygdala implies that it must also play a role in sexual behavior, but what it does is not yet known.

Overwhelming evidence links the sex hormones to sexual behavior. Experiments have been done in which the gonads of an animal were removed and the effects on its sexual responsiveness studied. Removal of the ovaries (ovariectomy) in many mammalian species abolishes the estrous cycle and sexual receptivity in females. Removal of the testes in many lower mammals either abolishes sexual behavior immediately or produces a gradual decline in sexual activity. Studies in which sex hormones were injected into or implanted in the brains of animals not yet mature or into mature animals from which the gonads had been removed once again show the indispensability of these hormones for normal sexual behavior.

Given the powerful effects of the sex hormones on the behavior of adult animals, it seems reasonable to assume that these hormones are involved in the differentiation of sexual structures during development, and so they are (Figure 6-11). Thus genetically male rats, if castrated within ten days of birth, display as adults the female behavior of squatting in the presence of a normal male. Administration of testosterone (male hormone) to five-day-old genetically female rats permanently impairs the regulation of the periodic sexual cycle of the adults and makes them sexually unresponsive to males. In one experiment, testosterone was injected into the mother of a genetically female monkey fetus for some period prior to birth. The result was a genetically female animal with a prominent and well-formed phallus, although no testes. On behavioral measures of dominance and aggression that clearly separate normal male and female monkeys, this animal rated as a male.

Rats castrated during development do not as adults respond to hormone injections with the sexual behaviors appropriate to their genetic sex. Moreover, the injection of an androgen, if it takes place during a critical development period, can impair the normal development of the hypothalamic–pituitary mechanisms responsible for the cyclicity of reproductive function in the female. These two facts imply that hormonal processes not only affect the differentiation of the internal and external reproductive structures but also are involved in the development and differentiation of the brain mechanisms that control reproductive cycles in females and sexual behavior in both males and females.

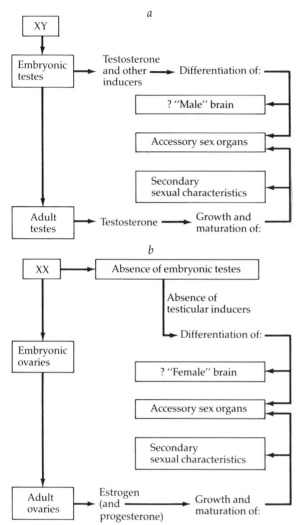

Figure 6-11 Summary of sex organ differentiation in development of (*a*) the male and (*b*) the female.

One additional implication of these studies is that the process of sexual differentiation involves both the suppression of the development of the female's neurobehavioral system and the enhancement of the male's. That is, in the absence of the male gonadal hormones, sexual differentiation proceeds according to a female ground plan. It seems that in the mammal the basic, genotypically determined sexual disposition (phenotype) is female. For differentiation to proceed according to the male pattern, the presence of male gonads and hormones is essential.

Sex Differences in the Brain

It has recently been discovered that there are in fact clear anatomical differen-ces between the brains of adult male and female rats. The brain follows the same rules as do the genital systems: the basic plan is inherently female. Male hormones cause the development of the male brain. In their absence, the genetic male will develop a female brain. Although these findings come from work done in the rat, it seems likely that similar sex differences exist in the brains of all mammals. There is one great advantage in using rats for studies of sex differences in the brain: although the reproductive systems in the rat develop before birth, the sexual brain changes develop after birth. In many species, including humans, it appears that both these processes of differentia-tion occur before birth.

The critical brain region is the *medial preoptic nucleus* of the hypothala-mus. This region controls the release of gonadotropin-releasing hormone, which, as we have seen, is the hypothalamic hormone that acts on the pitui-tary to cause the release of LH and FSH, the pituitary sex hormones. In adult rats, the structural difference between males and females in this region of the hypothalamus is so great that it can be seen in sections of the brain even without a microscope (Figure 6-12). The medial preoptic nucleus is four times larger in male brains than in female ones. The number of neurons per unit volume, however, is greater in the female, and so although the male nucleus is bigger, the female nucleus has more neural synaptic connections per unit size.

In the rat, at least, this difference in brain structure begins to develop shortly after birth. It is under the control of testosterone. This was shown in a series of experiments in which testosterone levels were altered in newborn animals. When an experimental drug is given, a substance called a *vehicle* is used to dissolve and so facilitate administration of the drug. In those experi-ments, the drug *testosterone propionate* (TP)—synthetic testosterone—was dis-solved in oil. Control females were given oil without TP for four days after birth. The vehicle is always given to the control animals to be sure that it does not have effects of its own. After the animals had reached maturity, the size of the medial preoptic nucleus was measured. Females given a small dose of TP on day 4 developed a larger brain nucleus than normal, and those given a larger dose developed a correspondingly larger nucleus. Females that are given TP in this way and develop a larger "sex" nucleus in the brain also develop more malelike sexual behavior patterns as adults. Males castrated at birth, thus losing their natural source of testosterone, developed a much smaller, more femalelike preoptic nucleus than did males castrated on day 21. It ap-pears that there is a critical period between birth and three weeks after birth

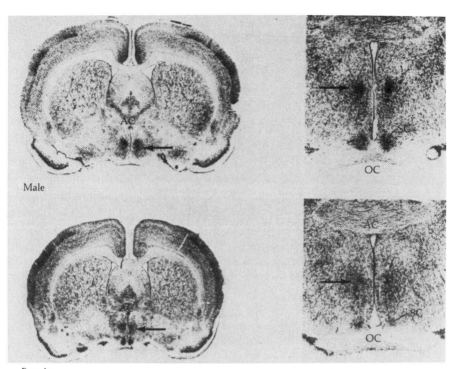

Male

Female

Figure 6-12 A clear structural difference can be seen in the sexually dimorphic nucleus (medial preoptic nucleus of the hypothalamus) between normal adult male and female rat brains (arrows). Left, low power; right, high power (AC, arcuate nucleus; SC, suprachiasmatic nucleus; OC, optic chiasm).

in the rat in which the male preoptic nucleus grows and develops to the normal male size.

The development of this permanent structural difference in the brain between males and females, brought about by early hormonal action, is of considerable importance. Behavior is controlled directly by the brain, and hormones must exert their influences on behavior by acting on the brain. This is a case where early hormonal action produces a permanent structural difference in the brain between the sexes. Such a difference can result in differential sexual behavior in the adult even in the absence of immediate hormonal actions.

The cover of a recent issue of *Time* magazine asked a particularly fatuous question: "Why are men and women different?" Men and women have suspected the answer to this question for several hundred thousand years.

Time referred to recent studies suggesting sex differences in the human brain but completely omitted reference to the classic work by Roger Gorski at UCLA, done some years ago, demonstrating the sexually dimorphic nucleus in the hypothalamus of the rat (Figure 6-12). This work is a completely noncontroversial demonstration of a sex difference in brain structure in mammals.

There is some evidence that certain regions of the adult human brain may be sexually dimorphic. A region of the corpus callosum, the massive band of fibers that connects the two hemispheres of the brain (Figure 1-7), seems to have more fibers in females than in males. The size of at least one region of cells in the hypothalamus appears to be larger in men. However, this finding is somewhat controversial. But the major and very controversial finding that led to *Time* magazine's question was a recent report by a scientist at the Salk Institute in San Diego that in adult homosexual males, this region of the hypothalamus, was smaller than in heterosexual males. This naturally leads to the conclusion that homosexuals are born, not made: developmental factors before birth, most likely hormone actions, result in a female rather than a male hypothalamus, which ultimately would determine behavioral patterns and sexual preferences.

This "homosexual brain" hypothesis has problems: (1) it is not clearly established that this hypothalamic region is truly sexually dimorphic in men and women; (2) this region of the human hypothalamus is not the same nucleus that is sexually dimorphic in rats; (3) nothing is known about the possible functions of this region of the hypothalamus. Clearly, much more work must be done before the hypothesis is established.

SUMMARY

The existence of receptors in neurons in the brain that are acted on by opium and its derivatives—morphine and heroin—is an intriguing recent discovery. Following this work, brain opioids were discovered—substances made by neurons and by the pituitary gland that act on the same receptors and produce effects very much like morphine: they alleviate pain and produce pleasurable sensations. These brain opioids are all peptides—chains of amino acids—and are derived from three superfamilies of peptides expressed by genes in the appropriate cells. These three very large peptides are cleaved to yield the much smaller opioid peptides: beta endorphin, met- and leu-enkephalin, and the dynorphins. The enkephalins are in neurons associated with the slow pain pathway; beta-endorphin is released by the pituitary gland.

There are three aspects to drug addiction: addiction, in which the drug is used with increasing frequency; tolerance, where increasingly large doses are needed to produce the sensations (usually pleasurable) that led to the drug use initially; and withdrawal, the unpleasant symptoms and feelings that develop when use stops. The severity of withdrawal symptoms is a major reason why addiction develops. The super-sensitivity theory, that repeated use of a drug causes marked changes in the receptors for the drug in the brain, accounts well for the phenomena of withdrawal.

The brain opioids are chemically parts of much larger molecules from which some hormones are made in the hypothalamus–pituitary gland. This endocrine system is the second major communication system in the brain and body (the first being nerve fibers). Many groups of neurons in the hypothalamus release peptide hormones that directly control hormone secretions from the pituitary gland. Actually, the posterior pituitary gland is simply a holding area for nerve fiber terminals from the hypothalamus; the hormones are released from these terminals directly into the bloodstream. The anterior pituitary is a true gland but is tightly controlled by hormones released from the hypothalamus into a local blood circulation system that carries them to the anterior pituitary to trigger release of its hormones. All the hypothalamic and pituitary hormones are peptides. Relatively new findings indicate that many peptide hormones and other substances are present in neurons together with the classical neurotransmitter chemicals we discussed in earlier chapters. They are colocalized. An example is substance P, contained in slow pain fibers along with the fast excitatory transmitter glutamate.

Hormones released from the pituitary into the general circulation act on target organs in the body (gonads, adrenal gland, stomach, and so on) to cause various reactions. Many of these target organs then also release hormones (some are peptides, others are steroid hormones derived from cholesterol) that cause many other effects, including important feedback control of hormone release in the hypothalamus and pituitary.

We used sexual development and behavior as the example of hormone actions. The hypothalamic hormone GnRH is secreted by neurons in the preoptic area of the hypothalamus and is transported via blood vessels to the anterior pituitary, where it triggers release of FSH and LH. In the adult female, they act on the developing egg cell and its surrounding tissues in the ovaries and cause release of estrogen from the ovary. In the adult male they act on the testes; LH causes testicular cells to release testosterone and FSH causes the development and growth of sperm cells.

Neurons in several regions of the brain—hypothalamus, amygdala, and midbrain—have specific receptors for estrogen and testosterone so these hormones can exert direct actions on brain systems and ultimately on behavior. In the development of sexual characteristics and behavior, the basic genetic plan is female. In the absence of testosterone in early development (prenatal in humans, postnatal in rats), a genetic male will develop as a female in terms of both bodily structure and hormone systems. Recent work in rats shows that in addition to producing males, testosterone causes a major increase in size of the so-called sexually dimorphic nucleus (medial preoptic nucleus in the hypothalamus) in males relative to females. Although the evidence is less clear, there also appear to be structural differences in human male and female brains. A very controversial recent report suggests that male homosexuals have the "female" rather than the "male" brain structures.

SUGGESTED READINGS AND REFERENCES

Books

Becker, J. B., Breedlove, S. M., and Crews, D. (1992). *Behavioral endocrinology.* Cambridge, MA: MIT Press.

Black, I. B. (1991). *Information in the brain: A molecular perspective.* Cambridge, MA: MIT Press.

Carlson, N. R. (1991). *Physiology of behavior* (4th ed.). Boston: Allyn and Bacon.

Cooper, J. R., Bloom, F. E., and Roth, R. H. (1991). *The biochemical basis of neuropharmacology* (6th ed.). New York: Oxford University Press.

Crews, D. (1987). *Psychobiology of reproductive behavior: An evolutionary perspective.* Englewood Cliffs, NJ: Prentice-Hall.

Harris, L. S. (1985). *Problems of drug dependence.* Washington, D.C.: U. S. Government Printing Office.

Julien, R. M. (1992). *A primer of drug action: A concise, nontechnical guide to the actions, uses, and side effects of psychoactive drugs* (6th ed.). New York: W. H. Freeman.

Knobil, E., and Neill, J. (1988). *The physiology of reproduction.* New York: Raven Press.

Martini, L., and Ganong, W. F. (1988). *Frontiers in neuroendocrinology.* New York: Raven Press.

Spitz, H. I., and Rosecan, J. S. (1987). *Cocaine abuse: New directions in treatment and research.* New York: Brunner/Mazel.

Vander, A. J., Sherman, J. H., and Luciano, D. S. (1990). *Human physiology: The mechanisms of body functions* (5th ed.). New York: McGraw-Hill.

Articles

Basbaum, A. I., and Field, H. L. (1984). Endogenous pain control systems: Brainstem spinal pathways and endorphin circuitry. *Annual Review of Neuroscience, 7,* 309–338.

Dougherty, P. M., Plaecek, J., Paleckova, V., Sorkin, L. S., and Willis, W. D. (1992). The role of NMDA and non-NMDA excitatory amino acid receptors in the excitation of primate spinothalamic tract neurons by mechanical, chemical, thermal, and electrical stimuli. *Journal of Neuroscience, 12,* 3025–3041.

Kelley, D. B. (1988). Sexually dimorphic behaviors. *Annual Review of Neuroscience, 11*, 225–252.

Marlatt, G. A., Baer, J. S., Donovan, D. M., and Kivlahan, D. R. (1988). Addictive behaviors: Etiology and treatment. *Annual Review of Psychology, 39*, 223–252.

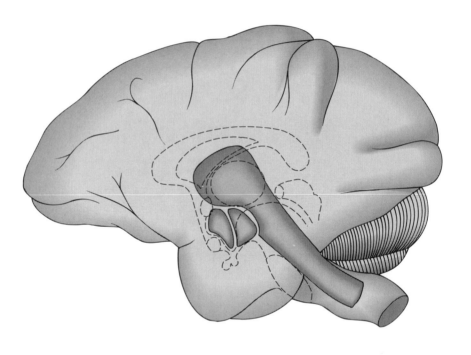

7

Biological Imperatives—The Hypothalamic Connection

Sex is a very basic and powerful drive. Yet as important as it is for the perpetuation of the species, it is irrelevant for the survival of the individual. Other basic drives—stress, sleep, temperature regulation, thirst, and hunger —are essential for the survival of the individual. Another way of looking at these basic drives, or motives, is that they seek to maintain the individual organism in an optimal condition. They arise as a result of internal conditions that are less than optimal, for example, lack of metabolic energy, and result in driving or forcing the organism back toward the optimal state, for example, by consuming food. This is the basic notion of *homeostasis*. Sexual behavior seems an exception: there is no "optimal condition," and the absence of sexual behavior in a sexually mature individual seems to have no relation to homeostasis. However, as we will see in comparing Chapters 6 and 7, the biological

Figure 7-1 Schematic of monkey's brain showing the general location of the hypothalamus in relation to the reticular formation. Both lie in the depths of the brain. The anterior and posterior portions of the hypothalamus are shown as two separate pie-shaped wedges lying just below the rostral portion of the tube-shaped reticular formation.

machinery driving sexual behavior is basically the same as the machinery that drives organisms to seek food, water, and other biological needs.

We used the term *drive* without really defining it. Everyone knows what it means to be hungry; the "hunger drive" hardly needs definition. There is something equally compelling about all the basic biological drives, including sex. This has led some scientists to use the term *motivation* to refer to generalized drive. It is certainly the case that when any of these drives is operative, the animal, including the human animal, becomes extremely active rather than sitting and doing nothing. We are driven to behave. When applied to humans, "motivation" of course has many meanings, from basic motives like hunger to complex psychological motives like avarice and idealism. Here we limit discussion to basic drives. The particular neural circuits that subserve different basic drives are different. But recent study of the biology of motivation suggests that a common brain system may operate for all drives. Pleasure, or reward, occurs when biological drives are satisfied. There appears to be a common pleasure system in the mammalian brain that functions for all basic drives and even for the "abnormal" drives that result from addiction. We consider the brain pleasure system at the end of the chapter.

Alan Epstein, a leading authority in the study of the biological substrates of basic motives, stressed that the basic reason large-brained, long-lived animals—mammals—engage in motivated behaviors is subjective feelings of needs. When you feel thirsty, you drink fluids; when you are hungry, you seek out and eat food; when you feel tired, you sleep. We do not yet know much about the brain mechanisms that produce these feelings, but we know a great deal about the neural machinery that controls these basic homeostatic motives.

THE HYPOTHALAMUS

The basic motives have in common the overridingly important actions of the hypothalamus. It is astonishing that this small amount of brain tissue, a few cubic millimeters containing a number of small collections of neurons (nuclei), can exert such profound effects on behavior and experience. The general location and relative size of the hypothalamus in the primate brain is indicated in Figure 7-1. There are about 15 nuclei in the hypothalamus. Functionally, they can be classed in three groups, the most important being the group lying close to the third ventricle—the *periventricular zone*. In this group are the "endocrine" neurons that control the pituitary gland (Chapter 6); the nuclei that control biological rhythms are also in this group. A second group of nuclei, the *medial zone*, receives input from the forebrain, particularly the limbic system (hippocampus and amygdala), and projects to the "endocrine" group of nuclei. The third group, the *lateral zone*, receives input largely from the major ascending dopamine pathway in the brain, the medial forebrain bundle, and appears to form a part of it, contributing both ascending and descending pathways. The medial zone nuclei also project to the lateral zone, conveying information to it from the forebrain limbic system.

A cross section through the brain shows the locations of some of the key hypothalamus nuclei and their relation to adjacent brain structures (Figure 7-2). Here I emphasize only the nuclei to be discussed later in the chapter. The organization of these nuclei into the three longitudinal zones is illustrated in Figure 7-3. In the periventricular zone, endocrine neurons at the anterior (front) end, the *preoptic nuclei*, contain gonadotropin-releasing hormone (GnRH) critical for sexual function (Chapter 6). In the middle of the zone are neurons in the *periventricular nucleus* (PVH) containing corticotropin-releas-

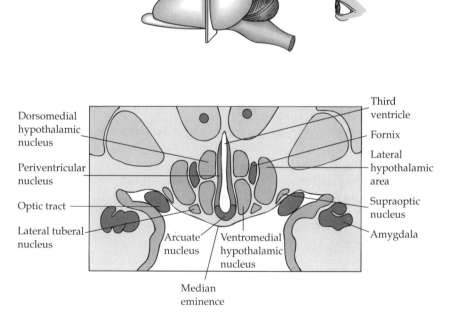

Figure 7-2 Cross section of the brain showing some of the hypothalamic nuclei. (The schematic showing the plane of section is a rat brain; the actual section is of a human brain.) The nuclei discussed in the text include the lateral area and the supraoptic, ventromedial, dorsomedial, and paraventricular nuclei. The fornix is a fiber bundle connecting the hippocampal system (limbic forebrain) to the hypothalamus and the amygdala is another major structure of the limbic forebrain with strong connections to the hypothalamus.

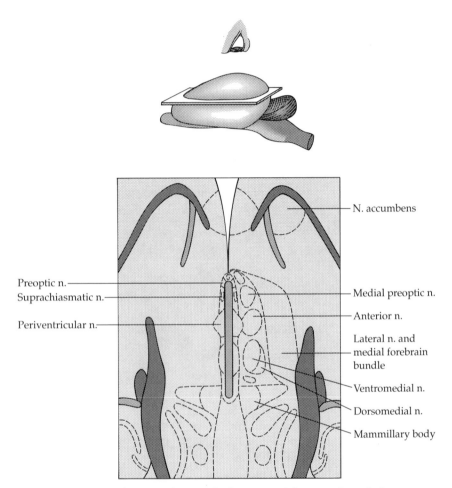

Figure 7-3 Horizontal section showing the locations of the major hypothalamic nuclei from the front (top) to the back of the brain. Only the periventricular nuclei are drawn at the left; the medial and lateral nuclei are shown at the right. Only the nuclei discussed in the text are labeled. Not shown is the supraoptic nucleus, which lies well below the periventricular nucleus and just above the optic nerves. The accumbens nucleus is not a part of the hypothalamus.

ing hormone (CRH), critical for coping with stress, thyrotropin-releasing hormone (TRH), critical for metabolism, as well as neurons containing oxytosin and vasopressin. Finally, at the back end, *dopamine-containing neurons* are found, together with *growth hormone-releasing neurons* (GRH) and two nuclei critical for biological rhythms.

The medial zone contains several very well-defined nuclei: *medial preoptic, anterior, dorsomedial,* and *ventromedial nuclei* and the *mammillary bodies.* Note that the names of these nuclei for the most part simply refer to their positions in the hypothalamus and are not at all helpful in terms of functions. This is unfortunately true for most brain structures. The early anatomists could see and name brain structures, including hypothalamic nuclei, long before any understanding of their possible functions developed.

The lateral zone of hypothalamic nuclei is very poorly defined anatomically—in the lateral zone it is hard to see individual nuclei—and many anatomists view it as the anterior continuation of the brain stem reticular formation. As we noted in Chapter 1, the lateral zone includes the medial forebrain bundle, the major ascending dopamine pathway in the brain. If any one function can be identified with the lateral zone of hypothalamic nuclei, it is general modulation of behavioral state—attention and arousal.

Finally, Figure 7-3 show a large and somewhat mysterious nucleus that lies anterior to the hypothalamus: the *nucleus accumbens*. The term accumbens, incidentally, means "lying next to," yet another position name. We will hear more about this nucleus later.

The nuclei in the periventricular zone are the major efferent, or output, neurons of the hypothalamus. In the discussion of stress we will focus on just one nucleus in this region to illustrate the basic principles of organization of the hypothalamus. The key point to note here is that these output nuclei of the hypothalamus have two quite distinct projection systems. One, of course, is to the pituitary gland. Hypothalamic endocrine neurons release hormones, either directly from the posterior pituitary gland or via the portal circulation, to trigger release of pituitary hormones from the anterior pituitary (Figure 6-7). The second system consists of descending axons from the hypothalamic neurons that act on the motor nuclei of the autonomic nervous system in the spinal cord and on brain stem nuclei. This system is not a hormonal system but a conventional neural pathway exerting synaptic actions on target neurons. These two hypothalamic output systems arise from different groups of neurons in the nuclei of the periventricular zone. The key point is that the hypothalamus exerts direct control over both the hormonal (pituitary) and neuronal (autonomic nervous system) substrates of the motivational and emotional aspects of behavior and experience.

STRESS

Most of us don't need to be told when stress is. We know it when we feel it, and we feel it a lot. Stress is the common coin of the human condition in this "age of anxiety."

Modern understanding of stress stems from classic work in the 1930s by Hans Selye, who developed the notion of the *general adaptation syndrome*. The basic point he made is that the body shows a common, integrated set of responses in an attempt to adapt to many different kinds of stress. Until his work, many scientists viewed different kinds of stress as having quite different effects on the body; for example, the effect of exposure to severe cold was thought to be very different from the effect of blood loss. Selye showed that different severe stressors all produce the same three stages. First is the *shock phase*, involving decreased blood pressure, body temperature, and muscle tone (the reader has no doubt experienced at least some degree of shock following a minor or not so minor injury, particularly if blood loss occurred). Selye termed the second phase of the adaptation response the *stage of resistance*, when the body fights back. But if the stress is severe and continues for a long period, the body defenses break down and the third stage, *exhaustion*, ensues. Among other things this stage includes a marked impairment of the immune system.

Selye focussed on physical stressors. We take blood loss as a simple and common example—even donating blood at the Red Cross can activate the general adaptation syndrome. Extensive blood loss causes an immediate drop in blood pressure and body temperature and the feeling of being faint—the shock stage. Shock triggers in the hypothalamus the release of corticotropin-releasing factor (CRH), which causes the pituitary to release adrenocortico-trophic hormone (ACTH), which acts on the cortex of the adrenal gland to release glucocorticoids (cortisol), which exerts a wide range of actions on body tissues, preparing the body to deal with stress. This is the stage of resistance, and all of these effects may occur the first time you donate blood. But they probably won't occur the second time you give blood.

But wait a minute! This simple and well-documented observation tells us that there is much more to stress than physical trauma. Blood loss is a clear physical stress—you donate the same amount of blood each time. Psychological factors are also critically important in causing stress, as we all know, and this is true in all mammals, not just humans. The humble rat can exhibit psychological stress as severe as that experienced by the complex *Homo sapiens*. In recent years the focus on stress has shifted from physical trauma, per se, to psychological, or more accurately, psychobiological factors— psychology and biology can never really be separated. Many types of stress, particularly chronic stress, do not produce the initial shock phase but to varying degrees they do cause the resistance phase and even, in the extreme, the exhaustion phase.

The Adrenal Gland

The adrenal gland is the major gland for coping with stress in humans. It actually consists of two almost completely independent glands, a central part called the *adrenal medulla* and an outer covering called the *adrenal cortex* (Figure 7-4). The adrenal medulla functions in the same way as sympathetic

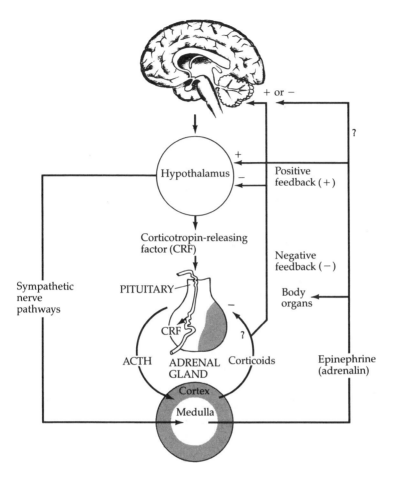

Figure 7-4 Schematic representation of interrelations of the pituitary gland and the adrenal gland, the pituitary–adrenal "axis" or system. The adrenal medulla releases epinephrine (adrenalin), which acts on body organs and back on the hypothalamus (and perhaps other brain regions) to facilitate the activity of the autonomic nervous system. The adrenal cortex releases corticoids, which act on body organs and act back on the pituitary gland, the hypothalamus, and other brain regions. The highest density of corticoid receptors in the brain is actually in the hippocampus.

ganglia. It is controlled by the axons of autonomic motor neurons from the spinal cord. However, there are no postganglionic neurons in the adrenal medulla. Instead, the motor axon terminals synapse with gland cells in the medulla called *chromaffin cells*. When chromaffin cells are activated by the motor neurons (release of ACh), they release norepinephrine (NE) and epinephrine (E) directly into the bloodstream. In humans, mostly E is released, but a small amount of NE is released as well.

Almost any type of sudden stress, either physical or psychological, will cause the sympathetic part of the autonomic nervous system, the *emergency system*, to increase its activity. This in turn causes the adrenal medulla to increase its secretion of E and NE into the blood. This is felt very rapidly: the heart immediately begins to pound. Other actions of E and NE include elevation of blood pressure, dry mouth, sweating from the palms of the hands and under the arms, and several metabolic changes that ensure an immediate supply of energy. Most of these effects are also produced by direct actions of the sympathetic nervous system on target organs. Release of E and NE by the adrenal medulla reinforces these effects.

The adrenal medulla is really a part of the sympathetic division of the autonomic nervous system, although it behaves in some ways as an endocrine gland. The adrenal cortex, on the other hand, is a typical endocrine gland. We shall look briefly at the autonomic nervous system before investigating the adrenal cortex.

The Autonomic Nervous System

The autonomic nervous system is primarily responsible for the maintenance of an optimal internal environment for the body. The system is generally involuntary and acts on the smooth muscle of the gastrointestinal tract, on cardiac muscle, and on the exocrine glands. The autonomic nervous system consists of two divisions, the sympathetic and the parasympathetic (see Figure 7-5). The *sympathetic division* of the autonomic nervous system acts as an arousal mechanism for the entire body and prepares it for vigorous action. It can act rapidly to prepare the animal to "fight or flee" in the face of perceived danger.

Activation of the *parasympathetic division* tends to produce effects opposite to those of the sympathetic division. Most of the visceral (body) organs have *dual antagonistic innervation*, which means that they are supplied with both sympathetic and parasympathetic nerves (see Figure 7-5). For the heart, increased sympathetic activity results in a faster than normal heart rate, whereas increased parasympathetic activity (transmitted by the vagus nerve) lowers the heart rate (Figure 5-8). The autonomic nervous system typically maintains a tonic level of output over both divisions, termed *tone*. Because of tone, the heart rate can be increased either by an increase in sympathetic input or by a decrease in parasympathetic input, since it is the algebraic sum of the inputs that determines the organ response.

The chemical neurotransmitters of the autonomic nervous system (ANS) are well understood. Indeed, both acetylcholine (ACh) and NE were first isolated and shown to be neurotransmitters in this system (Chapters 5 and 6: Figure 5-8). The motor neuron axons from both divisions, sympathetic and

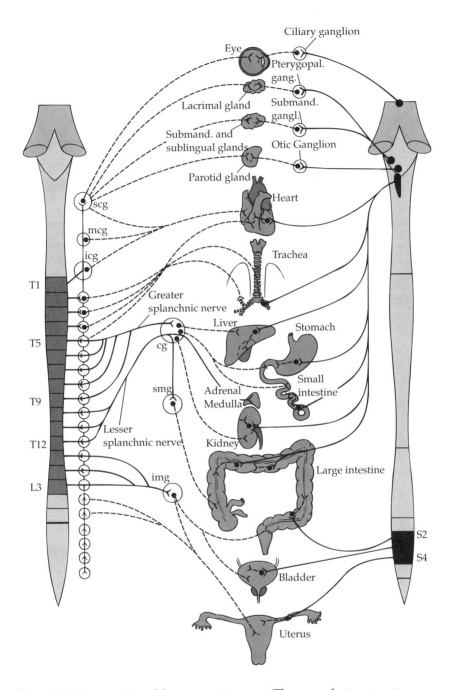

Figure 7-5 Organization of the autonomic system. The sympathetic system is shown at the left, the parasympathetic system at the right. Abbreviations for the names of sympathetic ganglia are as follows (from top to bottom): scg, superior cervical ganglion; mcg, middle cervical ganglion; icg, inferior cervical ganglion; cg, celiac ganglion; smg, superior mesenteric ganglion; img, inferior mesenteric ganglion. T1–T12, segments of thoracic spinal cord; L3, third lumbar spinal segments; S2, S4, sacral spinal cord segments. III–X, cranial nerves. The diagram represents the human but applies generally to vertebrate species.

parasympathetic, pass out from the brain and spinal cord and synapse in peripheral ganglia. Like all other motor neurons in vertebrates, they use ACh as their neurotransmitter. In the sympathetic portion of the ANS, the motor neurons synapse on a series of ganglia that lie next to the spinal cord, the *sympathetic ganglia*. The postsynaptic neurons in the sympathetic ganglia send their axons to all the various target organs, such as the heart, and form synapses: these are *neuromuscular junctions*. The muscle fibers of the viscera are not striated, skeletal muscle but rather smooth muscle (or cardiac muscle) fibers. The neurotransmitter is NE at the neuromuscular junctions between the postganglionic sympathetic neurons and smooth or cardiac muscle fibers.

In marked contrast, the parasympathetic motor axons, which come from the lower brain stem and from the bottom, or sacral, end of the spinal cord, travel to the vicinity of their target organs and synapse in ganglia close to the target organs. Their neurotransmitter, as we have said, is acetylcholine (ACh). The postganglionic neurons of the parasympathetic system in turn synapse on the target organ muscle fibers, either smooth or cardiac muscle. The neurotransmitter of the postganglionic neurons is also ACh.

The autonomic nervous system is under the direct control of various nuclei in the brain stem. These in turn are influenced by the hypothalamus and certain of the limbic forebrain structures. The autonomic nervous system is thus the peripheral motor system that mediates the actions of the brain structures most directly involved in the emotional and motivational aspects of behavior. The adrenal medulla is a part of the sympathetic nervous system, as we saw. The adrenal medulla and the sympathetic ganglia work together and reinforce each other to prepare the organism for action.

The Adrenal Cortex

The adrenal cortex is made up of glandular tissue and surrounds the adrenal medulla (Figure 7-4). It is the part of the adrenal gland that is a typical endocrine gland. Under certain conditions, neurons in a region of the hypothalamus (periventricular nucleus) release *corticotrophin-releasing hormone* (CRH) into the portal circulation. It is carried by the local blood supply directly to the anterior pituitary gland, where it causes the release of *adrenocorticotrophic hormone* (ACTH). ACTH is released into the general circulation. When it reaches the adrenal cortex, it causes endocrine gland cells there to release cortisol (corticosterone), a stress hormone, and a small amount of aldosterone. (ACTH does not stimulate the release of androgen, the third type of hormone of the adrenal cortex.)

Aldosterone regulates the body content of the basic ions sodium, potassium, and chloride. It does this by controlling the extent to which they are reabsorbed by the kidneys. The release of aldosterone by the adrenal cortex is primarily under the control of the blood concentration of potassium and the extracellular fluid volume. Consequently it plays an important role in causing thirst and drinking. If you are dehydrated, or low on water, the kidneys release angiotensin II, which stimulates the adrenal cortex to release aldosterone. ACTH has only a slight influence on the release of aldosterone.

The major action of ACTH is to cause the adrenal cortex to release *cortisol.* This is the only way cortisol can be released. Cortisol exerts powerful effects on all body tissues. It increases the level of glucose in the blood and also stimulates the breakdown of proteins into amino acids, inhibits the uptake of glucose by the body tissues but not by the brain, and regulates the response of the cardiovascular system to persisting high blood pressure (hypertension). All these actions are ideally suited to help an animal deal with stress. An animal faced with a threat usually must forgo eating but needs energy in the form of glucose in the blood. The brain, in particular, needs a good supply of glucose. The increased blood levels of amino acids help repair possible tissue damage. Increased vascular tone is also of great importance. For unknown reasons, an immediate effect of stress is to cause certain arteries to dilate, which reduces the blood pressure. Cortisol counteracts this and maintains the correct blood pressure.

The increased release of cortisol in response to stress is normal and very adaptive. However, as with most things in life, too much cortisol is a bad thing. Abnormally high levels of cortisol for prolonged periods can lead to high blood pressure, or hypertension. A bad life or job situation that gives rise to prolonged or chronic stress can lead to high blood pressure. Prolonged high levels of cortisol also lead to impairment in the immune system, a marked decrease in the ability of the body to resist infection, a fact of key importance in today's AIDS epidemic.

Hypothalamic Control of the Stress Response

The hypothalamic nucleus directly concerned with stress is the *periventricular nucleus* (PVH), illustrated in Figure 7-3. It is only about half a square millimeter of tissue and contains roughly 10,000 neurons. There are two groups of *endocrine neurons* in the PVH, large neurons that convey oxytocin and vasopressin to the posterior pituitary for release (not directly involved in the stress response) and smaller neurons that release CRH (corticotrophin-releasing hormone) into the portal circulation to activate secreting cells in the anterior pituitary to release ACTH into the general blood circulation. As we saw earlier, ACTH triggers release of cortisol from the adrenal cortex (Figure 7-4).

In addition to endocrine neurons, other neurons in PVH make axonal connections with neurons in the reticular formation, brain stem, and spinal cord. Most of these neurons terminate on motor neurons for the autonomic nervous system, one group on sympathetic motor neurons and another on parasympathetic motor neurons (the preganglionic neurons—see Figure 5-8).

Interestingly, in PVH there do not appear to be any interneurons, neurons that interconnect within the nucleus. Hence activity of the nucleus is under rather direct control by the input projections to the nucleus. Unfortunately, the inputs to PVH are complex; dozens have been described. We note here the four input systems that seem most important. First is an *"autonomic" input,* primarily from the vagus nerve (it contains sensory as well as motor fibers) that projects to PVH via autonomic nuclei in the brain stem. This system presumably conveys information about the state of the internal organs. The second input system comes from the *subfornical organ,* a little structure on the outside of the blood–brain barrier that has no such barrier itself—as we will see later this structure and its projection to PVH play a key role in thirst. The third class of inputs is relayed from the *forebrain limbic system,* particularly the hippocampus, amygdala, and prefrontal cerebral cortex. Finally, there are many projections to PVH from *other hypothalamic nuclei.*

Although our certain knowledge ends here, it is clear that "stress" neurons in PVH, those containing CRH, can be activated by alterations in the state of the body, as in blood loss—decreased blood pressure activates sensory fibers in the vagus nerve—and by perceived threat or danger, via forebrain structures. These CRH neurons also have receptors for cortisol, so they can continually monitor the activity of the adrenal cortex. As noted, cortisol decreases the secretion of CRH from these neurons (Figure 7-4). Interestingly, the other brain structures with high levels of cortisol receptors are the hippocampus and amygdala, the very regions that project to PVH.

The Biochemical Switching Hypothesis

We discovered in Chapter 6 that many neurons in the brain have more than one neuropeptide that might function as a neurotransmitter or modulator substance. This principle seems to be carried to the extreme in the hypothalamus. The CRH-containing neurons in PVH may contain as many as eight different neuroactive substances! Some of these are CRH, dynorphin, dopamine, and angiotensin. Larry Swanson, now at the University of Southern California, and his colleagues have developed clear evidence that a given neuron will express more or less of several of these neuroactive substances, depending on the kind of stress involved. Remember that these substances are expressed from the DNA in the cell nucleus, manufactured via the RNA, and conveyed to the terminals of the secreting PVH neurons. As an example, increased blood level of cortisol causes an increase in CRH but no change in vasopressin in one type of PVH neuron but a decrease in both types of peptides in another type of neuron. Other aspects of stress can produce quite different changes in the peptides expressed in PVH neurons.

Swanson suggests that different kinds of stress could produce differential production of different peptide hormones and neurotransmitters in the neurons, which could result in fine tuning of the most adaptive type of response to the particular stress involved. The biochemical switching hypothesis is illustrated in Figure 7-6. The key point about this hypothesis is that an anatomically fixed circuit can change its functions by altering the expressions of peptides in the neurons. This provides an intriguing example of biochemical plasticity without anatomical plasticity.

The Psychobiological Nature of Stress

Stress is in the eye of the beholder. The rate of cortisol secretion is astonishingly sensitive to psychological factors. Such a seemingly mild experience for a rat as being placed in a new environment can cause a massive increase in corticosterone release (corticosterone is the rat analogue of human cortisol). When a person boards an airplane there is often a massive increase in cortisol release. Cortisol release also means that CRH has been released from the hypothalamus and ACTH from the pituitary. As cortisol is released it acts back on the hypothalamus–pituitary to inhibit the release of CRH and ACTH. As ACTH release decreases, release of cortisol by the adrenal cortex

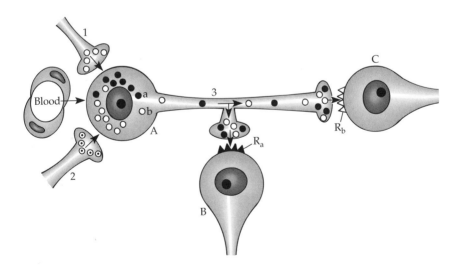

Figure 7-6 Biochemical switching in a neuroanatomically fixed circuit may be implemented by changes in the ratio of neuropeptides a and b within a particular neuron (A) if the neuron innervates two different cell types (B, C), each of which expresses receptors (Ra, Rb) for one neuropeptide or the other. The a/b ratio may be altered by substances released from neural inputs 1 and 2 or by steroid hormones entering from nearby capillaries.

decreases. The release of these substances appears to be much more finely tuned and sensitive to environmental and psychological factors than the increased activity of the sympathetic nervous system in response to a sudden stress or an emergency.

It has been known for many years that performance on various learning and skill tasks has an inverted U relation to degree of arousal in both humans and other mammals (Figure 7-7). At the extreme low end of arousal, for example, sleep, there is no performance. If you are exhausted and very sleepy, your performance will be poor. If you are alert, full of energy, and aroused, your performance will be optimal. However, if you are extremely aroused and under a great deal of stress, your performance will deteriorate. In general, stress impairs performance in proportion to the severity of stress—the right side of the inverted U.

It is now clear that stress cannot be identified simply with physical trauma. Recall the example of donating blood. The extent to which situations are stressful is determined by how the individual understands, interprets, sees, and feels about a situation. It is fundamentally a "cognitive" phenomenon depending more on how the individual construes the situation than on the nature of the situation itself. The key aspects are uncertainty and control—the less knowledge the individual has about a potentially harmful situation, the less control he or she feels can be exerted, the more stressful the situation is. Conversely, the more understanding and certainty the individual has about a situation, the more he or she feels in control and the less stressful it is. We and other mammals appear to be driven by nature toward certainty. This may in fact be the basis for the existence of various belief systems. A person firmly committed to a belief system does in fact "understand" the world and the nature of the controls that operate, even though this understanding may be quite wrong.

There are many examples of the cognitive nature of stess from both the human and the animal literatures. In an early study of a Harvard boat race, a decline in eosinophil count (a blood measure of stress) was marked in the crew

Figure 7-7 The inverted U function relating degree of stress and arousal to performance. Performance on a number of tasks, including learning, is optimal at some intermediate level of stress.

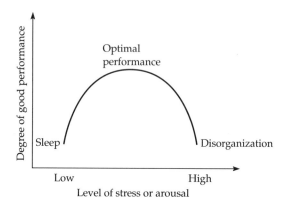

four hours after the race. This decline could have been due entirely to the physical stress of the race, but the coxswains and coaches had similar eosinophil drops, even though their stress was purely psychological.

A classic study was conducted on human beings in parachute training by Seymour Levine of Stanford University and Holger Ursin of the University of Olso, Norway. The hormonal and behavioral responses of a group of Norwegian paratroop trainees were examined after repeated jumps off a ten-meter tower on a guide wire. After the first jump there was a dramatic elevation of cortisol in the blood, but as early as the second jump cortisol dropped to basal levels, and basal levels persisted on subsequent jumps. It is also important to note that the fear ratings changed dramatically following the first and second jumps: the trainees expressed very little fear after the second jump, even though fear had had a very high rating prior to the first jump.

To take an example from the animal literature, dogs were subjected to a series of electric shocks that were either unpredictable or predictable. The predictable condition involved presenting the animal with a tone prior to the onset of shock. In the unpredictable condition, no such tone was presented. The adrenocortical response observed on subsequent testing of the animals clearly indicated the importance of reducing uncertainty by predictability. Animals that did not receive the signal preceding the shock showed an adrenocortical response that was two to three times that observed in animals with previous predictable shock experience.

It should be noted that the procedures used in this experiment are typical of those used in experiments examining learned helplessness. *Learned helplessness* refers to the protracted effects of prolonged exposure to unpredictable and uncontrollable stimuli of an aversive nature. It has been observed that organisms exposed to this type of experimental regimen show long-term deficits in their ability to perform appropriately under subsequent testing conditions. Furthermore, the experimental animals show a much greater increase in adrenocortical activity when exposed to novel stimuli than do control animals. Thus, an organism exposed to an uncontrollable and unpredictable set of aversive stimuli shows not only a dramatic increase in adrenocortical activity while exposed to these conditions but also long-term deficits in other, unrelated test conditions.

In a study done by Jay Weiss at Rockefeller University, rats were exposed to a strongly aversive shock. One group of the rats could terminate or postpone the shock by turning a wheel. The second group had no control over the shocks. They were wired up in series with the first group, so that they got a shock whenever the animals in the first group did, but there was nothing the second group could do to prevent it. Rats in the group that had no control over the shocks developed stomach ulcers at a much greater rate than the animals who could control the shocks.

In recent work in my laboratory, Seymour Levine, Michael Foy, and I found that sufficient stress in rats prevented the subsequent induction of hippocampal LTP, a possible mechanism of memory storage (see Chapter 4). In a further study, Tracey Shors found that LTP was impaired much less in rats that could control the shock stress than in rats that could not exert control, even though both groups of rats received identical physical stress.

The key is that the uncertainty exists in the organism. Situations are stressful if the organism views them as being unpredictable and uncontrollable. Studies of troops in Vietnam seem consistent with this view. Members of an experienced combat unit of Special Forces enlisted personnel, upon being informed of an impending attack, enthusiastically spent much time in task-oriented activities such as fortifying defenses. The concentration of a cortisol metabolite in their urine did not rise on the day of the expected attack. Although they could not directly control the behavior of the enemy, they felt in control of the situation. Their young captain, by contrast, was in a state of uncertainty about whether the orders he would receive would be considered inappropriate by his experienced soldiers. Concentrations of the cortisol metabolite in his urine were markedly higher on the day of the expected attack.

This research on stress implies that successful strategies for coping involve predictability, understanding, knowledge, and a sense of control. It may be helpful sometimes to simply be able to do something, even if that something does not really control the situation. In work done by Seymour Levine, rats allowed to fight after receiving strong, unpredictable shocks showed far less elevation of serum corticosterone than rats given the same shocks but not allowed to fight.

BIOLOGICAL REGULATION

Biological Rhythms: Sleep and Waking

There is no obvious reason why humans should have to sleep. Sleep certainly does not provide the body with rest; as far as metabolism goes, sleep is little better than quietly reading a book. Nor does the brain rest during sleep. In one phase of sleep it is more active than when a person is awake and sitting quietly. Yet all animals from the blue-green algae to humans function with a circadian rhythm, the 24-hour cycle.

For a long time it was thought that the circadian rhythm was determined simply by day and night. Rats, for example, are nocturnal, becoming active at night and sleeping during the day. The circadian rhythm of activity in rats is quite regular. Typically mammals and birds are on precise circadian schedules. Humans, most other primates, and some birds of prey all rely heavily on vision and are active by day. The prey of birds (such as mice) sensibly remain inactive by day. A number of human circadian rhythms are shown in Figure 7-8.

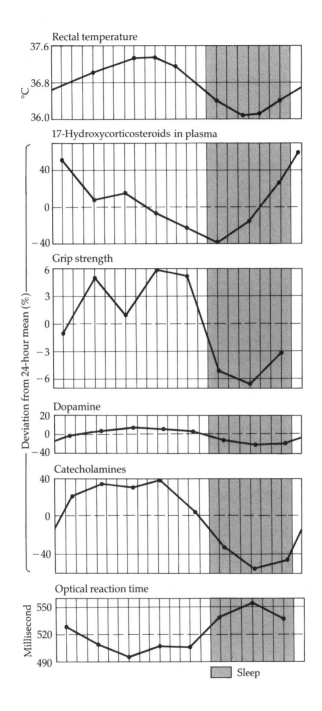

Figure 7-8 Many aspects of human physiology and behavior show circadian rhythms; a few examples are shown here.

The circadian rhythm of activity is not directly controlled by light or dark. If rats are kept in constant light or constant dark, they continue to show a normal circadian activity cycle for their entire lives. The cycle will drift in relation to actual day or night, since the animals have no way of knowing whether it is light or dark out. In some studies people have lived in caves with a constant moderate level of illumination for months. They show a normal circadian rhythm of sleep and waking, although it drifts relative to day and night outside the cave. Humans actually settle down to a circadian rhythm that is closer to 25 hours than 24, another mystery. Curiously enough, the cycle of the moon around the earth is also approximately 25 hours.

Some kind of internal clock must regulate the 24-hour cycle of an organism. Under the normal circumstances of life, the occurrence of day and night synchronizes the internal clock. If the light–dark cycle is reversed, rats gradually shift their cycle so that after a week or so they are again active in the dark and quiet in the light. When a person flies halfway around the world, it may take a week for his or her sleep–wake cycle to reverse completely. This forced shifting of the sleep–wake cycle undergone routinely by many people in the jet age is seen by a number of scientists as a serious biological stress.

The exact identification of the master clock in the brain was only recently accomplished. It is a structure in the hypothalamus called the *suprachiasmatic nucleus* (SCN). The SCN lies just above the *optic chiasm* (the crossing of the two optic nerves), as its name indicates. The relative size and structure of this small hypothalamic nucleus seems essentially identical in creatures as different as the mouse and the human; it apparently does its job in the same way in all mammals. Destruction of the SCN completely abolishes the circadian activity cycle in mammals (Figure 7-9).

Some of the optic nerve fibers projecting from the eye peel out of the optic nerve at the chiasm well before the thalamus is reached and innervate the neurons of the SCN (Figure 7-10). Light activates the optic nerve fibers and the neurons of the SCN; they are less active in the dark. However, this influence from the optic nerve serves to *entrain*, or modify, the activity of the SCN neurons, not simply to control them. If the optic nerves of an animal are severed, neurons in the SCN continue to show a circadian rhythm of activity, just as the animal does, although it will drift relative to outside light or dark.

It appears, therefore, that the SCN neurons have an inherent 24-hour cycle of increased and decreased activity. Although the inherent rhythm of the SCN neurons can be entrained by activity in the optic nerve, apparently it can exist in the absence of any neuronal input. Even if the SCN is surgically isolated from the rest of the brain, its neurons continue to show a circadian rhythm of activity. Thus it seems that the circadian rhythm is somehow coded in the genes of the SCN neurons (and perhaps in all other cells as well).

The SCN is the master clock controlling the 24-hour activity cycle. For a time it was thought that the SCN was the only such clock in the brain. Recent

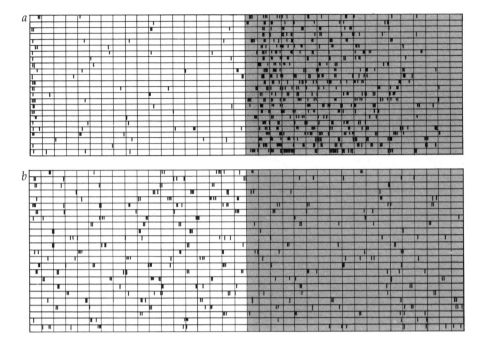

Figure 7-9 The normal activity cycle (water-drinking) of a hamster is shown in (a) The black marks are drinking bouts. Hamsters are nocturnal animals, or active at night—the drinking activity occurs almost entirely in the dark half of the 24 hour light–dark cycle. Effects of destroying the suprachiasmatic nuclei are shown in (b)—drinking now occurs entirely at random in light and dark periods, even though the animal can still see.

work, however, suggests that the 24-hour temperature cycle may have a clock that is at least partially separate. Normally, the temperature cycle is closely synchronized with the sleep–wake cycle: body temperature is lower during sleep. However, lesions of the SCN that completely abolish the circadian activity cycle in rats and monkeys do not abolish the circadian temperature cycle.

A number of bodily processes show circadian rhythms, for example, the secretion of many hormones (Figure 7-7). The extent to which these rhythms are under the direct control of the SCN remains to be determined. There are of course rhythms other than the 24-hour circadian rhythm. The estrous cycle, for example, has a much longer time constant, 4 days in female rats and 28 days in female humans. A separate nucleus in the hypothalamus, the *anteroventral periventricular nucleus*, lying just anterior to the SCN, appears critical for generating the estrous cycle (Figure 7-3). Humans also seem to have a much shorter rhythm, a cycle of about two hours. Attention and performance on tasks seems to wax and wane every two hours or so during our waking hours. The brain substrates of this attention cycle are not known.

Figure 7-10 (*a*) Location of the suprachiasmatic nuclei (SCN), lying just above the optic chiasm. Each nucleus receives visual input from both optic nerves. (*b*) Microscopic appearance of the SCN just above the optic chiasm (OC). The marker bar is 100 micrometers (100 millionths of a meter) long.

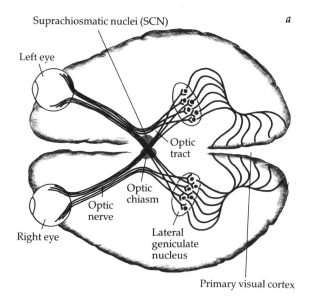

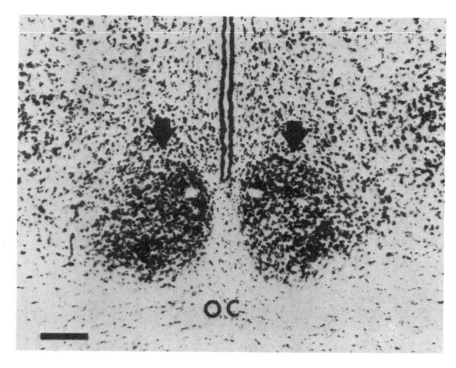

Sleep

In the 1950s the rather surprising fact emerged that there are two kinds of sleep. The two kinds of sleep have quite different properties and are easy to distinguish. One is called *rapid eye movement* (REM) sleep because it is characterized by continuous rapid movement of the eyes. In addition, an electroencephalogram (EEG), which measures electrical activity taken from the cortex during REM sleep shows a pattern of activity characteristic of the alert, awake brain. Another distinctive sign is a much lower degree of tension in the neck muscles (the head of a person who is sitting and dozing may suddenly drop). Penile erection also occurs in males during REM sleep but is due to reflexive changes in muscle tone and blood supply rather than to sexy dreams, or so we think.

The other kind of sleep is simply called *non rapid eye movement* (NREM) sleep. The cortical EEG shows the slow waves traditionally associated with sleep, and neck muscle tension is higher than in REM sleep. A normal night's sleep consists of regular cycling between periods of NREM and REM sleep. As the night wears on, the periods of REM sleep become more intense (Figure 7-11).

Another difference between REM and NREM sleep is the depth of sleep. A person can be more easily awakened from NREM sleep by external stimuli such as noises than from REM sleep, even though the cortical EEG of REM sleep is like that of an awake state.

The most intriguing difference between REM and NREM sleep concerns dreaming. Shortly after REM sleep was discovered, experimenters reported that if people were awakened from REM sleep, they almost always said they had been dreaming, whereas reports of dreams were much less common when people were awakened from NREM sleep. Subsequent work raised some question about this finding, but it is really a matter of degree. People do report dreams when awakened from either sleep state. However, dream reports are more frequent after REM than NREM awakenings. Perhaps more significant is that dreams reported by a person awakened from the REM state are much more vivid and fantastic, what we think of as typical dreams, than dreams during the NREM state. The dreams reported in awakenings from the NREM state are pale and have more the quality of thought, like daydreams.

The discovery of REM sleep and of its association with dreaming raised the exciting possibility of a new biological window on the mind. Previously, the only way dreaming could be studied was by asking people about their dreams, either on awakening or later. Memories of dreams are notoriously fleeting. Both REM and NREM sleep occur in all the mammals in which sleep has been studied and even in birds. It seems a reasonable supposition that dogs, for example, also dream. Owners of a dog have probably seen it twitch its paws in a regular rhythm during REM sleep, as though the dog is running in its dream.

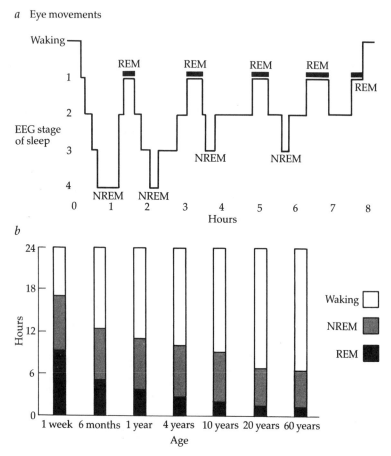

Figure 7-11 (*a*) Typical phases of REM and NREM in a night's sleep. The EEG and eye movement signs of the two states of sleep correspond closely. (EEG stages of sleep are determined from the pattern of brain waves recorded from the scalp.) Stage 1 is "awake" and REM sleep, and stage 4 is NREM sleep. Eye movements are indicated by *x*′ s. (*b*) Relative amounts of time spent in awake, NREM, and REM sleep at different ages.

In any event, REM sleep occurs in all mammals, whether or not they experience dreams. Researchers were initially hopeful that the problem of working out the brain systems and mechanisms that underlie REM sleep would be tractable, but it has proved much more difficult than anticipated.

A number of theories about brain mechanisms of sleep have come and gone, but only a few facts have been established. The reticular formation of the brain stem exerts a generally arousing or activating influence on the forebrain and seems to be involved in the general regulation of alerting or arousal. For a time it was thought that the major serotonin system of the brain, the many projections of the serotonin-containing neurons of the raphe nuclei in the brain stem, regulated REM sleep (see Chapter 5).

Destruction of these neurons with toxic drugs that act selectively on serotonin-containing neurons yielded animals that did not sleep much and showed no REM sleep at first. With sufficient recovery time, however, relatively normal sleep periods and REM sleep returned in the animals, even though the serotonin system in the brain was destroyed. A group of large neurons in the reticular formation shows characteristic increased patterns of discharge during REM sleep and appears to receive input from the serotonin neurons. The serotonin system has something to do with sleep, particularly REM sleep, but exactly what continues to elude researchers.

The greatest mystery about sleep is why it is necessary. Animals die if they are prevented from sleeping and normal humans go mad and, according to some reports, eventually die without sleep. The desire for sleep can become overwhelmingly powerful if a person has not slept for a long time. Yet sleep does not seem to serve any necessary physiological function in terms of rest, metabolism, or brain activity. Perhaps the simplest explanation is that there is a sleep substance that produces the sleeping states of the brain and that "substance S" increases in concentration as long as a person is awake. Although several candidates have been proposed for "substance S," none as yet has won the contest.

Temperature Regulation

The warm-blooded animals, the birds and mammals, have two quite different ways of regulating body temperature. One way is simply behavioral: the animal finds a warmer or a cooler place. The other involves a set of reflexes initiated by the hypothalamus and mediated mostly by the autonomic nervous systems: altered metabolism; sweating, panting, and dilation of blood vessels in the skin to cool the body; and shivering and contraction of blood vessels in the skin for warmth.

Behavioral temperature regulation has a much more ancient history. It is the only mechanism available to cold-blooded animals. Lizards, for example, prefer a sunny rock on a cool morning.

At present, evidence suggests that neurons in the hypothalamus in the preoptic region (Figure 7-3) act like thermometers. Their rate of activity is very sensitive to the temperature of the local blood supply. In mammals, local heating or cooling of this region produces both behavioral and reflex temperature-control activities. If the hypothalamic region is cooled, test animals will press a lever to increase the temperature of their test box and will shiver. These hypothalamic neurons have a very narrow range of preferred temperature, called the *set point*. When the temperature of the blood deviates from the set point, the neurons initiate the appropriate behavioral and reflex activities (Figure 7-12).

Sensory information from temperature receptors in the skin also influences the hypothalamic temperature-control system. Elegant studies by Eleanor Adair at the Pierce Institute in New Haven, Connecticut, have shown a very precise relationship between the controls exerted by temperature-sensitive neurons in the hypothalamus and skin temperature on both reflex and behavioral mechanisms of temperature regulation in monkeys (and by inference humans). She implanted a thermistor probe in the temperature-sensitive region of the hypothalamus in monkeys so that she could both record hypothalamic temperature (determined normally by blood temperature) and also change hypothalamic termperature slightly away from the normal 37° C. The monkeys could also precisely control the temperature of the air in the testing room by pressing a lever. If hypothalamic termperature was increased slightly, the monkeys lowered air temperature to just the level that would decrease the hypothalamus temperature to normal (by slight cooling of the blood) and vice versa. The relation between hypothalamus and skin temperature control of body temperature is amazingly precise.

Fever resulting from an infection is due to a change in the hypothalamic set point. Pyrogens, substances produced by infectious bacteria and other fever-causing agents, act to increase the set point. Normal body temperature is detected by the hypothalamic neurons in the feverish person as too low: a person feels cold, shivers, and the body temperature increases until it reaches the new and abnormally high set point. Aspirin is believed to act directly on the set point neurons to "reset" them to normal; hence it breaks a fever.

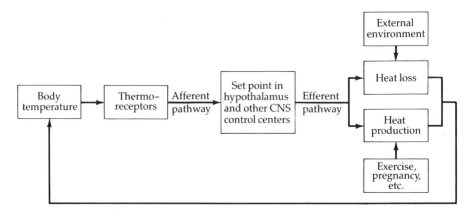

Figure 7-12 Schematic of temperature regulation. It is thought that there is a set point in the hypothalamus influenced directly by blood temperature and indirectly by sensory information from the skin and body that controls heating and cooling mechanisms (for example, shivering and sweating) to maintain a constant body temperature.

Interestingly, if pyrogens are administered to lizards they will seek out a warmer environment, as though they were trying to cause a fever. Work by Evelyn Satinoff at the University of Illinois suggests that in mammals the hypothalamic region controlling the more ancient behavioral form of temperature regulation, change of place, may differ in part from the region involved in reflex regulation, such as shivering and sweating.

Thirst and Drinking

Animals do an excellent job of regulating tissue fluid levels. In higher animals the primary mechanism seems to be the feeling of thirst, which serves as a strong motive for them to seek out and drink water.

The initial signal for thirst comes from the *supraoptic nucleus*, a group of neurons in the hypothalamus that detect a shrinkage in their size (volume). This occurs when water moves from inside the cells to the extracellular fluid outside. This, in turn, occurs when the osmolarity (salt content) of the extracellular fluid increases. This, yet in turn, occurs when you do not drink enough water to compensate for water loss or if you eat salt. The shrinkage-detecting neurons, when activated, activate endocrine neurons in the supraoptic nucleus to release vasopressin via the posterior pituitary. The thirst-detecting neurons also result in feelings of thirst (how, we do not yet know). Interestingly, the threshold for release of vasopressin is substantially lower than that for thirst. As the salt content of the extracellular fluid increases, vasopressin is released first, and only later do you feel thirst.

The organ in the body that directly regulates the amount of fluid in the blood is the *kidney* (see Figure 6-8). If the water content of the body drops, little urine is formed. If too much fluid is consumed, much more urine is formed. Vasopressin acts directly on structures in the kidney resulting in retention of water in the body. However, when the water level of the blood drops too low, more water must be drunk. In addition to exerting control over the amount of urine formed, the kidney signals the hypothalamus to initiate thirst and drinking when the fluid level drops and when it is activated by vasopressin. It does this by releasing into the blood a substance called *renin*, which is converted into the thirst hormone, *angiotensin II*. The kidney thus functions as an endocrine gland.

When angiotensin II was first discovered, it was assumed that it acted directly on the appropriate neurons in the hypothalamus. However, it was soon found that it does not cross the blood–brain barrier (see Chapter 2). Angiotensin II undergoes an intermediate step on its way to the hypothalamus involving a small structure in a ventricle of the brain called the *subfornical organ*. The brain ventricles contain cerebrospinal fluid, which exchanges freely with the blood. However, the cerebrospinal fluid in the ventricles is outside the blood–brain barrier. Glial-type cells line the ventricles and form the barrier, just as blood vessels in the brain are surrounded by the glial barrier cells. The subfornical organ lies on the lining of the ventricle and extends into it. Neurons from the subfornical organ project into the brain to act on the hypothalamus and have specific receptors for angiotensin II on their cell bodies in the ventricle (Figure 7-13).

The subfornical organ is one of the several such organs that lie outside the blood–brain barrier, collectively called *circumventricular organs* (they line the

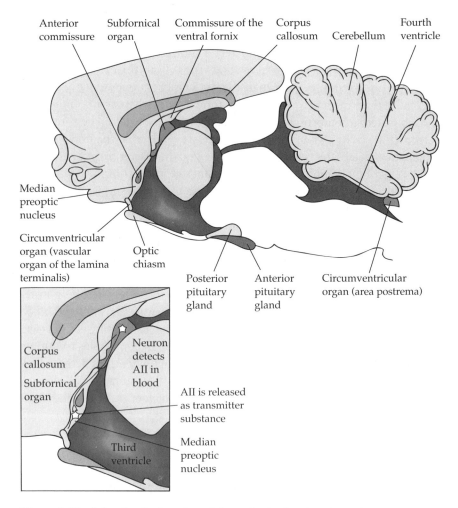

Figure 7-13 A longitudinal section of the rat brain showing the major components of the circumventricular (around the ventricles) organs. The insert shows the subfornical organ and its possible role in thirst (AII, angiotension II).

ventricles). They can all be activated directly by substances in the blood–cerebrospinal fluid and then exert neuronal actions on the brain. Another of these organs, in the area postrema, plays a key role in taste aversion learning. If an animal or human is made sick following the drinking or eating of a distinctive-tasting substance, they will avoid that taste in the future. This intriguing phenomenon was first demonstrated by John Garcia, then at UCLA. He injected poisons like lithium chloride to induce sickness after the animals (rats) had tasted saccharin, a taste they normally like. After this experience, the animals avoided saccharin as though it were poison. It appears that the actual poison, lithium chloride, may have exerted its actions on the brain by way of the circumventricular organ in the area postrema; destruction of this organ prevents the development of taste aversion.

In sum, angiotensin II is released via the kidneys into the blood when the blood fluid level is low. It passes into the cerebrospinal fluid and activates the subfornical organ neurons, which activate the hypothalamic thirst system.

There is another extracellular thirst-regulation system, which is triggered into action by a sudden drop in blood pressure, as with excessive bleeding. Pressure receptors in the heart decrease their activity, which influences the supraoptic nucleus in the hypothalamus to cause feelings of thirst and also triggers increased release of vasopressin from the posterior pituitary gland.

Hunger and Feeding

Thirst and hunger have quite different properties. No one ever becomes a water addict but, as we have said, many people suffer from addiction to food. Obesity is a serious medical problem as is its opposite, anorexia nervosa, or self-starvation.

It was established some years ago that lesions made on both sides in one region of the hypothalamus, the lateral hypothalamus (LH), caused animals to stop eating and die of starvation if not force-fed. Lesions made on both sides in another region of the hypothalamus, the ventromedial region (VMH), caused animals to be voraciously hungry, eat more than normal, and become obese. This led quite naturally to the two-centers theory of hunger, involving an LH hunger center and a VMH satiety center (Figure 7-14). It seems now that neither idea is correct.

The effective lesion in the LH in fact appears to destroy the ascending dopamine-containing pathway in the brain, the medial forebrain bundle. The result is a syndrome called sensory neglect, discovered by John Marshall and Phillip Teitelbaum, then at the University of Pennsylvania. If the lesion is made on just one side of the LH, the animal ignores all stimuli presented to it on that side. If the lesion is made on both sides of the LH the defect is massive: the animal ignores virtually all stimuli, including food. Actually, this dopa-

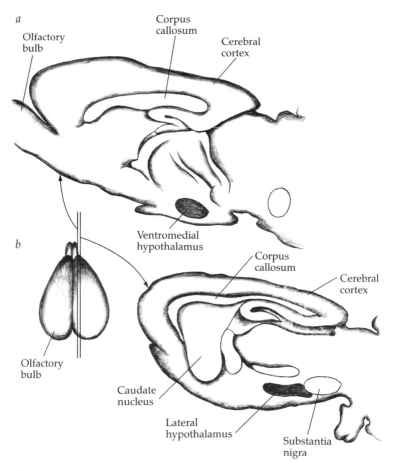

Figure 7-14 Location of (*a*) the ventromedial hypothalamic "satiety center" and (*b*) the lateral hypothalamic "hunger center" in the rat brain. The inset shows a top view looking down on the brain and the two planes of the sections shown in (*a*) and (*b*). Recent evidence casts doubt on this "two-centers" notion of the control of hunger and eating behavior.

mine lesion effect might be characterized as a massive loss of motivation, because the animal is no longer motivated to respond to anything.

Other lines of evidence suggest that neurons in the LH play some role in eating behavior. For one thing there are glucostatic neurons in the LH, neurons whose firing rates change very sensitively with changes in the concentration of glucose in the blood. These neurons could certainly signal hunger (low blood glucose) or satiety (high blood glucose). Furthermore, a long-lasting decrease in food intake is produced by chemical lesions of the LH that destroy neuron cell bodies but not the dopamine-containing axons passing through the VMH (forebrain dopamine is not decreased by this procedure, unlike LH lesions that destroy all the tissue in the region).

The effect of the VMH lesion has also recently been reinterpreted. First, a careful anatomical analysis by Paul Sawchenko and colleagues (at the Salk Institute in San Diego) indicated that the region critical for the lesion effect appeared to be not the VMH but rather a projection pathway from the periventricular nucleus (PVH), the hypothalamic stress nucleus we considered earlier at length. It was also found that if the vagus nerve is cut, lesion of the VMH (or the pathway from PVH) does not cause overeating and obesity. The vagus nerve has both motor-control nerves to and sensory nerves from the stomach and intestinal tract and also the heart and other organs, as we noted earlier. It seems that the VMH–PVH lesion somehow alters sensory–motor actions of the vagus nerves in such a way that more eating occurs. If the stomach feels hungry or experiences hunger contractions, the person or animal will eat more. Section of the vagus nerve might eliminate the feeling of hunger.

Many factors control hunger and eating, including neurons in the hypothalamus that are sensitive to the blood glucose level (blood sugar level), whether the stomach is empty or full, the taste of foods, the time of day (whether it is normal mealtime or not), and so on. However, at the moment it is not entirely clear what brain control systems are involved in controlling hunger and eating. It has recently been found that the intestinal tract also functions as an endocrine gland: it releases several peptide hormones into the blood. One of these, cholecystokinin (CCK), inhibits eating when injected systemically (into the blood stream) in hungry animals. Interestingly, the "satiety" effect of CCK is abolished if the vagus nerve is cut. But CCK might still be able to act indirectly on the hypothalamus by way of a structure like the subfornical organ that bypasses the blood–brain barrier. It seems likely that these "gut hormones" are important in the control of hunger and eating behavior.

Amphetamine also suppresses appetite, apparently through an action quite different from that of its effect as a stimulant. A whole family of similar drugs have been manufactured, some of which are much more effective in suppressing appetite than in acting as stimulants. (The use of amphetamines in appetite control is one of the factors that led to their abuse.) This specific action of amphetamine drugs led to the idea that there are amphetamine receptors on neurons in an "appetite suppression system" in the brain, and in fact such receptors appear to have been identified. As with the brain opioids, it is reasonable to assume that if there are receptors in the brain specific for the appetite-suppressive effects of amphetamine and related drugs, then the brain or body must make some substance or hormone that normally acts on the receptors, in this case to regulate hunger and eating. This substance has not yet been found.

It is interesting to note that the biological controls for sex, stress, and thirst all seem to work in the same basic way. The hypothalamus and pituitary release hormones that act on target organs to cause release of other hormones that in turn act on body tissues and back on the hypothalamus and pituitary to regulate their activities. Target hormones, substances released by body organs, are not yet known for sleep and hunger (CCK is a candidate for hunger), but we suspect that they exist. Evolution is very conservative. If a mechanism works well for the control of certain of the biological imperatives—the drives necessary to insure the survival of the individual and the species—it is likely to be operative for all such needs or drives.

THE BRAIN REWARD SYSTEM

One of the most extraordinary discoveries about the brain basis of behavior was made by James Olds and Peter Milner at McGill University in 1953, electrical self-stimulation of the brain. The discovery was serendipitous; they discovered something they were not looking for, but it proved to be far more important than what they had hoped to find. They were delivering small electric shocks to regions of the brain in freely moving rats in the hope of stimulating a sleep-control system.

> In the test experiment we were using, the animal was placed in a large box with corners labeled A, B, C and D. Whenever the animal went to corner A, its brain was given a mild electric shock by the experimenter. When the test was performed on the animal with the electrode in the rhinencephalic nerve, it kept returning to corner A. After several such returns on the first day, it finally went to a different place and fell asleep. The next day, however, it seemed even more interested in corner A.
>
> At this point we assumed that the stimulus must provoke curiosity; we did not yet think of it as a reward. Further experimentation on the same animal soon indicated, to our surprise, that its response to the stimulus was more than curiosity. On the second day, after the animal had acquired the habit of returning to corner A to be stimulated, we began trying to draw it away to corner B, giving it an electric shock whenever it took a step in that direction. Within a matter of five minutes the animal was in corner B. After this, the animal could be directed to almost any spot in the box at the will of the experimenter. Every step in the right direction was paid with a small shock; on arrival at the appointed place the animal received a longer series of shock.
>
> After confirming this powerful effect of stimulation of brain areas by experiments with a series of animals, we set out to map the places in the brain where such an effect could be obtained. We wanted to measure the strength of the effect in each place. Here Skinner's technique provided the means. By putting the animal in the

"do-it-yourself" situation (i.e. pressing a lever to stimulate its own brain) we could translate the animal's strength of "desire" into response frequency, which can be seen and measured.

The first animal in the Skinner box ended all doubts in our minds that electric stimulation applied to some parts of the brain could indeed provide reward for behavior. The test displayed the phenomenon in bold relief where anyone who wanted to look could see it. Left to itself in the apparatus, the animal (after about two to five minutes of learning) stimulated its own brain regularly about once every five seconds, taking a stimulus of a second or so every time. After 30 minutes the experimenter turned off the current, so that the animal's pressing of the lever no longer stimulated the brain. Under these conditions the animal pressed it about seven times then went to sleep. We found that the test was repeatable as often as we cared to apply it. When the current was turned on and the animal was given one shock as an *hors d'oeuvre* it would begin stimulating its brain again. When the electricity was turned off, it would try a few times and then go to sleep. —(J. Olds, Pleasure centers in the brain, *Scientific American*, 195: 107–108, 1956).

This discovery triggered a massive field of research mapping the brain reward system. There were even some studies of self-stimulation of the brain in human patients. Many regions of the brain are susceptible to rewarding self-stimulation, and some regions are clearly aversive, for example, the slow pain system. The region that yielded the most consistent and positive results appeared to be the *lateral hypothalamus* (LH). This is the region we discussed earlier that contains the medial forebrain bundle, the large ascending dopamine pathway in the mammalian brain. Further work indicated that the critical system was the medial forebrain bundle itself; the dopamine system was the "pleasure center." From this, most workers concluded that it was activation of the dopamine projections to the forebrain that subserved pleasure or reward.

A few words are in order about what animals actually do when self-stimulating their medial forebrain bundle (MFB). They exhibit consummatory behaviors such as eating, drinking, chewing on wooden blocks, copulating, and so on, depending on where the stimulating electrode is in the MFB and what objects are present in the test cage. In other words, the animals are behaving as though they are being rewarded with biologically relevant rewards, food, water, sex, and so on.

Meanwhile, other studies showed that drugs antagonistic to dopamine, for example, the antipsychotic drugs that block dopamine receptors (Chapter 5), block electrical self-stimulation and also appear to block the rewarding effects of food and water. Conversely, agonists of dopamine that activate dopamine receptors seem to enhance electrical self-stimulation and the rewarding effects of natural rewards.

Yet other studies provided much evidence that one particular dopamine pathway was critical for both self-stimulation and the rewarding effects of natural appetitive stimuli like food and water. This pathway arises in the brain stem, in the ventral tegmental area, and projects to the nucleus accumbens, lying anterior to the hypothalamus (Figure 7-3). Local treatment to block or enhance dopamine actions in the nucleus accumbens produces all the effects of both electrical self-stimulation and natural rewards.

All these findings seemed to fit together nicely into a theory that brain reward is due to activation of the dopamine pathway to the nucleus accumbens. At this point several investigators threw a big monkey wrench into the works. They showed that stimulation of the MFB did not in fact activate the dopamine axons projecting from the ventral tegmental area to the nucleus accumbens. These dopamine axons are small and unmyelinated and have high thresholds to electrical stimulation. The phenomena of electrical self-stimulation are elicited by stimulus intensities too low to activate the dopamine axons!

A current working hypothesis in the field is that electrical self-stimulation of the MFB activates larger, lower-threshold myelinated axons from the LH and preoptic areas of the hypothalamus that project down to activate the ascending dopamine axons in the ventral tegmental area, and these in turn project to and activate the nucleus accumbens (Figure 7-15). There is some evidence to support this "indirection" hypothesis. On the other hand, animals will still self-stimulate the LH after the forebrain, including the nucleus accumbens, has been removed.

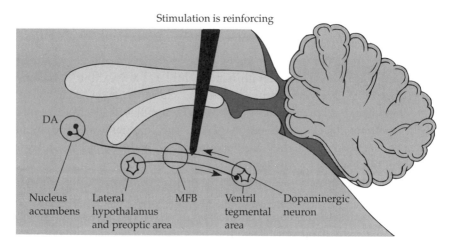

Figure 7-15 The "indirection" hypothesis to account for electrical self-stimulation of the brain: effects of medial forebrain bundle stimulation. When the medial forebrain bundle is electrically stimulated, axons of dopaminergic neurons are indirectly stimulated by way of the ventral tegmental area. MFB, medial forebrain bundle.

Much of course remains to be learned about the brain reward system. Even if the hypothesis of the brain reward system schematized in Figure 7-14 is partly correct, it is only a beginning. The nucleus accumbens is not an island unto itself. In addition to the ascending dopamine projection it receives input from the hippocampus and amygdala, and its outputs go largely to midbrain motor systems. This does not help us much in understanding pleasure and reward. A further question might occur to you—why do drugs that block the nucleus accumbens "pleasure center" treat the positive symptoms of schizophrenia? Recall that dopamine pathways projecting to the forebrain are thought to play a key role in schizophrenia (Chapter 5). Too much dopamine action in this system is hypothesized to cause the positive symptoms of schizophrenia and too little dopamine action the negative symptoms. At least the negative symptoms—lack of affect or feeling—seem to be consistent with the dopamine-to-nucleus accumbens pleasure system hypothesis.

A final note that may remind you of our discussion of drug addiction in Chapter 6. There is at least some evidence that drugs of addiction cause an increase in release of dopamine in the nucleus accumbens! This has been reported for opiates, cocaine, amphetamine, nicotine, caffeine, and alcohol. If the nucleus accumbens system is indeed a key brain substrate for pleasure and reward (very hypothetical), it might account for the rewarding effects of addicting drugs. As we noted in Chapter 6, pleasurable sensation seems a key reason why people begin using the drugs. As addiction develops, the negative feelings of withdrawal come to dominate and the addict is "hooked."

SUMMARY

Organisms are driven to meet basic biological needs: hunger, thirst, sleep, sex. The hypothalamus, a small collection of about 15 nuclei (collections of nerve cells) at the base of the forebrain, is the master neural control system that deals with these basic needs, together with response to stress and expression of emotions. There are three zones of hypothalamic nuclei: the periventricular group, which control the pituitary gland, the medial nuclei, concerned with some specific needs, and the lateral zone, which contains the medial forebrain bundle, the ascending dopamine system.

Stress involves both physical and psychological factors: uncertainty and lack of control in potentially harmful situations appears to be the major cause of stress and understanding and ability to control such situations the most successful coping strategy. Stress, either physical injury or perception of stress, results in activation of the hypothalamus to release corticotropin-releasing hormone (CRH), which acts on the anterior pituitary gland to release adrenocorticotrophic hormone (ACTH) into the bloodstream. ACTH acts on the cortex of the adrenal gland to release cortisol, the stress hormone, that mobilizes the body to deal with stress. In stress, the hypothalamus also acts directly on the autonomic nervous system to prepare the body for emergencies and via forebrain structures to prepare the organism for "fight or flight." Simultaneously, forebrain structures act to evaluate situations as potentially harmful or stressful, in other words, uncontrollable and act via limbic structures to activate the hypothalamus.

The circadian rhythm of sleep and waking activity is under the direct control of the suprachiasmatic nucleus of the hypothalamus. This nucleus has its own built-in 24-hour pacemaker that controls activity. It is "set" and modulated by incoming visual (light) activation and maintains a 24-hour cycle in the absence of visual input. We do not yet know why sleep occurs and why it is necessary. There are two forms of sleep, nonrapid eye movement (NREM) and rapid eye movement (REM); dreaming is associated with REM sleep. Regions of the brain stem reticular formation appear to play a critical role in sleep, particularly REM sleep.

Temperature regulation is controlled by the proptic region of the hypothalamus. There are two aspects to temperature regulation, behavioral and reflex. The behavioral mechanism, going to a colder or warmer place, is more ancient (it is the only mechanism available to cold-blooded animals). In warm-blooded animals there are thermostat neurons in the hypothalamus exquisitely sensitive to blood termperature that trigger appropriate reflex responses, shivering or sweating. These neurons appear to have a "set point" temperature and attempt to maintain blood temperature at that value.

Thirst is the basic mechanism for regulating body fluid level in higher animals. If the water content of the blood decreases, cells in the supraoptic nucleus of the hypothalamus shrink by losing water (as do all other cells). But they very sensitively detect this shrinkage and activate two systems, hormone release and feelings of thirst. The more sensitive of the two systems causes release of vasopressin at the nerve terminals of these neurons in the posterior pituitary. Vasopressin via the bloodstream acts directly on cells in the kidney to release a substance that becomes angiotensin II, which activates the hypothalamus and other brain systems via the subfornical organ, leading to thirst and fluid consumption. Shrinkage of the fluid-level-detecting neurons in the hypothalamus can also lead directly to feelings of thirst by as yet unknown processes.

Brain substrates of hunger and eating are less well understood today than they seemed to be a few years ago. The notion of two hypothalamic centers (one for hunger and one for satiety) is no longer believed. The so-called hunger center, in the lateral hypothalamus, actually seems to involve the medial forebrain bundle (dopamine pathway)—lesions here not only prevent eating but cause sensory neglect to all kinds of stimuli. The ventromedial "satiety" center (lesions cause animals to overeat and become obese) seems rather to involve incoming sensory information from the digestive organs via the vagus nerve.

The brain reward system is seen by many as a unifying system that integrates feelings of pleasure or reward for all the basic sources of need. In brief, electrical stimulation of the medial forebrain bundle region (lateral hypothalamus) yields self-stimulation. Animals will deliver electrical stimulation to this region of their brain. A current view of how this system works hypothesizes that electrical stimulation in the lateral hypothalamus activates descending neurons that activate neurons in the brain stem that are the origin of the medial forebrain bundle (dopamine) system. This system in turn projects up to a nucleus in the forebrain, termed the nucleus accumbens. Interestingly, dopamine-blocking drugs that help in treating the symptoms of schizophrenia block electrical self-stimulation of the brain when infused in the accumbens.

SUGGESTED READINGS AND REFERENCES

Books

Becker, J. B., Breedlove, S. M., and Crews, D. (1992). *Behavioral endocrinology.* Cambridge, MA: MIT Press.

Carlson, N. R. (1991). *Physiology of behavior* (4th ed.). Boston: Allyn and Bacon.

Cooper, J. R., Bloom, F. E., and Roth, R. H. (1991). *The biochemical basis of neuropharmacology* (6th ed.). New York: Oxford University Press.

DeCaro, G., Epstein, A. N. and Massi, M. (1986). *The physiology of thirst and sodium appetite.* New York: Plenum.

Druckman, D., and Bjork, R. A. (1991). *In the mind's eye: Enhancing human performance.* Washington, DC: National Academy Press.

Groves, P. M., and Rebec, G. V. (1992). *Introduction to biological psychology* (4th ed.). Dubuque, IA: William C. Brown.

Horne, J. (1988). *Why we sleep: The functions of sleep in humans and other mammals.* Oxford: Oxford University Press.

Kruyger, M. H., Roth, T., and Dement, W. C. (1989). *Principles and practices of sleep disorders in medicine.* New York: W. B. Saunders.

Logue, A. W. (1991). *The psychology of eating and drinking.* New York: W. H. Freeman.

Moore-Ede, M. C., Sulzman, F. M., and Fuller, C. A. (1982). *The clocks that time us.* Cambridge, MA: Harvard University Press.

Stricker, E. M. (1990). *Handbook of behavioral neurobiology.* New York: Plenum.

Walsh, B. T. (1988). *Eating disorders.* Washington, DC: American Psychiatric Press.

Articles

Keesey, R. E., and Powley, T. L. (1986). The regulation of body weight. *Annual Review of Psychology, 37,* 109–134.

Shors, T. J., Foy, M. R., Levine, S. and Thompson, R. F. (1990). Unpredictable and uncontrollable stress impairs neuronal plasticity in the rat hippocampus. *Brain Research Bulletin, 24,* 663–667.

Swanson, L. W. (1991). Biochemical switching in hypothalamic circuits mediating responses to stress. *Progress in Brain Research, 87,* 181–200.

Wise, R. A., and Rompre, P. -P. (1989). Brain dopamine and reward. *Annual Review of Psychology, 40,* 191–225.

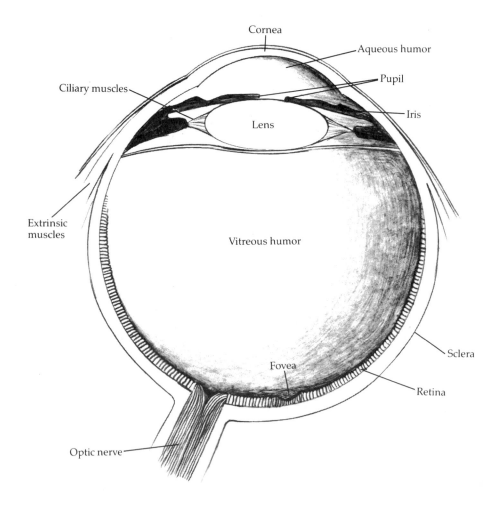

Cornea

Aqueous humor

Pupil

Ciliary muscles

Iris

Lens

Extrinsic
muscles

Vitreous humor

Sclera

Fovea

Retina

Optic nerve

8

Sensory Processes

Humans and other animals are remarkably sensitive to stimuli. The human eye and ear are as sensitive as the physical limits of light and sound permit. At certain wavelengths, the human eye can detect a single photon of light energy, the smallest amount of light that exists. The human ear can hear sounds much fainter than can be detected with any physical instrument.

The sensory systems show the molding pressure of evolution with striking clarity. The eye of an octopus is similar in many ways to the human eye because, although the octopus and the human have very different evolutionary histories, apparently such an eye represents the best solution to the problem of detecting visual stimuli. There are numerous examples of such convergent evolution in sensory receptors. In general, animals are the most sensitive to the stimuli that are important for the adaptive behavior they need to live in their particular environment. Bats and porpoises echolocate, building a picture of objects out of the darkness and turbidity of their worlds from the reflections of high-frequency sounds they emit. They can hear sounds five

Figure 8-1 *Human eye. The lens focuses images on the retina at the back of the eye. The fovea is the region on which the center of gaze is focused, and it provides the best detail vision.*

or six times higher in fi quency than humans. Honeybees can see ultraviolet light. Many flowers thai look dull to us reflect large amounts of ultraviolet light and may be much m re attractive to a bee.

Here we shall focus n the visual system as an example of a sensory system. The reason for this choice is twofold: more is known about the vertebrate visual system than about other vertebrate sensory systems, and it is the most important sensory modality for adaptive behavior in primates.

VISUAL SYSTEM

The ultimate job of the eye is to transmit information about the visual world to the brain. It does this through the fibers of the *optic nerves*. The cell bodies of the optic nerves, the *ganglion cells*, are situated in the retina of the eye and send their axons to the brain. The ganglion cells are the final output system of the eye proper, and they appear to work like standard neurons. When they are depolarized to threshold by inputs from other neurons in the retina, an action potential develops at the initial segment of the axon and travels rapidly (the axons are myelinated) to the brain. We shall examine presently how ganglion cells code visual stimuli.

The *lens* of the eye works much like the lens of a camera: it focuses a rather clear image of the visual world on the *retina*, the sheet of photoreceptors and neurons lining the back of the eye (Figure 8-1). As in a camera, the image on the retina is reversed. Objects to the right of center project images to the left part of the retina and vice versa, and objects above the center project to the lower part and vice versa. The shape of the lens is altered by the muscles of the *iris* so that near or far objects can be brought into focus on the retina. The amount by which the lens must be altered also provides cues about the distance of nearby objects.

A complete, although reversed, visual image of the world is projected on the retina of each eye in the human (Figure 8-2). The two eyes see the world from slightly different angles and the slight disparity of the images formed on the retina provides additional cues about the distances of objects, particularly objects that are more than a meter or so away.

The advantage of two eyes over one in distance vision or depth perception can be appreciated by examining a scene with both eyes open and then with one eye shut. Depth can be seen with one eye, but the sense of it is much less striking than when both eyes are used. The facts that each eye sees the entire world and that the images brought back to the retina from each are slightly different has important consequences for the organization of the visual regions of the brain and for their normal development in humans and other higher mammals, a matter we shall discuss shortly.

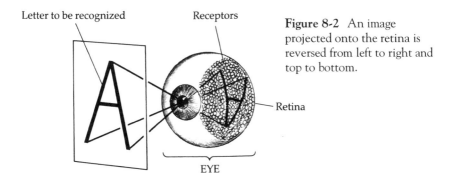

Letter to be recognized   Receptors

Retina

EYE

Figure 8-2 An image projected onto the retina is reversed from left to right and top to bottom.

Photoreceptors

All visual systems begin with photoreceptors, which are cells that respond to light energy (see Figure 8-4). Photoreceptor cells all contain one or more pigments that respond chemically to light, and much is known about the biochemistry of these pigments. Structurally, the visual chemical, called *retinal*, is a variation on the vitamin A molecule (which explains why one should eat foods containing vitamin A for good eyesight) and is associated with proteins.

There are two types of photoreceptors in the vertebrate eye, rods and cones. In general, the *rods*, which mediate sensations of light versus dark and shades of gray, are much more sensitive to light than the cones: they have much lower thresholds and can detect much smaller amounts of light. The rods of the human eye contain a single pigment, called rhodopsin. *Rhodopsin* is a combination of retinal and one variety of the protein *opsin*. *Cones* mediate acute detail vision and color vision. In the human eye there are three types of cones: one type that is the most sensitive to red light, one that is the most sensitive to green, and one that is the most sensitive to blue. In each of the three types of cones is a pigment containing retinal and a kind of opsin protein that is most sensitive to one of the three wavelengths of light.

The cones function poorly at low light levels. If you happen to be outside at twilight, watching the night advance, you might notice that the world gradually loses all its color and objects take on shades of gray. The cones cease in the growing darkness to function and finally you are seeing only with rods. The *fovea*, the region of the retina where the center of the visual field projects, is made up entirely of densely packed cones. When you look at something, the point at which you look projects to the center of the fovea, the part of the retina that gives the best detail vision. Cones become less dense farther away from the fovea and rods become more populous. You can see a faint star best if you look a few degrees away from it so that its image projects away from the fovea to the part of the retina where the rods are the densest.

Some animals, particularly nocturnal animals, have mostly or entirely rods, and others have mostly or entirely cones. Humans, apes, and monkeys have both rods and cones. Indeed, the retina of the macaque and other old-world monkeys appears to be identical to the human one: both macaques and humans have rods and three types of cones. It is now thought that the genes for the cone pigments and rhodopsin evolved from a common ancestral gene. Analysis of the amino acid sequences in the different opsins suggest that the first color pigment molecule was sensitive to blue. It then gave rise to another pigment that in turn diverged to form red and green pigments. Unlike old-world monkeys, new-world monkeys have only two cone pigments, a blue and a longer wavelength pigment thought to be ancestral to the red and green pigments of humans and other old-world primates. The evolution of the red and green pigments is thus quite recent; the new-world and old-world continents separated only about 30 million years ago. The new-world monkey retina, with only two color pigments, provides a perfect model for human red–green colorblindness. Genetic analysis of the various forms of human colorblindness suggests that some humans may someday, millions of years from now, have four cone pigments rather than three and see the world in very different colors than we do now.

Evidence that the three cone pigments code all of the visible colors has come from behavioral studies of color matching by humans. In one type of study a subject is presented with a circular field, half of which has been made any color the experimenter wishes, the other half consisting of three light sources tuned to emit the wavelengths of light to which the three cone pigments are the most sensitive. (The light sources can be lasers, virtually single wavelengths of light). The subject attempts to match the colored half of the circle by increasing or decreasing the intensity of each of the three colored lights. By doing so the subject can, to his or her way of thinking, match identically any color under the sun. Our entire experience of all color is built up from the relative excitation of the three types of cones.

Phototransduction — From Photon to Neuron

Virtually all the steps in the visual process, from photons of light landing on the rod photoreceptor to synaptic activation of neurons in the retina, have now been worked out. It is an extraordinary story. First, a further word about retinal—it is a relatively simple molecule embedded within the hugely complex protein molecule rhodopsin, the latter embedded in and crossing the membrane of the rod cell (Figure 8-3). Retinal is in a particular structural form, called *11-cis-retinal*. When a photon bombards the rod, the retinal changes its actual structural shape and is now described as *all-trans-retinal*. This process occurs in a few picoseconds (a picosecond is one billionth of a

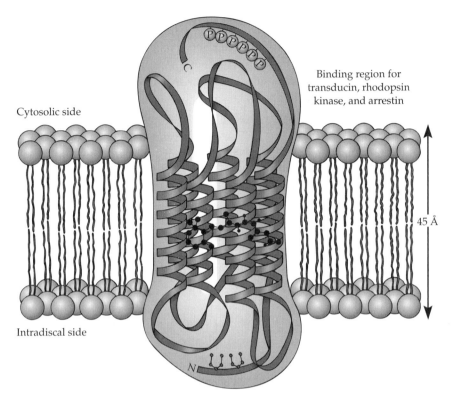

Cytosolic side

Binding region for
transducin, rhodopsin
kinase, and arrestin

45 Å

Intradiscal side

Figure 8-3 Entire rhodopsin molecule embedded in the membrane of the rod cell in the retina. It is a hugely complex protein molecule. However, the key photosensitive part of the molecule, retinal, is a very simple molecule (black dots and lines) embedded in the depths of rhodopsin molecule.

second). So the basic process is the conversion of a photon into atomic motion. Both retinal and its protein opsin continue to change shape through several intermediate forms until they become *metarhodopsin II*. The molecule then dissociates into all-trans-retinal and the protein opsin, which are recycled.

The total time from photon to metarhodopsin II is a few milliseconds, a time domain comfortable for the nervous system. Metarhodopsin II is the key actor. It activates a substance called *transducin* that in turn results in the activation of *cyclic GMP*, one of the common second-messenger systems in neurons (Chapter 5 and 6). This process in the rod directly alters ion channels in the rod membrane. This is a most unusual action of a second-messenger system; typically, second-messenger systems influence ion channels only indirectly, via the intracellular machinery, or not at all. The next step in the story also comes as a surprise. The action of the activated cyclic GMP on ion channels is to close sodium channels! If you were to do this in a neuron you would block action potentials and EPSPs (see Chapter 3). There is an extraordinary amplification in the process from photon to sodium channel closing. A single photon exciting one rhodopsin molecule activates about 500 molecules of transducin, which in turn results in cyclic GMP closing many hundreds of sodium channels, which blocks the entry of about one million sodium ions into the rod. One photon thus blocks one million sodium ions.

The rod cells form synapses on neurons in the retina. These resemble conventional fast excitatory synapses in some ways, and *glutamate*, the workhorse fast excitatory transmitter, appears to be the neurotransmitter released by the rods. The key to the synaptic action of the rod is the fact that in the dark, many of its sodium (Na^+) channels are open, a situation just the opposite of the Na^+ channels in a neuron at rest. Hence the rod membrane is markedly depolarized. In the dark, the resting rod membrane potential is about -30 mV. When photons act on the rod, Na^+ channels are closed, leading to a more negative membrane potential—in the direction of hyperpolarization. Unlike a conventional synapse, the rod synapse appears to release glutamate continuously. In the dark the synapse is depolarized and releases a maximum amount of glutamate. When light photons act on the rod to close Na^+ channels and the membrane becomes hyperpolarized, less glutamate is released.

A semirealistic drawing of the elements in the retina is shown in Figure 8-4a and the basic wiring diagram is given in Figure 8-4b. The most direct connection from rod and cone receptors to ganglion cells is via the bipolar cells. Remember that the ganglion cells send their axons to the brain, forming the optic nerve. We think of the eye as being a peripheral structure outside the brain, and most of it is. But the key part of the eye, the retina, is actually a part of the brain. In embryological development the retina grows out from the brain to join the other tissues—lens, cornea, and so on—that form the eye. The retina should be viewed as a miniature peripheral brain designed to process visual information.

We left the rods releasing less glutamate onto the bipolar cells when activated by light than they do in the dark. This should result in more hyperpolarization of the bipolar neuron dendrites at the rod synapse on it, and indeed it does. The bipolar neurons (and the horizontal neurons) in the retina are peculiar in that they do not generate action potentials. In this regard they are like the rods—if they are depolarized they release more neurotransmitter on to the ganglion cells, and if they are hyperpolarized they release less. This appears to be a great advantage in terms of the amount of information they can transmit—they are very sensitive to small gradations of transmitter release from the rods, due in turn to small changes in the amount of light falling on the rods. The result of all this information processing ought to be that the ganglion cell will generate many action potentials in the dark and cease generating action potentials when light shines on the rods, and indeed it is. This follows logically from the excitatory synaptic action of glutamate.

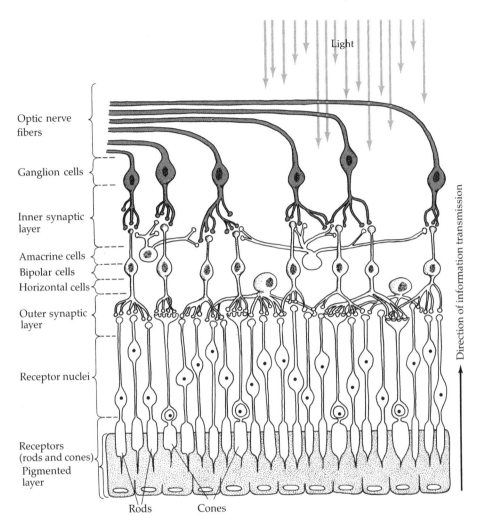

Figure 8-4 (*a*) The retina has three basic layers of cells, the light-sensitive photoreceptors (rods and cones) at the back, a middle layer of interneurons, and an outer layer of ganglion cell neurons whose axons make up the fibers of the optic nerve. Oddly, light must pass through the layers of nerve fibers and cells to reach the photoreceptors at the back of the retina. This actually improves vision by reducing the amount of scattered light in the eye that reaches the rods and cones.

But there is also an opposite kind of response shown by many other ganglion cells—they generate more action potentials when light strikes the rods that influence them and fewer action potentials in the dark. It turns out that glutamate actually hyperpolarizes many bipolar neurons. How this occurs is not yet known. But given this, it follows that the ganglion cells controlled by these hyperpolarizing bipolar cells will respond to light and not to dark.

Figure 8-4 (*b*) Very schematic wiring diagram of the neuronal connections in the retina. The G_1 ganglion cell (ganglion cell axons form the optic nerve fibers) receives direct activation from the rod via the bipolar interneuron and is characteristic of higher mammals. The G_2 ganglion cell receives direct connections only from amacrine interneurons, which are involved in complex synaptic processing within the retina. The G_2 ganglion cells are characteristic of lower vertebrates (for example, the frog).

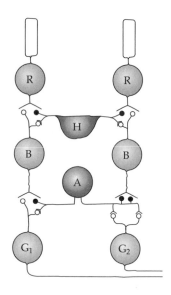

Receptive Fields

When a small spot of light enters a vertebrate eye, the lens focuses it on a particular place on the retina. As the spot of light is moved about, its image moves about on the retina. Suppose you are recording the action potentials from a single ganglion cell, perhaps by placing a microelectrode near it or its axon in the optic nerve. In darkness it will have some characteristic rate of discharge, say one action potential every second. When the light strikes the retina, it activates some rod and cone receptors. If these recptors are in the vicinity of the ganglion cell that is being monitored and are connected to it through the neural circuits in the retina, then the light will have some influence on the rate of firing of the ganglion cell. Depending on the neural circuits, the ganglion cell will be excited (fire more often than the spontaneous rate) or inhibited (fire less often). The complete extent of the retinal surface that can so influence the ganglion cell is called the ganglion cell's receptive field.

In mammals, most ganglion cell receptive fields on the retina are simple circular or oval patches. There are, in fact, only two major types of receptive field that a ganglion cell can have, and each ganglion cell has only one type: on-center/off-surround or off-center/on-surround (Figure 8-5). In the on-center/off-surround type, a spot of light on the central region of the receptive field excites the ganglion cell, making it fire more frequently. If the spot of light is moved onto the off-surround region, it will inhibit the ganglion cell from firing. Just the reverse holds for the off-center/on-surround type of field.

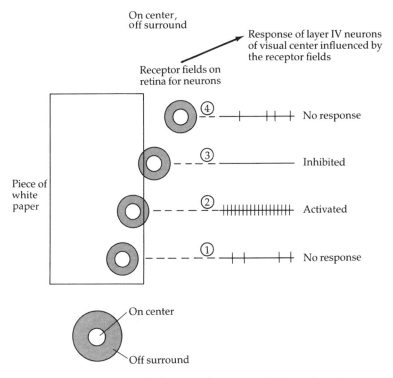

Figure 8-5 The on-center/off-surround receptive fields on the retina are most activated when an edge, a light-dark boundary, falls across the receptive field (2 in the figure).

Except for color information, the simple patterns of ganglion cell response are all that the brain sees from the eye. The intensity of light seems to be coded by the frequency of firing of the ganglion cells: a bright light causes them to fire more. Since a complete image of the visual environment is projected onto the retina, if one recorded the activity of all the one million plus ganglion cells from the eye, a rather complete representation of the retinal image would be found. However, the ganglion cells would simply indicate whether more or less light was present at each receptive field, nothing else.

Although the mechanisms by which the rods and cones and interneurons in the retina convert light into activation of the ganglion cells is an intriguing topic, from the point of view of the animal and behavior what the brain sees is the output of the ganglion cells. A most interesting reverse trend occurred in the evolution of the vertebrate retina. Reptiles and amphibians have the same basic neuronal elements in the retina as mammals, but the wiring diagrams are different. In the frog visual system virtually all information processing is done in the retina. In mammals very little information processing occurs in the retina (except for color vision, in which the key initial coding is done there). Given this we might expect that the receptive fields of ganglion cells in lower vertebrates would be very much more complicated than in mammals, and such is the case.

In the frog a number of different types of receptive fields are found. In fact, the frog's visually guided behaviors can be predicted rather well just from these receptive fields. One type of receptive field was dubbed the "bug detector" by its discoverer, Jerome Lettvin at the Massachusetts Institute of Technology. One class of ganglion cells responds only to a small, dark object moving irregularly. When a normal frog is presented with such a stimulus, the frog, hoping a bug is flying by, will snap its tongue out and attempt to capture the object. This prey-catching behavior is triggered by the activation of the "bug-detector" ganglion cells. The analysis of the meaning of the visual stimulus has been done at the retina; the frog does not need to process the information any more in the brain.

Over the course of evolution the retina became wired up in very specific and specialized ways in various reptiles. Dinosaurs are thought to have been highly visual animals with very small brains. The retina probably functioned as a rather complete visual brain. Just the opposite trend developed in mammals. Higher mammals such as carnivores and primates have the simplest on–off receptive fields. Visual information processing is done in the brain rather than in the retina.

If complex visual information processing is to be done, as is the case if experience and learning are involved, it must occur in the brain. If the retina did all visual stimulus coding, we could never learn to read, because the retinal ganglion cells do not have receptive fields that respond selectively to the letters of the alphabet. We must learn to see letters and words.

The responses of the ganglion cells in the mammalian retina are actually somewhat more complicated than I have indicated. In most current texts, three types of ganglion cells, X, Y, and W, are described. John Dowling at Harvard University, a leading authority on the retina, argues that a simpler classification into two types is more appropriate. We will follow Dowling's classification but to avoid confusion will term one class XY and the other class W. The XY *ganglion cells* have the typical relatively simple mammalian on-center/off-surround or off-center/on-surround receptive fields. The receptive fields of the W *ganglion cells* are quite different. They respond poorly to diffuse light but are very sensitive to movement, particularly of dark stimuli, for example, an edge of an object or a "bug," and they are direction sensitive— they respond better to movement of an object in one direction than another. These much more complex receptive fields are believed to be due to the actions of the amacrine neurons in the retina. These are the only interneurons in the retina that generate action potentials, and they can exert complex influences on the ganglion cells. As indicated in Figure 8-4*b*, some ganglion cells receive input only from amacrine cells.

It appears that over the course of vertebrate evolution, the more primitive retina consisted primarily of amacrine cell actions on ganglion cells. Frogs, turtles, and other cold-blooded vertebrates (including dinosaurs?) have mainly W ganglion cells, whereas the XY type predominates in mammals. Primitive vertebrates did what visual processing they needed in the retina, as we noted. More complex processing has to be done in the brain and is ultimately more adaptive. There must have been strong pressure from natural selection for more complex and successful visual processing and hence for a bigger brain. Dowling gives a particularly apt example. Frogs capture and eat only moving prey. Bugs that have recently died would make a perfectly fine meal for a frog, but the frog retina is so wired that frogs do not respond to stationary objects. A frog would starve to death amidst a field of dead bugs. In mammals, the evolutionary pressure toward brain processing of visual information is evident. Simpler mammals like the squirrel and rabbit have many more direction-sensitive W type ganglion cells than do cats and monkeys.

Visual Pathways

In mammals, the anatomical relations of projection from the visual field to the retina to the brain are a bit complicated. In lower vertebrates such as the frog there is complete crossing of input: all input to the right eye (the right visual field) goes to the left side of the brain, and vice versa. Such animals have no *binocular vision*. In lower mammals, such as the rat or the rabbit, the visual fields from the two eyes partially overlap. Here there is incomplete crossing; about 80 percent of the fibers from the left retina and 20 percent of the fibers from the right retina project to the right side of the brain. The projections from the two retinas overlap, so perhaps 30 percent of the visual area of the cerebral cortex receives input from both eyes and hence can mediate binocular vision. In the dog and the cat there is about 80 percent overlap so they have considerable binocular vision. Primates, including man, have virtually total binocular vision; the left half of each retina projects to the left visual cortex and the right half of each retina projects to the right visual cortex (Figure 8-6). This means, of course, that the right cortex receives all of its input from the left visual field, and the left visual cortex receives all of its input from the right visual field. Removal of the left visual cortex eliminates all visual input from the entire right half of the visual field of both eyes.

Although a single eye can use various cues to obtain some information about depth, or the distance of objects, much better cues are provided by binocular vision, in which input from the two eyes can be compared by cells in the visual cortex. Among mammals, predators such as cats and wolves have

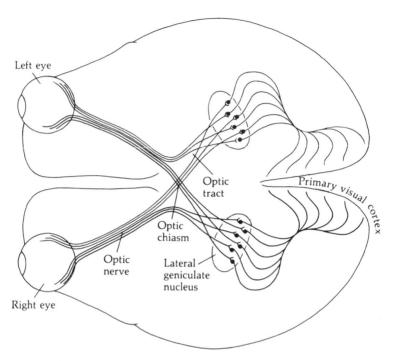

Figure 8-6 The major visual pathway from the eye to the visual cortex. Optic nerve fibers re-sort at the optic chiasm so that all input from the left half of each retina (the right half of the visual field) projects to the left lateral geniculate nucleus (thalamus) and left visual cortex, and vice versa.

good binocular vision; hence they can judge the distance to prey very accurately. Many animals that are prey, such as rabbits and deer, have much less binocular vision. Instead, their eyes are far to the sides of the head so that they can see movements behind them. The excellent binocular vision of primates is probably due to the fact that they live in trees, or at least their ancestors did. If one mistakes the distance to a branch one is leaping for, one's genes will not be propagated.

In primates, optic nerve fibers from the left half of each retina (representing the right half of each visual field) project to the *left lateral geniculate body* of the thalamus and fibers from the right half of each retina project to the *right lateral geniculate body* (Figure 8-6). The crossing of the fibers takes place at the *optic chiasm*, the point at which the two optic nerves come together. The fibers from the retinas to the chiasm are called *optic nerves* and those from the chiasm to the central nervous system are called *optic tracts*. The optic tracts synapse in the lateral geniculate body, the thalamic relay nucleus, and projections continue to the visual region of the cerebral cortex. The projections from the optic tract to the lateral geniculate body and hence to the cerebral cortex constitute the main visual pathways in higher vertebrates; there are several other pathways of importance in lower vertebrates.

The lateral geniculate body that relays information from the optic nerve to the visual cortex consists of six layers in the monkey and human. These layers are completely segregated in terms of the input from the two eyes. The top, third, and fifth layers of the left lateral geniculate body receive input from the left half of the left retina and the second, fourth, and sixth layers receive input from the left half of the right retina, and vice versa for the right lateral geniculate body. All six layers of the left lateral geniculate body project to layer IV of the left visual cortex, and all six layers of the right lateral geniculate body project to the right visual cortex. The inputs from the different layers of the lateral geniculate body to the visual cortex are segregated so that a given cell in layer IV of the visual cortex receives input from one eye or the other but not from both. In fact, as we shall see, the cells of layer IV of the visual cortex are organized in columns in such a way that one column will respond to the left eye, an adjacent column will respond to the right eye, and so on.

The projections from the retina to the cerebral cortex are highly organized and orderly. Neighboring regions of the retina make connections with neighboring geniculate cells. Even cells in the different layers of the geniculate are laid out in such a way that those cells receiving input from a given region of the retina are closest to one another.

THE VISUAL CORTEX

The primary visual area of the cerebral cortex, termed the *striate cortex*, is in the occipital lobe in the posterior region of each cerebral hemisphere. Essentially there is a point-to-point representation of the retinal regions on the occipital cortex. However, nearly half of the primary visual cortex is occupied by the representation of the foveal area of the retina. The fovea, although it is only a small region of the retina, is the central focal point of the eye and mediates detail vision, as we noted earlier; consequently a considerable amount of cortex is devoted to it.

Studies by David H. Hubel and Torsten N. Wiesel have provided a great deal of information about the way cells in the visual cortex of higher mammals code visual form. (They received a Nobel prize in 1981 for their work.) The relatively simple receptive fields and response patterns described earlier for the ganglion cells of the optic nerve fibers of mammals (on-center/off-surround and off-center/on-surround) seem to be maintained even at the level of the lateral geniculate body in cats, monkeys, and humans. Complex information-coding processes occur in the cells of the visual cortex.

One group of cells in the visual cortex has the same type of receptive field as do the ganglion cells in the retina and the relay cells in the lateral geniculate body. These cells are the primary receiving neurons in layer IV of the cortex; they are the cells that receive input from the lateral geniculate body. These cells are also monocular, meaning that they receive input from only one eye. They are spatially laid out in layer IV as alternating patches of cells activated by the right eye or the left eye. These patches of monocular cells in layer IV provide the basic information to other neurons in the visual cortex (Figure 8-7).

It is relatively easy to imagine how the more complex receptive fields of most of the neurons in the visual cortex could be built up from the basic on-center/off-surround receptive fields of the primary receiving cells in layer IV. Suppose you look at a piece of white typing paper on your desk. The white paper reflects light and is projected to a fairly large region of your retina. Most of the primary receiving cells that have their receptive fields in the part of the retina receiving light from the paper will do nothing at all. The center and surround fields balance each other out. Yet you clearly see a white piece of paper. The key is the edges. Consider the four examples shown in Figure 8-5, which is a schematic of the projection region of the piece of paper on the retina. Cell 1 has its entire receptive field inside the region and does nothing: excitation and inhibition balance out. Cell 4 has its entire receptive field outside the region and also does nothing. Cell 2 is along the edge, so the on-center part of its receptive field is just inside the region of the paper projection but part of its off-surround field is outside. It is fully excited but only partly inhibited. The net result is that it will be excited and increase its firing. Cell 3 has only a part of its off-surround field inside the paper projections and none of its on-center part, and so it will be inhibited. The edges of the paper will cause a row of retinal cells to be excited and a row to be inhibited. Consequently, in the visual cortex a rectangular-shaped border of activated and inhibited cells will be represented.

Most neurons in the visual cortex show more complex patterns of response than the primary receiving cells of layer IV. They respond as though they are detecting features. It is easy to see how such "feature-detector" cells can be built from the simple on-center/off-surround cells in layer IV. Suppose that all the cells that are excited by the right edge of a piece of typing paper— the cells activated from primary receiving cells, such as cell 2 in the previous example—connect to another neuron in the visual cortex. This neuron will then be activated by the right edge. It will be a "vertical-edge-detector" neuron. Suppose we tilt the paper. A different set of primary receiving cells will now be activated by the oblique right edge. If they all project to another neuron, it will be an "edge detector" for an edge that tilts away from the vertical. In this way, the complete spectrum of orientations can be built up in the cortex.

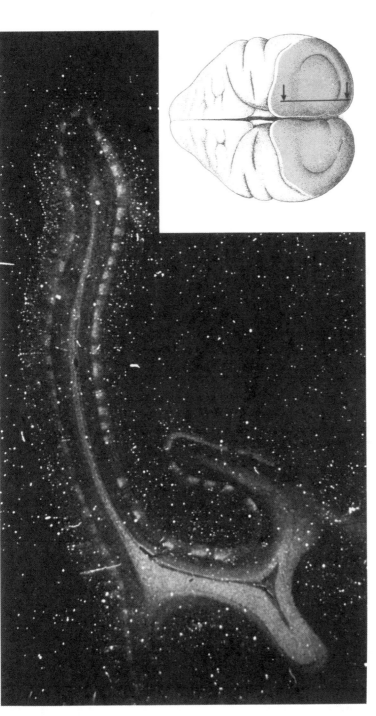

Figure 8-7 Section through the visual cortex of a monkey (the inset shows the region from which the section was taken). The bright patches running along the cortex represent input from the right eye, and the interspersed dark patches are input from the left eye, all in layer IV of the cortex. The two eyes thus project (by way of the lateral geniculate body) to alternating patches or columns of cells in layer IV of the visual cortex. This picture was obtained by injecting a radiolabeled substance in one eye that was transported to the lateral geniculate and on to the visual cortex. There it "lit up" the neurons in layer IV to which it was transported.

Cell Columns in the Visual Cortex

A striking finding by D. H. Hubel and T. N. Wiesel is the existence of a columnar organization in the visual cortex. If a microelectrode is pushed through the cortex in a path perpendicular (at right angles) to the surface, all the cells that are encountered will respond only to a stimulus edge of the same orientation. Different columns of cells respond to stimuli having different orientations. A small region of the retina projects to each small region of cortex. Within that area of cortex are many different columns of cells, each column consisting of cells that respond to a different stimulus orientation. This vertical columnar organization appears to be a very general principle in cortex; it was first discovered by Vernon B. Mountcastle at Johns Hopkins University. A great many different types of columns in the visual cortex are responsive to different stimulus orientations. Further, the neural organization required for this columnar "abstraction" of stimulus orientation in the visual system occurs at the cortex. No such organization is found for cells of the lateral geniculate body. Presumably, orientation coding by the columns of cells in the visual cortex plays a role in the neuronal reconstruction of visual space.

In sum, the receptive fields of most of the cells in the primary visual cortex are not concentric or circular, except for layer IV cells; most fields tend instead to be rectangular or "edge shaped." In addition to shape, the orientation of the receptive field and the movement of the appropriate shape across the field are crucial variables. The cell fires when the stimulus edge is at a particular orientation; movement of the edge in one direction through one angle is the most effective stimulus. In more general terms, most of the cells of the primary visual cortex respond to edges or boundaries of particular orientations, often only if they move in particular directions.

Most of the cells in the primary visual cortex are binocular for the corresponding receptive fields of the retina for each eye, meaning that they can be activated by stimuli presented to either eye (the exception to this is again the primary receiving cells in layer IV). Remember that comparable regions of each retina project to the same region of the visual cortex. If you look at a given point, a small object somewhat to the right of that point projects to the same small region of the left retina of each eye, and these two regions in turn project to the small region of the left visual cortex.

Although most of the cells in the primary visual cortex are binocular, a given cell will prefer one eye over the other, responding more if the stimulus is given to that eye. This reaction is called *ocular dominance*. The functional columns of cells in the visual cortex are organized in terms of ocular dominance as well as by orientation. An elementary functional unit of the visual cortex is indicated by shading in Figure 8-8. In this unit are two adjacent rows of columns; one row consists of cells that prefer information from

RECEIVE FIELD CELLS

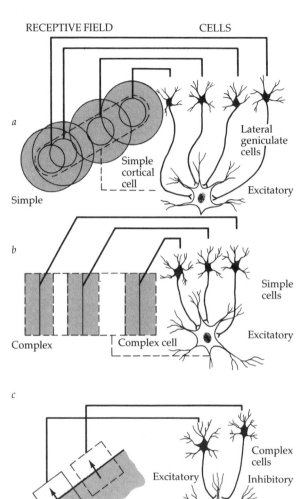

Figure 8-8 How more complex receptive fields might be built up in the visual cortex. (*a*) Each of a group of simple on-off receptive fields activates a neuron in the lateral geniculate body, and these neurons all connect to a cortical cell such that a straight edge on the retina will cause maximal activation of the cortical cell. (*b*) Several of these "edge" simple cells connect to another cell (complex), so that edges over a region of the retina will all activate the complex cell. (*c*) These complex cells interconnect on still another cell (hypercomplex), so that it responds best to a corner.

the left eye and the other row of the cells that prefer information from the right eye. Each vertical slab within a row represents a somewhat different orientation of movement. The entire set of slabs represents movement in all of the directions around a compass, that is, from up–down (zero degrees) through left–right (90 degrees) through down–up and right–left back to up–down. This functional unit thus contains complete information about the orientation of a stimulus and the input from each retina. Hubel and Wiesel stressed that the cell column is the dynamic unit of function in the visual cortex.

The neurons that respond to an edge at a particular orientation, the "edge detectors," are said to have simple receptive fields (Figure 8-9). It is easy to see how a row of concentric or circular cells in layer IV could all connect to an edge-detector cell so that it would be activated only by an edge of a particular orientation, an edge falling on a particular row of receptor cells in the eye. A given simple edge-detector neuron will respond only if the edge falls on an exact location on the retina of the eye.

Another type of neuron in the primary visual cortex is called complex (Figure 8-9). A *complex neuron* also responds best to an edge of a particular orientation, but the image of the edge does not have to fall on just one location on the retina. If the edge falls anywhere within a given region of the retina, the complex neuron will fire.

Other types of neurons found in visual cortex have been called *hypercomplex*. They tend to respond to particular sizes and forms of objects over wider regions of the retina. An example of a hypercomplex cell is shown in

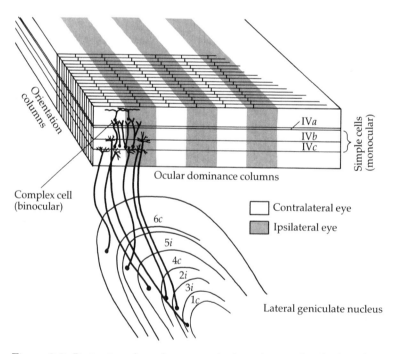

Figure 8-9 Projections from the eyes to the lateral geniculate body to layer IV of the visual cortex. The top layer and fourth layer of the lateral geniculate (6c and 4c) receive input from the opposite side (contralateral) eye and project to one column of cells in layer IV of the visual cortex (IVc), whereas the same side eye (ipsilateral) projects to layers 5i and 3i, which in turn project to the next column of cells in layer IV of the cortex (IVb).

Figure 8-10. This cell is a "right-angle detector"; it responds best to a right angle anywhere within its field and at two different orientations, but it will not respond to a straight edge.

A word of caution is necessary. Single cells in the visual cortex respond to certain and sometimes abstract aspects of visual stimuli. In some ways these responses are analogous to our perceptual experience. Both we and the cell in Figure 8-9 seem to respond to right angles. It is tempting to conclude that these cell receptive-field properties are "perception," but cannot yet make such inferences. To again quote Hubel and Wiesel:

> What happens beyond the primary visual area, and how is the information on orientation exploited at later stages? Is one to imagine ultimately finding a cell that responds specifically to some very particular item? (Usually one's grandmother is selected as the particular item, for reasons that escape us.) Our answer is that we doubt there is such a cell, but we have no good alternative to offer. To speculate broadly on how the brain may work is fortunately not the only course open to investigators. To explore the brain is more fun and seems to be more profitable. (D.

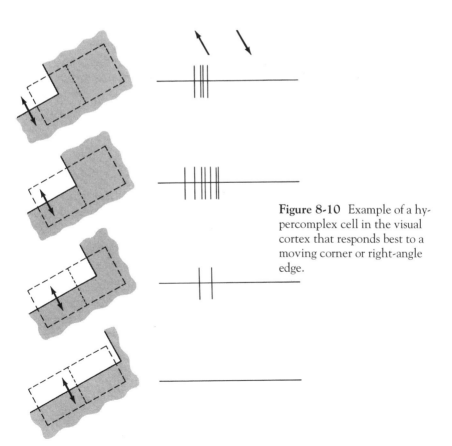

Figure 8-10 Example of a hypercomplex cell in the visual cortex that responds best to a moving corner or right-angle edge.

H. Hubel and T. N. Wiesel, Brain mechanisms of vision. In *Scientific American*, New York: W. H. Freeman, p. 96, 1979.)

We are just beginning to gain some understanding of how the basic patterns of connections form in the primary visual cortex during the growth and development of the brain. The visual cortex is astonishingly plastic in the infant brain and very sensitive to visual experience. This topic will be taken up in detail in Chapter 10.

Additional Visual Areas in the Cortex

Although we have spoken of the visual cortex as though it were one area, in fact it is made up of many visual areas. A *visual area* is defined as a complete map of the retina, the receptive surface of the eye. (Actually a visual area in the left visual cortex would have a complete map of the left half of each retina and vice versa for the right area, but we can ignore this detail here.) A complete map is just that: if a small light strikes each different part of the retina, a corresponding part of the visual area will respond.

At last count there were thought to be perhaps 20 visual areas in the visual cortex of the monkey, and presumably the human visual cortex has more (Figure 8-11). For convenience I shall simply refer to the visual areas as V1, V2, and so on. Area V1 corresponds to the original primary visual cortex. The cells we have described so far—the ones in layer IV that detect spots, the layers of simple cells in the column that respond to oriented edges, much more from one eye than the other, and the complex cells—are found in area V1. This area receives its visual input from the eye by way of the thalamus (the lateral geniculate body), which connects with the cells in layer IV. Most of the input to area V2 is from V1, most of the input to area V3 is from V1 and V2, and so on—a progressive funneling of visual information. Most of the cells in

Figure 8-11 Highly schematic representation of some of the visual areas in the cerebral cortex of the monkey. Each visual area has a retinal projection: a map or layout of the visual field (actually of the left half of the visual field since the right hemisphere is shown).

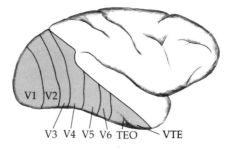

FRONT

V1 V2
V3 V4 V5 V6 TEO   VTE

Surface of cerebrum covered with cerebral cortex

area V2 are of the complex type, and more than half of the cells in area V3 are of the hypercomplex type.

Perception of Three Dimensions   In addition to the funneling effect, another major difference between the neurons in area V1 and those in areas V2, V3, V4, and V5 is that the most of the latter respond equally well to input from both eyes. In many of these binocular cells the response differs a bit for each eye, which may be the neuronal basis of depth perception. We see a three-dimensional world because we see it with both eyes. If an object is far away, the two eyes look at it almost in parallel. As the object moves closer to the face, both eyes point more and more toward the nose. The image of the object falls over a slightly different region of the retinas of the two eyes. This retinal disparity, reflected in differing responses of the binocular cells of the secondary visual areas, is the major visual cue of three dimensions. Three-dimensional movies are made using two side-by-side cameras with different color filters. When you put on cardboard glasses with a different-colored filter over each eye to view the movie, it suddenly becomes three-dimensional because you are seeing it through both cameras, just as you normally see the world through both eyes.

Perception of Movement   Why are there so many visual areas in the cerebral cortex? It seems that several of the secondary visual areas may play special roles in particular aspects of seeing, such as the perception of movement. Cells in all of the visual areas tend to respond better to moving objects than to objects at rest. However, the cells in area V5 respond particularly well to the movement of an object in front of either eye. Neither the shape of the object nor the direction of movement matters, only the movement itself. Area V5 may also play a key role in depth perception. There are reports in the human clinical literature of very localized brain damage that abolishes the ability to see movement, although color and form perception is normal.

Perception of Color   Color is the most immediate visual sensation. Imagine describing what it is like to see colors to a person blind from birth. The sizes and shapes of objects can be described in words easily enough, but there is no way at all to describe colors. Color is an experiential given. Infants can match colors to samples long before they learn the names of the colors. Early experiments on English-speaking adults who were shown a variety of colors revealed that their memory for colors was much better for the primary ones—red, green, and blue—than for in-between colors, which are harder to describe. At first better memory for the primary colors was thought to be learned: in the English-speaking world, the primary color names are set by the language. In fact, just the opposite is true. Anthropological studies of a people who have only two color terms in their language have shown that they also remember the primary colors best, even though they do not have words to describe them all. The primary colors are set by the color receptors in the eye, not by language and culture.

Color does not exist in the world; it exists only in the eye of the beholder. Objects reflect many different wavelengths of light, but the light waves themselves have no color. Animals developed color vision as a way of telling the difference between the various wavelengths of light. The eye converts different ranges of wavelengths into colors in a very simple way. We have seen that in the human eye there are three types of cones, or color receptors, which have one of three different light-sensitive pigments: red, green, and blue. The cones connect to different neurons and send color information to the brain.

A given color-sensitive ganglion cell sending its axon from the eye to the brain will respond to, say, red light entering the eye but will be inhibited by green. Another will respond to green and be inhibited by red. Still another class of color neurons will respond to yellow and be inhibited by blue, and a fourth group will respond to blue and be inhibited by yellow. Russell De Valois of the University of California at Berkeley first discovered these opponent responses of color neurons in the eye and brain. In the nineteenth century two major theories of color vision were put forward. The Young–Helmholtz theory argued for three primary color receptors in the eye: red, green, and blue. The Hering theory (now called the Hering–Jameson-Hurvich theory) argued for opponent pairs of receptors: red–green and yellow–blue. De Valois's work placed him in the unusual position of showing that two theories disagreeing strongly with each other were both correct. There are indeed three primary color receptors in the eye, but the neural interconnections in the eye and the neurons that convey color information to the brain convert information from these receptors into opponent color messages.

DeValois determined that many neurons in the visual thalamus, the lateral geniculate body, were also opponent-process color-coding cells. Hence, detailed information about the colors of objects is projected to the visual cortex. But it was only recently that we gained some understanding of how color is coded in the cortical visual areas. Margaret Livingston and David Hubel at Harvard treated area V1 of the monkey cortex with a substance that stains the enzyme cytochrome oxidase. The reader may recall that biological energy in the form of ATP is made in the mitochondria of cells from glucose and oxygen in the process known as *oxidative metabolism*. Cytochrome oxidase is one of the key enzymes in the process, and the more metabolism that occurs in a neuron, the more cytochrome oxidase is present. It seems that some neurons are much more active and require more ATP than others and hence have higher levels of cytochrome oxidase. When area V1 is stained for this enzyme, regular little dark blobs appear, particularly in the upper layers of the cortex. Each blob is about 0.15 millimeter across and the blobs are about 0.5 millimeter apart.

The dark blobs are scattered through the various receptive field columns in area V1 (Figure 8-12). When Livingston and Hubel recorded from neurons in the center of a blob, they found that the cells had no orientation selectivity. Furthermore, most of them had opponent-process color-receptive fields. They did not respond to white light, but small colored spots made them respond vigorously. Actually their color-receptive fields were more complex than those in the lateral geniculate body; they exhibited "double" opponent processes. Thus a cell would respond to red and be inhibited by green in the center of its field but be excited by green and inhibited by red in the surround portion of the receptive field. Similar color responsive fields were found in certain regions of cortical area V2 as well.

The regions of area V2 containing color-responsive cells (Figure 8-12) project preferentially to yet another visual area termed V4. Semir Zeki, at

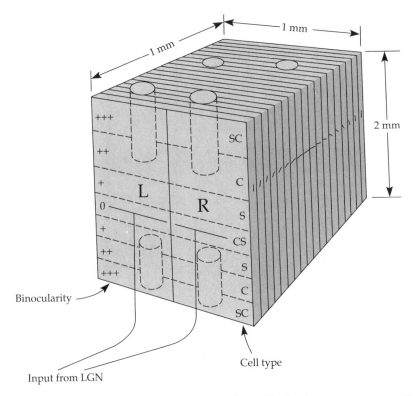

Figure 8-12 Hypercolumn: 1 mm × 1 mm × 2 mm block of cortex containing all the cells required to analyze a bit of visual space. In a hypercolumn, input from both eyes is represented. Furthermore, all types of simple and complex cells are present, and the cells have all possible orientation preferences and varying degrees of binocularity. In addition, color-sensitive cells are found in the pegs or "blobs" inserted into the hypercolumn. Compare with Figure 8-9.

University College, London, first reported that neurons in area V4 responded preferentially to color. Most of these cells appear to be highly selective and respond only to a narrow range of wavelengths of light. Overall, different cells respond to all the wavelengths of light we see as colors. These cells are concerned only with color not the shape, size, or movement of stimuli. Clinical reports of patients who have suffered damage to area V4 indicate that their ability to see colors is impaired but not their ability to see shapes and movement.

Shape Perception   A secondary visual area (V6 or TEO in Figure 8-11) may specialize in deciphering the shapes of objects. When area V6 is damaged in monkeys, they lose the ability to tell different two-dimensional patterns apart. However, they can still see simpler aspects of objects, such as size.

Perhaps the most remarkable visual area of all does not appear to have a map of the retina, and for a long time it was not thought to be a visual area. This structure, called the visual–temporal (VTE) area, lies in the association cortex of the temporal lobe and receives the complex and highly processed input from area V6 and other secondary visual areas. When the VTE area is damaged in monkeys, they have great difficulty in learning certain kinds of visual tasks.

The discovery that the VTE area receives prominent visual input is a classic case of serendipity. According to the story, Charles Gross and his associates at Harvard University were studying the responses to visual stimuli of monkey cells in the VTE area. They used spots of light, edges, and bars, the standard elementary visual stimuli. Neurons in the VTE responded a bit to these simple stimuli and not to sounds or touches, and so it seemed to the experimenters to be a visual area but not a significant one. After studying one particular cell for a long time with minimal results—the cell did not respond very much to their stimuli—they decided to move on to another cell. As a gesture, the experimenter said farewell to the cell by raising his hand in front of the monkey's eye and waving goodbye. The cell fired wildly in response to his moving hand. Needless to say, the experimenters stayed with the cell. They immediately cut out different paper shapes of hands and tried them on the cell. The cell apparently liked best the upright shape of a monkey's hand. The cells in visual area VTE seem to respond best to specific complex shapes. However, our understanding of this visual area is still quite fragmentary.

Work has really just begun on many of the secondary visual areas. To the extent that we have information, it can be said that each area has the basic columnar organization: clusters of cells running from surface to depth have common functional properties. The great advantage of columnar organization is that several dimensions of information can be unfolded. Take visual area V1 as an example. Its two-dimensional surface area represents the spatial map, or layout, of the retina, the receptive surface of the eye, and hence the spatial extent of the visual world we see. The large columns running through the cortex are right-eye-dominant or left-eye-dominant for input. Within each large eye-dominant column are many small columns, each having cells that respond to a different orientation on the compass. Superimposed on the columns of area V1 are the blobs containing color-coding neurons. Thus area V1 is a "five-dimensional" array, with two dimensions for the areal extent of the retina, two dimensions running at right angles through the cortex that respond to input for one or the other eye and orientation of line, and finally, a dimension for color.

SOMATIC SENSORY SYSTEM

The organization of the cerebral cortex into columns was first discovered by Vernon Mountcastle, at Johns Hopkins, who was studying the somatic sensory area of the cortex of cats and monkeys, which receives information from the skin and the rest of the body. The body surface is represented part by part along the somatic cortex, forming a homunculus, or little person, on it (Figure 8-13). This remarkable topographical projection was discovered by Clinton Woolsey and others in the United States and by Lord Adrian in England. Within each small region of body surface map—for example, the region corresponding to the right forefinger—were very small columns of cells running through the cortex that responded to different modalities of stimulation. One column of cells would respond only to light touch and another only to deep pressure. The various dimensions of the skin senses are coded in columns at right angles to the map of the body surface extending over the surface of the cortex.

The primary somatic sensory pathway, often termed the *lemniscal system*, conveys information about touch, pressure, and joint position (Figure 8-14). The pain pathways (described in Chapter 6) convey information from the skin and body about pain and temperature.

The skin and body are equipped with a variety of specialized sensory receptors. The *Pacinian corpuscles* are receptors specialized to convey pressure and other pressure receptors convey joint-movement information. At the base of each body hair are pressure receptors to detect its movements, and the skin is amply serviced by still other pressure and touch receptors. Specialized receptors appear to register temperature, whereas pain seems to be detected by free nerve endings in the skin and other body tissues. It is not entirely clear how many different types of receptors there are in the skin, or to what extent the different dimensions or modalities of experience correspond to different receptors.

In the lemniscal system, the sensory fibers enter the spinal cord, turn upward in the dorsal column of the cord, and make their first synapse on cells

a

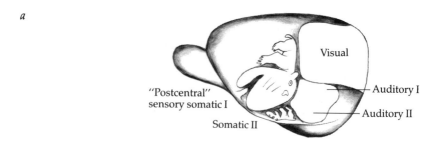

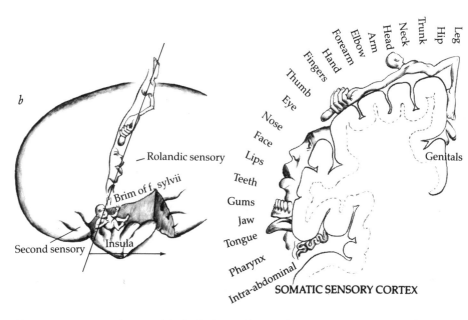

Figure 8-13 Map or layout of the body skin surface on the somatic sensory area of the cerebral cortex of (*a*) the rat and (*b*) the human. The "ratunculus" is more recognizable and less distorted than the homunculus. The projection is mostly crossed: the right half of the body projects to the left hemisphere of the cerebral cortex, and vice versa.

in nuclei at the posterior end of the brain stem. Fibers from the nuclei cross and ascend in a pathway called the *lemniscal tract* to synapse in the thalamic relay nuclei, the *ventrobasal complex*. These thalamic nuclei project to the primary somatic sensory area of the cerebral cortex. The fast pain pathway is somewhat similar to the lemniscal pathway (see Chapter 6). The representation of the body surface on the primary somatic sensory cortex (SI) was shown in Figure 8-13 for the rat and the human. Although the general or-

Primary somatic sensory (lemniscal) pathway

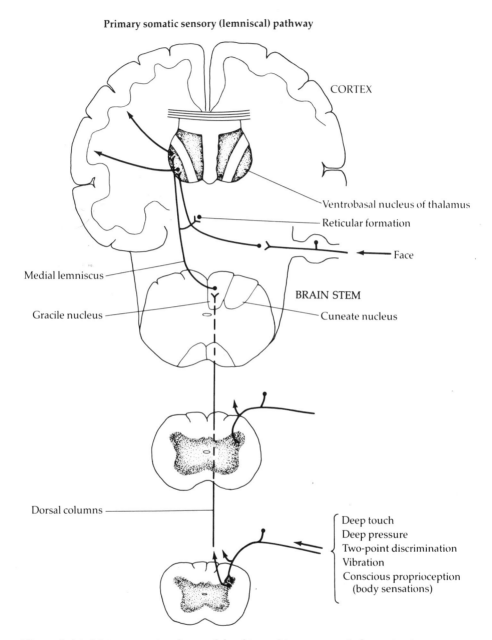

Figure 8-14 Major central pathway of the skin and body senses. Information is relayed up the spinal cord on the same side of the body it comes from to the gracile nucleus at the back end of the brain stem. Fibers from here then cross and ascend in the medial lemniscus all the way to the thalamus (ventrobasal nucleus) and from there to the cerebral cortex. The fast pain pathway follows a somewhat similar course but differs in some details (see Figure 6-4).

ganization of the SI is comparable for all mammals, details differ considerably. Figure 8-13 is not to be taken literally. It is designed to indicate the relative amount of cortex devoted to each region of skin surface, and their topographical relations.

A fundamental generalization may be made concerning the projections of body surface onto the cortex: the amount of cortex devoted to a given region of body surface is directly proportional to the amount of use and the sensitivity of that region. In the monkey, the amount of cortex devoted to the hand and foot areas is so great that other skin representation regions in a cortex map have been pushed aside. The hand area has enlarged so much that it has split the head area into two spatially separate fields, the ear and the back of the head are above the hand area and the face area is below it.

In humans, the exaggerated size of the area of cortex servicing the fingers is even more pronounced than the hand area in the monkey, and the face area is also much enlarged. So far as the cortex is concerned, the human appears to be mostly fingers, lips, and tongue, which corresponds well with the behavior of *Homo sapiens*. The relative development of cortical projections of skin areas can be traced from the rat, in which there is less distortion in the cortical representation, or "ratunculus," to the human, in whom differential enlargement of skin regions produces considerable distortion of the cortical representation, or homunculus (Figure 8-13).

The generality of the principle that the relative amount of sensory cortex (and thalamus) is proportional to the amount of use and the sensitivity of a given body region has been strikingly illustrated in a series of studies by Wally Welker at the University of Wisconsin. He determined the relative amount of tissue in the thalamus and cortex devoted to different regions of the body for four different mammals, the spider monkey, raccoon, rat, and sheep and the characteristic behavior of each animal (Figure 8-15). For example, the spider monkey makes good use of its tail for feeling, the raccoon is a forepaw feeler, the rat is a whisker feeler, and the sheep is a lips and tongue feeler.

Welker carried the generalization one step further by comparing in various animals the relative sizes of the three major sensory relay nuclei of the thalamus: those concerned with vision, touch, and hearing (Figure 8-16). The relative sizes of these thalamic nuclei correspond to the relative amount of cerebral cortex devoted to the particular sense relayed by the nuclei, but the relation is perhaps easier to see in the thalamus. The largest of the three nuclei and its corresponding cortical region will be the unit corresponding to the primary sense the animal uses to explore its environment. Primates (including humans) are visual animals, or "beholders," and so have a relatively large visual thalamus and cortex. "Feelers," such as the raccoon and the rat, have a larger somatic sensory thalamus and cortex. Animals such as bats and porpoises are predominantly "listeners" and have a large auditory thalamus and cortex.

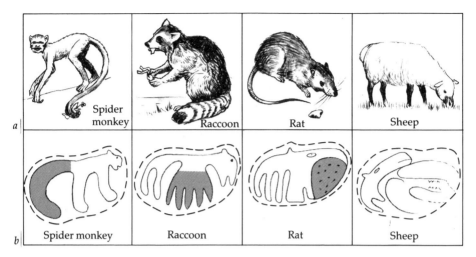

Figure 8-15 Within the modality of touch, in animals that are "feelers" the behaviorally most used and sensitive area of the body touch sense (upper panel) is much expanded in its representation on the somatic sensory area of the cerebral cortex (lower panel). The spider monkey explores with its tail, the raccoon with its forepaws, the rat with its whiskers and the sheep with its lips and tongue.

Thomas Woolsey and Hendrick van der Loos, working at Johns Hopkins University, discovered that in the somatic sensory thalamus of the rat and mouse, each whisker appears to have a separate region devoted to receiving information from it, which corresponds to the rat's extensive use of its whiskers to explore the world. Each whisker (vibrissa) connects to pressure receptors, which are very sensitive to movements of the whisker. They convey pressure information to the somatic sensory thalamus, which transmits it to the face region in the somatic area of the cerebral cortex. Each whisker is represented in the cortex by an individual *whisker barrel*, a column of neurons in layer IV that literally is barrel shaped. A whisker barrel consists of a cylinder of neurons surrounding a central area with many fewer neurons. In the small space between barrels there are almost no neurons. When you look at

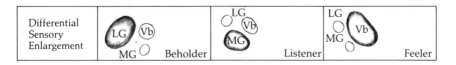

Figure 8-16 Relative sizes of the visual (LG) auditory (MG) and somatic sensory (Vb) thalamic relay nuclei in animals that can be classified in terms of their behavior as "beholders" (e.g., monkeys), "listeners" (e.g., rats) or "feelers" (e.g., raccoon).

this cortical tissue you can actually see the barrels (Figure 8-17). Each barrel is a column of neurons coding movement of a single whisker. Cortical columns are not merely abstractions from studies of nerve cell activity. At least in the case of whisker barrels, the columns are actual little structures in the brain.

There are actually several somatic sensory areas in the cortex. The primary, or SI, region can be subdivided into several areas in which different aspects or modalities of somatic sensory stimulation predominate. The middle or core region of SI receives cutaneous tactile information for fine discriminations of touch, whereas a surrounding shell region both anterior and posterior

Figure 8-17 A separate column of cells in the somatic sensory cortex of the rat and mouse serves each whisker. In layer IV , the neurons for a whisker form a barrellike structure. (*a*) Snout of a mouse with the vibrissae (whiskers) marked by dots. (*b*) Section running along layer IV of the somatic sensory cortex, which receives input from the snout. Note the ring of cells (whisker barrels), each corresponding to a single whisker. (*c*) Schematized pattern of the barrels.

a

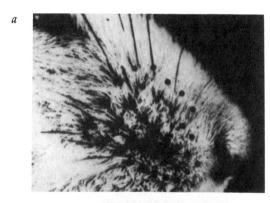

b

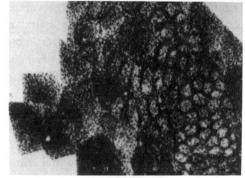

c

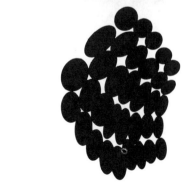

to the core area receives kinesthetic information (about limb positions and movements) and more diffuse pain and temperature information. There is also a small secondary region, SII, where the representation of the body surface is bilateral, in contrast to the contralateral, or opposite side, representation in SI. Little is known about the possible functional importance of SII. Finally, there is also somatic sensory representation in the primary motor cortex (see Chapter 9, particularly Figure 9-15).

AUDITORY SYSTEM

The degree of sensitivity in the human ear is such that a movement of the eardrum of less than one-tenth of the diameter of a hydrogen atom can result in an auditory sensation. If the ear were any more sensitive, the random Brownian movements of air molecules would produce a constant roaring sound masking other sounds. As a matter of fact, people with very good hearing are able to detect Brownian movement under ideal listening conditions, for example, in a soundproof, echo-free room.

In contrast to the million or so fibers in the optic nerve of humans, each auditory nerve consists of only 28,000 fibers. Nevertheless, the total number of single tones the ear can discriminate on the basis of frequency and intensity is about 340,000, approximately the total number of single visual stimuli discernible on the basis of frequency (wavelength) and intensity of light. Investigators have puzzled for years over the nature of the mechanisms underlying this efficiency in the auditory system.

Two important terms in hearing, pitch and frequency, are often confused. *Frequency* is the number of physical vibrations or sound waves in the air or another medium during some unit of time, commonly expressed in cycles per second (cps), or Hertz (Hz). (Cycles per second is the older term; 1 cps equals 1 Hz. Heinrich Hertz was a pioneering scientist in acoustics.) *Pitch*, on the other hand, is a subjective sensation correlated with the frequency of a sound. Middle C on the piano is 261.6 Hz and the C one octave above it is 523.2 Hz, or twice as high in frequency. However, the higher C sounds a good deal less than twice as high in pitch.

A similar distinction exists between the physical and subjective scales in the case of sound intensity. The relation between the subjectively judged loudness of a tone and the amount of physical energy in the tone is approximately logarithmic. The decibel scale, based on the logarithm of the sound energy level, relates the subjective and physical measures of sound intensity. The auditory system compresses a very wide range of stimulus energies, from the sound of a leaf blowing in the wind to a thunderclap, into a range of loudnesses that can be managed perceptually (Figure 8-18).

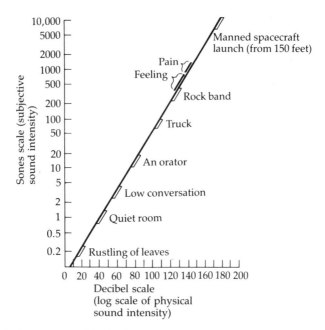

Figure 8-18 Comparison of the loudness of sounds. The decibel scale (abscissa) is a log scale of physical sound intensity and the sone scale (ordinate) is a scale of the subjective intensity of sounds: how loud we judge they sound. Our subjective experience of loudness is thus related to the logarithm of physical intensity—we compress a wide range of sound intensities into our perception of loudness.

The external ear canal ends in the *tympanic membrane*, or *eardrum*. The eardrum connects through the three small bones of the middle ear to a membrane covering the end of the *cochlea*, a coiled tube shaped much like a snail shell (Figure 8-19). The cochlea is actually a tube within a tube filled with fluid; the smaller tube, the *cochlear duct*, contains the sense organ proper. A cross section through the cochlear duct is also shown in Figure 8-18. Sound vibrations cause movement of the fluid in the cochlear duct, which in turn produces vibrations of the *basilar membrane*. This rather stiff membrane bends, activating hair cell receptors. These receptors are innervated by fibers of the auditory nerve, which enters the central nervous system and connects with the cochlear nuclei in the medulla. In humans, the total range of audible frequencies is from about 15 to about 20,000 Hz. The ear is the most sensitive, however, to tones between 1000 Hz and 4000 Hz. As the frequency increases or decreases beyond this range of maximum sensitivity, increasingly greater sound energy is required to make the tone audible (Figure 8-20). Several lines of evidence indicate that the physical characteristics of the external and middle ear structures, such as their elasticity and inertia, determine the form of the frequency-threshold curve.

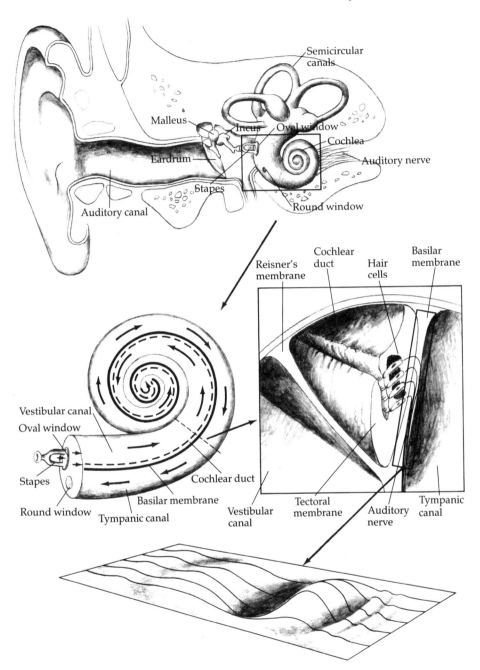

Figure 8-19 Key parts of the ear. Middle-ear bones transmit sounds from the eardrum to a membrane covering one end of the fluid-filled cochlea. The cochlea is a coiled tube containing the basilar membrane, which runs the length of the coiled cochlear tube and contains the hair cell receptors. A given sound sets up a pattern of standing waves in the cochlea so that only certain areas of hair cells are bent and thus activated. They in turn activate fibers of the auditory nerve.

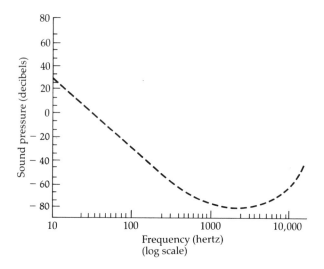

Figure 8-20 Absolute auditory threshold curve for humans. We are most sensitive to sound between about 1000 and 4000 hertz (infant cry). Smaller animals tend to be most sensitive to higher-frequency sounds. The elephant has the best low-frequency hearing.

Among mammals, elephants can hear sound at the lowest frequencies and small animals such as the rat are sensitive to extremely high frequencies. Humans, as one might suppose, have a frequency range somewhere between those of the elephant and the rat. Cats can hear sounds ranging from about 30 to 70,000 Hz. Bats and porpoises can hear exceptionally high-frequency sounds, to about 100,000 Hz. As we have seen, these animals emit high-frequency pulses of sound and determine the position of objects from the reflected sound pulses.

The movements of the basilar membrane in the cochlea in response to auditory stimuli were analyzed in a series of elegant experiments by Georg von Bekesy, who was awarded the Nobel prize in 1962 for his work. In essence, he showed that a tone of given frequency causes a standing-fluid wave to develop in the cochlea. The wave brings about a maximum displacement of a region of the basilar membrane, the location of which is related to the frequency of the tone.

The auditory pathways in the brain are much more complicated than the visual or somatic sensory pathways (Figure 8-21). Auditory information is relayed and processed through several nuclei before it arrives at the auditory nucleus of the thalamus (medial geniculate body), which relays it to the auditory cortex. Note that each cochlear nucleus sends ascending pathways up on each side of the brain stem; the pathways are bilateral.

What are the most important jobs of the auditory system? What aspects of sounds are the most important to animals and humans? At first, investigators

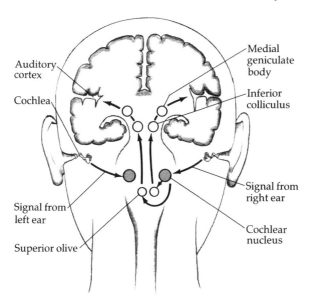

Figure 8-21 Simplified sketch of the auditory pathways. Auditory nerve fibers project to the cochlear nucleus. From here many fibers cross and ascend on the opposite side of the brain but many also ascend on the same side. Above the level of the cochlear nucleus, the auditory system is bilateral: each side of the brain has input from both ears. There are several relay nuclei in the auditory pathways, but the major pathway is from the cochlear nucleus to the inferior colliculus in the roof of the midbrain, from here to the medial geniculate body nucleus in the thalamus, and from the medial geniculate to the auditory region of the cerebral cortex.

focused on how the auditory system codes the frequencies of sounds, or pitch. Animals can of course distinguish many different sounds on the basis of pitch, a useful ability. However, prey animals or predators might find the ability to tell where a sound is coming from even more important.

Many neurons in the auditory system are exquisitely sensitive to differences in the properties of sounds at the two ears. If a sound occurs to one side or the other of an animal, the sound waves reach the two ears at slightly different times, and the sound is slightly more intense at the ear closest to it.

Neurons in a region called the *superior olive* (there is one on each side in the brainstem) have two large dendrites: a right dendrite that has input by way of the right ear and right cochlear nucleus and a left dendrite that has input from the left ear and left cochlear nucleus. These neurons can detect differences in the time of activation from the two ears on the order of microseconds (millionths of a second) (Figure 8-22).

Animals that hunt at night must find their way almost exclusively using sound cues, and they have developed remarkable specializations in the audi-

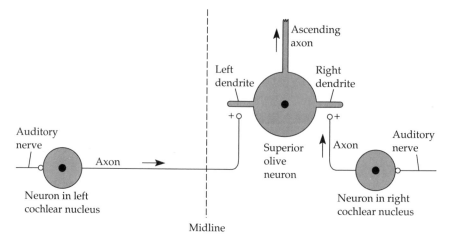

Figure 8-22 Schematic of a superior olive neuron receiving synaptic activation from sounds presented to the two ears via the cochlear nuclei. These neurons can detect time differences on the order of microseconds between activation of the right and left ears.

tory system. The barn owl, for example, has developed a special type of feathers around the face and ears that help it to detect sounds; it can localize sounds better than any other animal. The midbrain auditory nucleus (analogous to the mammalian inferior colliculus) is very large. The neurons in it respond to sounds from the two ears in such a way as to provide the bird with a very detailed and precise map of the space in front of it. The barn owl literally "sees" the world with its ears.

How does the auditory system code the pitch of sounds? Two major theories were developed in the nineteenth century, the place theory (Helmholz) and the frequency theory (Rutherford). The *place theory* argued that frequencies are coded by the place of activation of the hair cell receptors in the cochlea; the *frequency theory* favored the idea that pitch was coded by the frequency of discharge of neurons in the auditory system.

From the work of von Bekesy and others, it is now clear that the place of activation on the cochlea is the major mechanism. Different frequencies of sounds cause the greatest activation of different regions along the basilar membrane of the cochlea. The frequency theory is in part refuted because a given neuron cannot fire much more than about 1000 times per second (a frequency of 1000 Hz) in response to sound, yet we can hear frequencies of up to 20,000 Hz. The rate of cell discharge does appear, however, to be involved in our perception of low-frequency sounds, sounds below about 1000 Hz.

Less is known about the functional organization of the auditory cortex than about the visual or somatic sensory areas. The receptor surface, in this case regions of the basilar membrane and the corresponding hair cells, is mapped in the auditory cortex, and so there is frequency representation. Recent evidence suggests that there may be functional columns of cells in the primate auditory cortex that respond selectively to tone frequency, that is, pitch-detector columns. As is true of somatic sensory and visual areas, there appear to be a number of cortical auditory areas—six have been described in the monkey. Although much less is known about the auditory areas, they are likely to be at least as complex as the secondary visual areas, particularly in humans, who abstract from the basic properties of sounds to speech and language.

SUMMARY

Animals, including humans, are most sensitive to the stimuli impinging upon them from the external world that are most important for adaptive behavior in their environment. In humans and other primates, vision is the most important sense. The human eye can detect the smallest unit of light energy, a single photon. Most of the steps in this remarkable feat of detection by the rod receptors in the retina have been worked out. When a photon impinges on the rod it activates a simple chemical substance, retinal (similar to vitamin A), that is embedded in the complex protein rhodopsin. Retinal undergoes complex changes in its structure that result in activation of a second messenger (cyclic GMP) that closes sodium ion channels in the rod membrane, such that 1 million sodium ions are blocked from entering the rod. This in turn decreases glutamate release from the rod synapse on interneurons in the retina. These interneurons process the information and carry two kinds of messages to the ganglion cells, whose axons project to the brain as the optic nerve: on-center/off-surround and off-center/on-surround receptive fields (a receptive field for a ganglion cell is the total extent of the retina where visual stimuli influence the cell). Color is coded by three types of cones in the human (and old-world monkey) retina, each most sensitive red, green, or blue.

The visual pathways are so organized that the left half of each retina (right half of visual field) projects to the left visual thalamus and visual cortex and vice versa. The two hemisphere regions of visual cortex are interconnected by the corpus callosum. In the primary visual cortex (V1), the simple receptive fields of the retinal ganglion cells are built up into edge-, orientation-, and binocular-sensitive neurons, which exist in columns. In addition, color information is projected to "blob" regions in V1. There are a number of additional visual areas, receiving input ultimately from V1, that seem specialized for particular visual functions. Area V5 seems specialized for movement and depth perception, area V4 for color perception, and area V6 for shape perception.

The discovery that sensory areas of the cerebral cortex are organized into columns was first made for the somatic sensory area of the cortex. The representation of the body surface is projected via the thalamus to the primary somatic sensory area. Within each region of this area, columns of neurons are selectively sensitive to light touch, deep pressure, joint movement, and so on. Different types of receptors in skin, muscle, and joints are especially sensitive to those types of stimuli. In general the body surface map, or animunculus, is distorted in that the most sensitive regions have the greatest representation—judging by the cortex, humans are mostly fingers, lips and tongue. There are also other somatic sensory cortical areas.

The basilar membrane containing the hair cells in the inner ear is the receptive surface for auditory stimuli. Tone frequency is coded by standing wave patterns on the basilar membrane, tone intensity by amplitude of the wave patterns. The auditory nerve fibers are activated via the hair cells laid out along the basilar membrane. Different frequencies of sound activate different nerve fibers and different intensities activate more or fewer discharges in the fibers. Complex sounds like speech are thus coded by complex wave patterns on the basilar membrane and corresponding complex patterns of activation of auditory nerve fibers.

The projection pathways in the auditory system are more complex than in the visual system, involving several relay nuclei, and are largely bilateral (in contrast to the somatic sensory system, which is contralateral). The auditory system seems to be specialized to detect the locations of sound sources in the environment and, at least in humans, to analyze and differentiate very complex sounds, as in speech. There are several auditory areas in the cerebral cortex, but little is known about their possible functions.

The most important principle of organization in the cerebral cortex appears to be the cell column. All of the sensory areas of the cerebral cortex are organized into columns, which appear to code the different aspects or dimensions of sensory experience. What about the association areas? The visual temporal area that has cells that respond preferentially to an upright monkey hand is an association area, but not enough work has been done on it to know if it is organized into columns. There do appear to be complex functional columns of neurons in certain association areas of the cortex that have to do with voluntary, or intentional, movements. We shall consider these further in the next chapter.

SUGGESTED READINGS AND REFERENCES

Books

Aitkin, L. (1990). *The auditory cortex: Structural and functional bases of auditory perception.* London: Chapman and Hall.

Boynton, R. M. (1979). *Human color vision.* New York: Holt, Rinehart and Winston.

De Valois, R. L., and De Valois, K. K. (1988). *Spatial vision.* New York: Oxford University Press.

Dowling, J. E. (1987). *The retina: An approachable part of the brain.* Cambridge, MA: Harvard University Press.

Dowling, J. E. (1992). *Neurons and networks: An introduction to neuroscience.* Cambridge, MA: Belknap Press of Harvard University Press.

Edelman, G. M., Gall, W. E., and Cowan, W. M. (1988). *Auditory functions.* New York: John Wiley & Sons.

Gulick, W. L., Gescheider, G. A., and Frisina, R. D. (1989). *Hearing: Physiological acoustics, neural coding, and psychoacoustics.* New York: Oxford University Press.

Hubel, D. H. (1988). *Eye, brain, and vision.* New York: W. H. Freeman.

Articles

Darian-Smith, I. (1982). Touch in primates. *Annual Review of Psychology, 33,* 155–194.

Hudspeth, A. J. (1985). The cellular basis of hearing: The biophysics of hair cells. *Science, 230,* 745–752.

Livingstone, M., and Hubel, D. (1988). Segregation of form, color, movement, and depth: Anatomy, physiology, and perception. *Science, 240,* 740–749.

Lund, J. S. (1988). Anatomical organization of macaque monkey striate visual cortex. *Annual Review of Neuroscience, 11,* 253–288.

Maunsell, J. H. R., and Newsome, W. T. (1987). Visual processing in monkey extrastriate cortex. *Annual Review of Neuroscience, 10,* 363–402.

Schnapf, J. L., and Baylor, D. A. (1987). How photoreceptors respond to light. *Scientific American, 256,* 40–47.

Stryer, L. (1986). Cyclic GMP cascade of vision. *Annual Review of Neuroscience, 9,* 87–119.

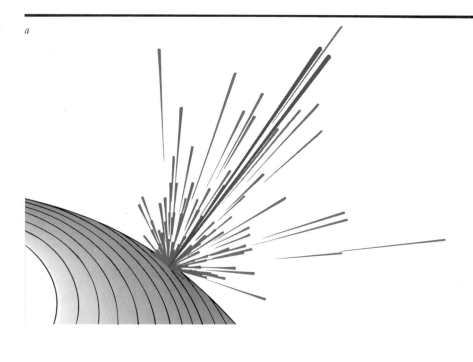

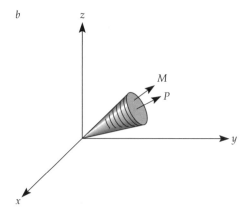

9

Motor Control Systems

The purpose of the brain is to produce behavior. Virtually all behavior consists of movements resulting from the actions of the skeletal muscles; the only other observable behavior comes from the actions of smooth and cardiac muscles and glands. All these behaviors are generated and controlled by the motor neurons. There is, of course, much more to the behavior of complex organisms, particularly humans, than the overt muscle and gland actions we can measure. Hormone actions, learning and memory, consciousness, and many other processes and events transpire inside the body and brain that can have consequences for behavior. These processes and events, however, can be seen or expressed only through their products, muscle movements and gland secretions.

The skeletal musculature, the striated muscles attached to the bones of the body that produce most of our behavior, will be the focus of this chapter. Thanks to our skeletal muscles, we can perform any number of complicated

Figure 9-1 (a) Cluster of the "movement vectors" of 224 cells in monkey motor cortex. Each of these cells responded when the monkey reached in a number of close directions but tended to respond most for a particular direction, which was not necessarily very close to the actual direction (thick line). However, when all the individual direction vectors were added together, the population vector (thickest line) predicted the actual direction of movement precisely. (b) Schematic of the 95% "confidence cone" (statistical significance) around the population vector P shown. The direction of movement vector M falls within the cone.

behaviors: play tennis, speak, and initiate the intricate eye movements that make reading possible. The skeletal muscles are all innervated by or connected by, the axons of the alpha motor neurons. The cell bodies of these neurons lie in the spinal cord gray matter, where they are collected into groups, or nuclei, one serving each muscle, and also in the cranial nerve motor nuclei of the brain stem.

The notion of levels of organization or hierarchies of function is useful in considering the brain systems that generate and control movement. At the spinal level, local feedback circuits control each muscle. Stretch receptors in the muscle send information about muscle tension and degree of stretch back to the spinal cord and there synapse directly on the alpha motor neurons that innervate the muscle. The *gamma motor neurons*, another class of motor neurons, go to the special fibers in the muscle that contain stretch receptors and control the fibers, making them more or less active. The only way that the descending pathways from the brain can produce or influence muscle activity is by acting on the alpha or gamma motor neurons. More will be said about the gamma system later on in the chapter; for now, the important point is that only the alpha motor neurons can produce measurable contraction of a muscle.

A variety of local circuits in the spinal cord control reflex movements, and there are motor control systems at every major level of the brain: in the brain stem, midbrain, and forebrain. Two brain structures seem to be almost entirely concerned with movement: the cerebellum, an evolutionarily very old structure, and the basal ganglia in the forebrain. A substantial part of the cerebral cortex, the motor and somatic sensory region, is also much involved in movement control. Indeed, it has been said that the fundamental purpose of the brain is to produce movement.

NEUROMUSCULAR SYSTEM

In terms of structural characteristics there are three general types of muscle tissue: striated, smooth, and cardiac (Figure 9-2). *Smooth muscle* and *cardiac muscle* are under the control of the autonomic part of the nervous system. These muscles continue to function after all neural control is eliminated, whereas *striated muscle* is useless after the nerves connecting with it are cut. Biologists sometimes classify striated muscle activity as "voluntary" and smooth and cardiac muscle activity as "involuntary." The label voluntary could almost be used for all the muscle actions a person can make on request. Some people can learn to control certain smooth muscle actions, such as the heartbeat rate, and some striated muscle responses are involuntary or at least unconscious, such as postural adjustments.

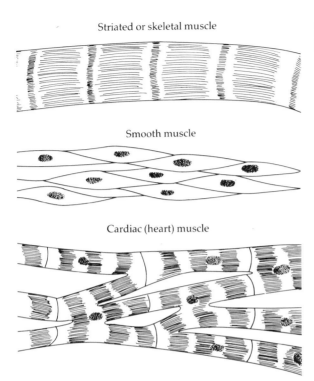

Striated or skeletal muscle

Smooth muscle

Cardiac (heart) muscle

Figure 9-2 Types of muscle fibers.

In gross appearance striated muscle seems to be made up of many small fibers all running lengthwise. A striated muscle is attached to a bone at each end by tendons and tough connective tissue. Each muscle fiber is a separate entity but not necessarily a single cell, as there are a number of cell nuclei in each fiber. Striated muscle fibers are of two types, extrafusal and intrafusal. The *extrafusal fibers* are those that actively contract, and they make up most of the muscle. The *intrafusal fibers* contain the spindle organs, which send signals back to the spinal cord about the degree of stretch of the muscle.

In the normal animal striated muscles are activated by nerve fibers. Each efferent (output) nerve fiber to a muscle branches and innervates several of the muscle fibers. The basic unit of action of the neuromuscular system is the *motor unit*, which consists of a single efferent nerve fiber that comes from a single motor neuron together with the muscle fibers it innervates (Figure 9-3). The number of muscle fibers per nerve fiber (the innervation ratio) ranges from about three to one for small muscles concerned with fine movement control, as in the fingers, to over 150 to one for large muscles such as the back muscles. A spike discharge conducted along the axon of a single motor neuron

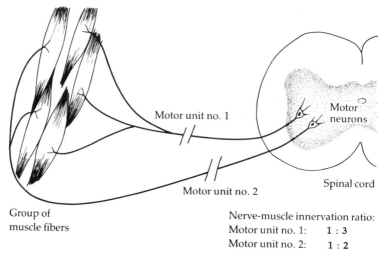

Motor unit no. 1

Motor unit no. 2

Motor
neurons

Spinal cord

Group of
muscle fibers

Nerve-muscle innervation ratio:
Motor unit no. 1: **1 : 3**
Motor unit no. 2: **1 : 2**

Figure 9-3 A motor unit consists of a single motor neuron axon and all the muscle fibers it innervates. A given motor neuron axon can innervate from as few as two or three muscle fibers, as is the case for the muscles controlling the fingers, to more than 100, as in the back muscles. A given striated muscle fiber never receives input from more than one motor neuron.

travels out all the axon branches and activates all the muscle fibers receiving its branches. The whole set of muscle fibers acts as a unit; all fibers contract or none does.

The neuromuscular junctions where motor neurons synapse on striated muscle fibers involve the fast ACh synaptic transmission, discussed at length in Chapter 4. When the action potential arrives at the motor axon terminal, calcium channels open, Ca^+ rushes in, and molecules of ACh are released at the synapse from vesicles, diffuse across to the muscle, and attach to ACh receptors, activating the muscle fiber. The ACh is then broken down by AChE. The initial step in the contraction of the muscle is the depolarization of the muscle membrane by the activated ACh receptors (Figure 9-4).

Each striated muscle fiber is made up of many smaller fibers called *myofibrils*, which are the basic units of action (Figure 9-5). The myofibrils appear striated under the light microscope. Each myofibril consists of a series of contractile elements, the *sarcomeres* (Figure 9-5). The sarcomeres are made up of still smaller subunits containing the contractile proteins *actin* and *myosin*. These proteins are present in all cells and provide the basic mechanism for cell movement or mobility. In striated muscle, actin and myosin are organized so that they can move bones at joints and hence move the entire animal rather than merely individual cells.

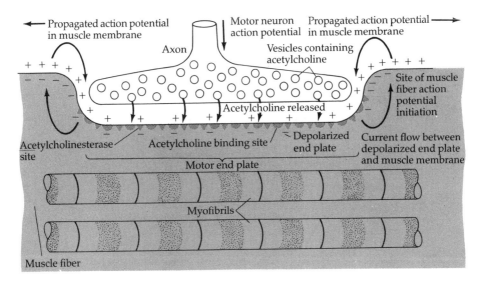

Figure 9-4 Neuromuscular junction on a striated muscle fiber.

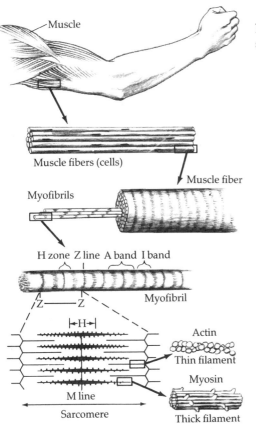

Figure 9-5 Components of a striated muscle fiber.

The contraction of the skeletal muscles is thought to be well described by the *sliding-filament model*. (What follows may be more than some readers will want to know about muscle contraction, but muscles are intimately connected with behavior, and it is a straightforward story.) Filaments of actin and myosin are interlocked within each muscle fiber. The thicker myosin filaments have large "heads" at right angles to the rest of the filament, which stick out toward the adjacent and much thinner actin filaments (Figure 9-6). The ends of these heads bind to the actin filaments when the muscle contracts. The energy for muscle contraction comes from ATP, which attaches to the myosin heads and is broken down into ADP, releasing energy. (As you know, muscle contractions use considerable amounts of energy.)

The thin actin filaments are actually composed of actin molecules wrapped around by chains of another protein, *tropomyosin*, which is bound up with still another kind of protein, *troponin*. Troponin is the calcium binding site (Figure 9-6). The sites on the actin molecules to which the myosin heads bind are covered by the tropomyosin chains when the muscle is not contract-

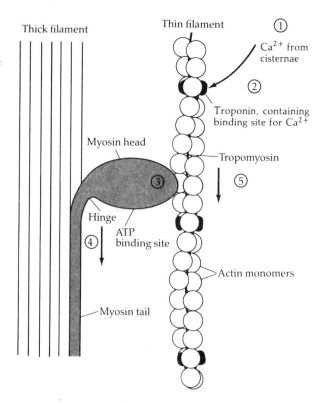

Figure 9-6 The myosin heads connect the thick and thin filaments of the muscle fiber and slide them across each other when activated.

Thick filament

Thin filament

① Ca²⁺ from cisternae

②

Troponin, containing binding site for Ca²⁺

Myosin head

Tropomyosin

③ ⑤

Hinge

ATP binding site ④

Actin monomers

Myosin tail

ing, preventing myosin from binding. When calcium ions bind to the troponin molecules, the tropomyosin chains move aside, exposing the myosin-head binding sites and allowing the myosin heads to bind to the actin molecules (Figure 9-7). At this point the ATP energy reaction at the myosin heads occurs, and the myosin heads bind, moving or sliding the actin and myosin filaments across each other. This results in contraction of the muscle fiber. The breakdown of ATP into ADP triggers the binding of more ATP to the myosin heads, which causes them to let go of the actin binding sites, and the muscle relaxes.

How does the nerve impulse trigger this series of events? When ACh molecules are released from the motor neuron terminal by an action potential and attach to the ACh receptors on the muscle fiber, the muscle fiber membrane becomes depolarized, as we noted. The outer membrane depolarization is conducted by tubules into the internal region of the muscle fiber called the *sarcoplasmic reticulum*, which is a system of tubules, or *cisternae*, surrounding each muscle fiber (Figure 9-8). When the cisternae are depolarized they release free calcium ions. The calcium ions bind to receptors on troponin and trigger the chain of events that leads to contraction of the muscle fiber.

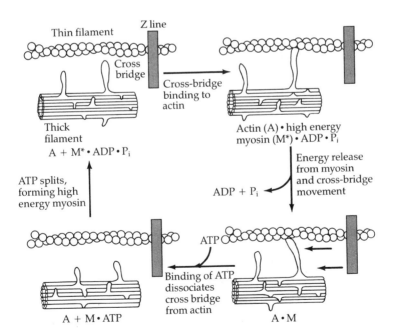

Figure 9-7 The sequence of events that result in the muscle fiber contracting. The sequence begins with the relaxed fiber at the upper left of the drawing.

Figure 9-8 Muscle contraction by synaptic activation of the muscle fiber (Figure 9-4). When the action potential develops in the muscle fiber membrane and sodium ions rush in, it triggers the release of bound calcium in a region of the fiber called the sarcoplasmic reticulum. The free calcium binds to the troponin molecules of the thin filament (Figure 9-6) and triggers the sequence of events shown in Figure 9-7.

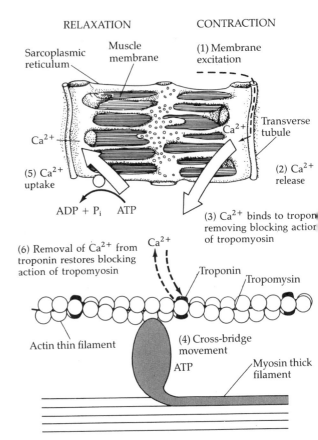

RELAXATION CONTRACTION

Sarcoplasmic reticulum Muscle membrane (1) Membrane excitation

Ca^{2+} Ca^{2+} Transverse tubule

(5) Ca^{2+} uptake (2) Ca^{2+} release

$ADP + P_i$ ATP

(3) Ca^{2+} binds to troponin removing blocking action of tropomyosin

(6) Removal of Ca^{2+} from troponin restores blocking action of tropomyosin Ca^{2+}

Troponin Tropomysin

Actin thin filament

(4) Cross-bridge movement

ATP Myosin thick filament

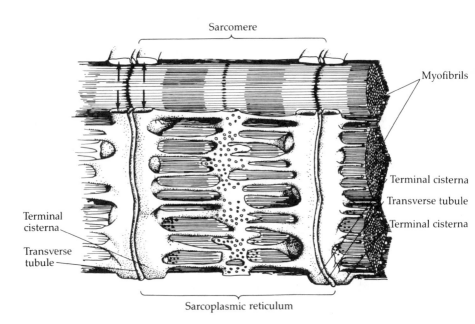

Sarcomere

Myofibrils

Terminal cisterna

Transverse tubule

Terminal cisterna

Terminal cisterna

Transverse tubule

Sarcoplasmic reticulum

The muscle contraction process is what happens when a muscle fiber is activated by one nerve impulse. Such a contraction, a "twitch," can be produced in the laboratory by giving a single electric stimulus to a motor nerve in, say, a frog's leg. The depolarization of the muscle fiber by a single nerve impulse lasts only a few milliseconds, but the contraction process takes much longer. For about 10 milliseconds after the nerve impulse nothing happens. Then the muscle fiber begins to contract, reaching a peak about 70 milliseconds after the depolarization. Normally, however, motor nerve fibers do not fire just once and then remain inactive. They fire at some slow rate, causing the contractions of the muscle fibers to add together over time and so yield some average level of contraction. As the firing rate of the motor nerve fiber increases, so does the contraction of the muscle, and vice versa.

SPINAL REFLEXES

The nervous systems of the most primitive vertebrates, such as a lamprey, are essentially a rudimentary spinal cord with a little brain tissue at the top to handle sensory information from light and chemical receptors. The human spinal cord is a complicated assemblage that can bring about adaptive behavior. An animal with its spinal cord severed from its brain (a spinal animal) can maintain muscle tone and some degree of posture and movement; it can remove its paws from painful stimuli, scratch an itch, and even learn very simple conditioned reflexes.

The spinal cord is a vital structure in movement. It contains the motor neurons that innervate all the muscles of the body below the head. In order for you to execute any body movement, whether running a race or performing microsurgery, many of these groups of motor neurons must be activated in very precise and controlled ways. The motor systems of the brain are in large part the activators of the motor neurons in the spinal cord, but spinal reflexes have an important share in the control of movement. The connections of some of the major types of motor neurons in the spinal cord are indicated in Figure 9-9.

Stretch Reflex and Flexion Reflex

We shall consider briefly two simple examples of spinal reflexes: the stretch reflex and the flexion reflex. The *stretch reflex* is a *monosynaptic reflex*, meaning that there is only one set of synapses between the sensory fibers and the motor neurons involved in the reflex (Figure 9-9). When a muscle is stretched,

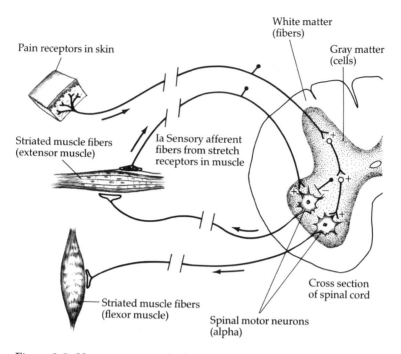

Pain receptors in skin

White matter
(fibers)

Gray matter
(cells)

Striated muscle fibers
(extensor muscle)

Ia Sensory afferent
fibers from stretch
receptors in muscle

Cross section
of spinal cord

Striated muscle fibers
(flexor muscle)

Spinal motor neurons
(alpha)

Figure 9-9 How motor control of muscles reacts to sensory information from the skin and muscles. If an extensor muscle is stretched, the large Ia fibers in the spindle organ receptor in the muscle (see Figure 9-10) are activated and connect directly to the alpha motor neurons to that same muscle to cause it to contract (stretch reflex). However, if the skin overlying this same extensor muscle is pinched, afferents from the skin act through interneurons to inhibit the motor neurons that connect to this extensor muscle and excite motor neurons to flexor muscles that will move the body part away from the pinch (flexion reflex).

sensory fibers connected to it act through the spinal cord directly on the motor neurons that control the same muscle, causing it to contract. The knee-jerk reflex is an example of a stretch reflex. A tap to the patellar tendon just below the kneecap stretches leg extensor muscles and activates the stretch receptors, which in turn activate their alpha motor neurons in the spinal cord. The alpha neurons then signal the muscle to contract, extending the leg. The general function of the stretch reflex is not to cause knee jerks, however, or other quick muscle contractions. Rather, it maintains posture and the overall tone of muscles while you are engaged in movements. Instead of thinking of it as a reflex, think of it as a system that tends to increase the contraction of muscles that are stretched.

The *flexion reflex* is a basic defensive tactic against bodily injury. If your finger touches a hot stove, your arm jerks away before you even feel the heat or the pain of the burn. Flexion is a *polysynaptic reflex*, meaning that more than one set of synapses occur between the sensory fibers and the motor neurons that make up the reflex pathway (Figure 9-9). Touching the hot stove activates fast pain fibers in the skin of the fingers. These fibers connect through interneurons in the spinal cord to act powerfully on flexor motor neurons, which activate flexor muscles. These muscles flex the arms and legs and pull them away from injury.

All of the higher motor systems in the brain act on the motor neurons of the reflex machinery of the spinal cord, by way of pathways that descend through the brain and spinal cord. Spinal reflex activity, particularly the stretch reflex, is always going on, determined by sensory input from the muscles, joints, skin and other sources in the body.

Sensory Information from Muscles

Sensory control of reflex activity is of two forms. The first is the control provided by the sensory receptors in the muscles and tendons, which transmit rather complete information to the spinal cord and brain concerning the state of muscles: the degree of tension, the rapidity, extent, direction, and duration of changes in tension, and so on. The other form of control is provided by the gamma motor neurons in the spinal cord, which exert direct control on the sensory receptors in muscles. The gamma motor neurons do not produce direct changes in muscle tension but instead modify the degree of activity of certain of the stretch receptors in the muscles. In a sense this action is the opposite of the traditional reflex; instead of sensory input determining motor output, motor output determines sensory input. The sensory input from the muscles, of course, induces alterations in the motor output as well, which in turn modifies sensory input, and so on. The system represents a rather complex and elegant example of feedback control (Figure 9-10).

Individual muscle bundles are of two types, regular muscle bundles made up of extrafusal fibers, which are the contractile elements of the muscles discussed above, and sparser bundles made up of intrafusal fibers, which contain the spindle organs. Throughout muscles, the occasional *spindle organs* are intermingled with regular muscle bundles and are attached to tendons or to regular muscle bundles. Spindle organs always lie parallel to the regular muscle bundles. Although the intrafusal fibers of the spindle organ are muscle fibers and do contract, they contract very weakly and contribute nothing to the overall pull of the muscle, which is left entirely to contractions of the ex-

Figure 9-10 Arrangement of intrafusal and extrafusal fibers in muscle. All of the pull exerted by the muscle is by the extrafusal fibers. The intrafusal fiber is connected in parallel. When the muscle is pulled or stretched, it is stretched and activated. When the muscle actively contracts, the stretch on it is actually relaxed so that it is not activated. The tendon organs in the tendons where the muscle fibers attach to the bone, on the other hand, are in series, so that they are stretched and activated whether the muscle is stretched or contracted.

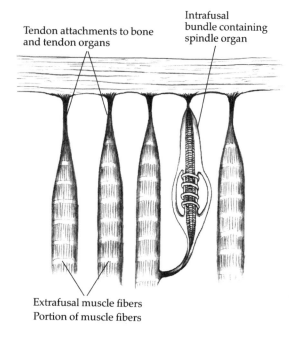

Tendon attachments to bone and tendon organs

Intrafusal bundle containing spindle organ

Extrafusal muscle fibers
Portion of muscle fibers

trafusal fiber bundles. The gamma motor neurons of the spinal cord activate and cause contraction of the intrafusal fibers of the spindle organ, which in turn stretch and activate the spindle afferent fibers. These fibers in turn play back on the alpha motor neurons to the muscle to cause changes in muscle tension (Figure 9-10).

Because the spindle organ is connected in parallel with the muscle bundles, tension on the spindle organ is reduced when the muscle bundles contract, which reduces the activity of the spindle afferent (sensory) gamma motor neurons connecting with the spindle. When the muscle is stretched, the spindles also stretch and hence are activated. The spindle afferents have a moderately high spontaneous discharge rate, but the rate of spontaneous firing of spindle afferent fibers is directly related to the degree of muscle tension. The afferent fiber terminals from the spindle organ are found in its enlarged central region (Figure 9-11).

The gamma motor system has a general significance that extends beyond its role in spinal reflex activity. A number of descending pathways from the brain and upper regions of the spinal cord exert excitatory and inhibitory control on the gamma motor neurons. In this way many higher control systems can exert influence on muscle tension without necessarily causing direct

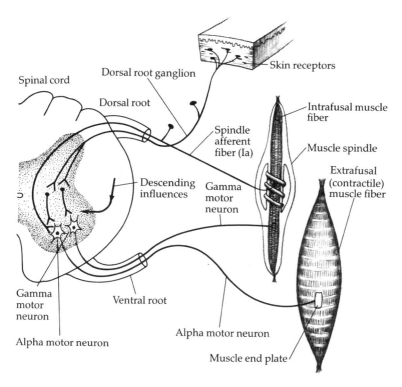

Figure 9-11 Spindle organ in its specialized intrafusal muscle fiber (see also Figure 9-10) sending stretch information via its Ia sensory fiber. The spindle organ in turn is controlled by a special type of motor neuron—the gamma motor neuron—that, when active, causes the intrafusal fibers to contract and activate the spindle organ, thus activating the Ia sensory fiber from the spindle. This in turn activates the alpha motor neuron that causes the extrafusal fibers of the same muscle to contract (see Figures 9-9 and 9-10).

contraction or relaxation of the contractile muscle fibers. An increase or decrease in the degree of contraction of the muscle spindle fibers alters the degree of spindle afferent activity and hence the probability that the contractile muscle fibers will respond. This occurs to some extent independently of what state of contraction the muscle fiber is in: just before the starting gun, the runner has a high level of readiness to respond, even though he or she is motionless.

Another type of muscle receptor of importance is the *Golgi tendon organ*, or receptor. This is simply an afferent nerve fiber whose terminals lie in the tendons joining muscle and bone. The terminals proliferate in the tendon fibers close to the muscle-tendon connection (Figure 9-11).

In physical terms the tendons and their tendon organs are in series with the muscle bundles. They are activated when a muscle contracts because the muscle pulls on the tendon attachments when it contracts, which compresses and activates the tendon organs. If the muscle is stretched by a passive pull (as when muscles with an action antagonistic to a muscle contract), the tendon organ is also activated. However, the tendon organ has a relatively high discharge threshold and is not activated by moderate resting tension in a muscle. Hence only a fairly rapid change in the muscle tension, either a contraction or a relaxation, will cause a burst of activity in the fibers from the Golgi tendon organ. Its spontaneous discharge rate is lower than that of the spindle organ for a muscle under a given amount of tension.

The complex and elaborate sensory feedback systems for muscles suggest that movements might be crucially dependent on such feedback. It has been known for many years that if all the dorsal roots that convey sensory information from one arm of a monkey are cut, the animal simply does not use that arm. More recent observations indicate, however, that in monkeys a striking degree of movement control can develop even if sensory information from both arms is abolished. Such monkeys can learn to move an arm to a particular extent to ward off shock to the ear, even when they are prevented from seeing their arms. Thus, a learned arm movement can develop in the complete absence of all sensory information regarding the position and movement of the arm. There are higher-order feedback systems within the brain itself that provide information back to the brain motor systems about where the body and limbs ought to be for a given movement, as we shall see.

CEREBELLUM

The cerebellum is one of the oldest structures in the history of the vertebrate nervous system. It is well developed in fish and reptiles and very much elaborated in birds and mammals. In mammals, the cerebellum consists of a very large number of neurons. It has been said, tongue in cheek, that if the brain consists of 10^{11} neurons, 10^{12} of them are granule cells in the cerebellum. The general function of the cerebellum is clearly motor in nature, but the detailed mechanisms of its action are only now beginning to be understood.

The overall structure of the cerebellum is somewhat analogous to that of the cerebrum; the cellular layers form a *cortex* of *gray matter* that covers *white matter* and several deep *nuclei* (collections of neuron cell bodies). The cerebellum is highly convoluted in appearance, with considerable areas of cortex buried in fissures. The general location of the cerebellum is dorsal to (above) the brain stem and posterior to the cerebrum (Figure 9-12). In primates it is

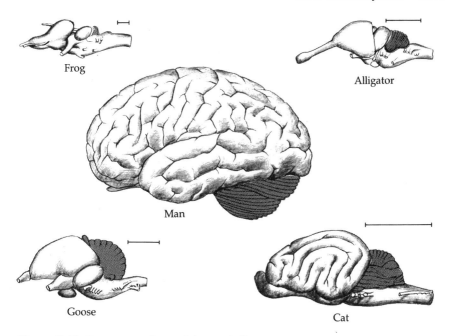

Frog

Alligator

Man

Goose

Cat

Figure 9-12 Location and size of the cerebellum in several species.

almost completely covered over by the occipital lobes of the cerebral hemispheres.

Input to the cerebellum includes all varieties of sensory information. On the cortex of the cerebellum there are detailed somatic sensory maps projected from the skin and body, just as on the cerebral cortex. In addition, strong input from the spindle organs and other muscle receptors provide the cerebellum with detailed information about the state of contraction of the muscles. Powerful vestibular input conveys information about head position. Neurons carrying auditory and visual information also project to the cerebellum, but not in nearly as much detail as is the case for the cerebral cortex. The major outputs of the cerebellum are relayed through a variety of brain structures concerned with the control of movement. Of particular importance are detailed reciprocal interconnections between the cerebellum and the sensory-motor areas of the cerebral cortex.

Masao Ito, a neuroscientist at Tokyo University, made a most important discovery that changed many of the ideas previously held about the functional organization of the cerebellum. All output from the cerebellar cortex occurs via the axons of the *Purkinje cells*, which are large neurons in the cerebellar cortex (Figure 9-13). Purkinje cell axons go mostly to the *cerebellar subcortical nuclei*, with a portion going to the *vestibular nuclei*. Ito demonstrated that all

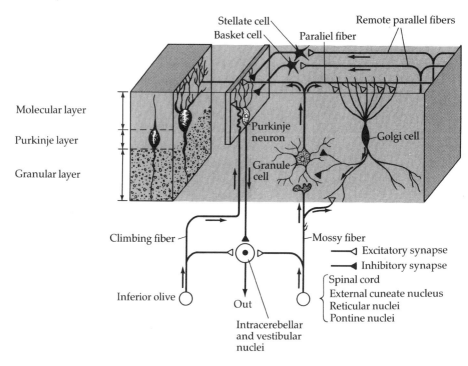

Figure 9-13 The basic wiring diagram of the cerebellar cortex is common to a wide range of species. Purkinje cells are excited directly by climbing fibers and indirectly by the mossy fibers, by way of the granule cells and parallel fibers. Stellate and basket cells are excited by parallel fibers and are inhibitory interneurons, acting to inhibit Purkinje cells. The Golgi cells act to inhibit the granule cells when excited by parallel fibers. The output of the Purkinje cells is inhibitory on the cells of their target structures (cerebellar and vestibular nuclei). See also Figure 9-1.

Purkinje cells exert inhibitory actions on all the cells on which their axons terminate. More specifically, they induce postsynaptic inhibition on all their target cells. Evidence is strong that the chemical inhibitory transmitter released by the axon terminals of Purkinje cells is gamma-aminobutyric acid (GABA), the inhibitory amino acid transmitter (see Chapter 4).

It may seem somewhat puzzling that the Purkinje cells are exclusively inhibitory. Since Purkinje cells are the only output from the cerebellar cortex, the cerebellum might seem to be a large mass of neural tissue whose only function is to inhibit. Actually, this is not quite the case. The major outputs from the cerebellum as a whole come from the cells that constitute the subcortical cerebellar nuclei. Sensory input to the cerebellum goes to both the cerebellar cortex and the underlying nuclei. The cells in the subcortical nuclei normally exhibit high levels of activity. The Purkinje cells from the cerebellar cortex for the most part terminate on these cells, and consequently, the inhibitory actions of the Purkinje cell axons can function as a higher-order loop to modulate and tune temporal patterns of activity in the cells of the subcortical cerebellar nuclei. The cerebellar cortex thus becomes a system that exerts its influence by continuously and selectively modulating or damping the ongoing activity of the subcortical cells that act on the motor systems of the brain.

The neuronal circuitry of the cerebellum is among the best understood in the brain. The basic wiring diagrams are relatively simple, as indicated in Figure 9-13. The cerebellum is organized into a large and convoluted cortex and a group of deep nuclei, as we saw. There are two major input pathways to the cerebellum: the climbing fibers and the mossy fibers. The *climbing fibers* come from a brain stem nucleus called the *inferior olive*, which in turn receives input from several brain regions and spinal cord pathways. The *mossy fibers* come from several sources in the brain and spinal cord. Both the climbing fibers and the mossy fibers pass the deep nuclei and project to the cerebellar cortex. In passing, they give off synapses onto neurons of the deep nuclei. Thus there is a pathway from other brain structures to neurons of the deep nuclei and back out to other brain structures. The vast cerebellar cortex lies above the deep nuclei, acting only on them and only to inhibit them.

The climbing fibers from the neurons in the inferior olive have a very precise and localized projection to the cerebellar cortex. Each Purkinje neuron has one and only one climbing fiber forming a synapse on it. The axon from each inferior olive neuron branches and sends climbing fiber terminals to several Purkinje neurons. The climbing fiber wraps around the Purkinje neuron dendrites close to the cell body and exerts a powerful excitatory synaptic action. Indeed, this climbing fiber synapse is the exception to the rule that a single excitatory synapse cannot evoke an action potential in a brain neuron (Chapter 3). It does.

The possible functions of the inferior olive climbing fibers have proved an interesting puzzle. The olive neurons, and hence their climbing fiber axons, have a very low spontaneous discharge rate, 2 to 4 seconds, much too low to provide information about, for example, the positions or movements of the limbs. Activity seems to be evoked in climbing fibers particularly when mistakes in movements are made, for example, you are walking down a flight of stairs, not paying enough attention, and think there is one more stair than there is. In aversive learning—learning with an unpleasant unconditioned stimulus such as a shock—the climbing fiber system appears to convey unconditioned stimulus information to the cerebellum (see Chapter 11). So in general terms, the inferior olive climbing fiber system appears to convey error signals—signals to the cerebellum that an error in a movement has occured.

The mossy fibers synapse on the ubiquitous granule cells, which give rise to parallel fibers. A given parallel fiber may synapse, in passing, on the dendrites of up to 100 Purkinje neurons and exerts a weak excitatory action. But each Purkinje neuron receives about 200,000 parallel fiber synapses! The cerebellar cortex also has several types of interneurons and they are all inhibitory (Figure 9-13). The mossy fiber-granule cells provide detailed information to the cerebellum about the positions and movements of limbs, about what parts of the skin surface are being stimulated, and about auditory and visual stimuli. You will recall from Chapter 8 that the somatic sensory and motor areas have multiple "maps" representing the skin surface. The cerebellar cortex has maps as well, but they are fractured and broken up—a bit of face may be represented next to a finger. The topology of the body surface is not maintained, whereas the topology is maintained on the skin surface maps on the cerebral cortex. This *fractured somatotopy* on cerebellar cortex was worked out in detail by Wally Welker at the University of Wisconsin.

The cerebellar cortex differs from the cerebral cortex in another way as well. The wiring diagram, the cytoarchitectonic organization, is the same everywhere in the cortex of the cerebellum. You may recall from Chapters 1 and 8 that this is not the case in the cerebral cortex—layer IV is much expanded in sensory areas, layer V is expanded in motor areas, and so on.

Another striking fact about cerebellar cortex is that its cytoarchitectonic organization is identical in all mammals from mouse to human. But the size of this extraordinarily uniform structure has expanded apace with the expansion of the cerebral cortex in evolution. The area of human cerebellar cortex is vast, rivaling the area of the cerebral cortex in extent—it is much more fissured than the cerebral cortex. The *neocerebellum*, the most recent region of the cerebellar cortex to evolve, is interconnected with the most recently evolved association areas of the cerebral cortex.

The extraordinary organization of the cerebellar cortex—the fact that the only output neurons, the Purkinje cells, receive only one climbing fiber per cell, but 200,000 parallel fibers per cell—led scientists who develop theoretical models of neural systems, most notably David Marr at the Massachusetts Institute of Technology, to speculate that the cerebellum is a learning machine par excellence whose job is to learn, store, and remember memories for skilled movements. The pioneering neuroscientists who worked out the basic functional organization of the cerebellum, Sir John Eccles, Masao Ito, and János Szentágothai, put it this way:

> The immense computational machinery of the cerebellum with a neuronal
> population that may exceed that of the rest of the nervous system gives rise to the

concept that the cerebellar cortex is not simply a fixed computing device, but that it contains in its structure the neuronal connexions developed in relationship to learned skills. We have to envisage that the cerebellum plays a major role in the performance of all skilled actions and hence that it can learn from experience so that its performance to any given input is conditioned by this "remembered experience." (Eccles, J. C., Ito, M., and Szentágothai, J. 1967. *The cerebellum as a neuronal machine*. New York: Springer-Verlag, p. 314.)

Recent work in my laboratory has established that this is indeed the case for the learning of elementary skilled movements (Chapter 11).

Perhaps the most important functional interconnection of the cerebellum is to the motor–sensory area of the cerebral cortex. The cerebellum and motor cortex form a massive loop system that is continuously active in the control of movement. The major pathways of the system are shown in Figure 9-18. Fibers from the deep cerebellar nuclei cross and ascend to terminate in a large nucleus in the thalamus. This nucleus projects to the motor areas of the cerebral cortex. There is a very precise region-to-region projection from the cerebellum to the motor cortex. The motor cortex sends fibers in descending pathways to control motor neurons and sends many fibers to nuclei in the pons of the brain stem—the *pontine nuclei*. These in turn project to the cerebellum via the mossy fibers.

When an animal is engaged in making a voluntary movement, neurons in both the cerebellum and the motor cortex are massively activated. Edward Evarts and his associates at the National Institutes of Health in Washington compared the activity of neurons in the two structures when a trained monkey makes a movement. Interestingly, neurons in the cerebellum increase their activity before neurons in the motor cortex do. This suggests that the cerebellum is in some way "closer" to whatever mechanism initiates a voluntary movement.

BASAL GANGLIA

The functions in mammals of the group of brain nuclei called the basal ganglia are not entirely clear (Figure 9-14). We do know that they have something to do with the control of movements. Parkinson's disease is the best known of several clinical syndromes that occur in humans following damage to the basal ganglia. Parkinson's is a chronic and progressive disorder of movement. Its incidence is about 100 per 100,000 of the total population, but the incidence is much higher in older people. The severity of the disorder varies a great deal,

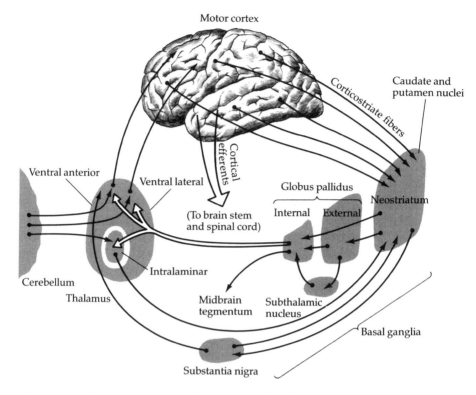

Figure 9-14 Major connections of the basal ganglia: the caudate, putamen, and globus pallidus. The dopamine-containing pathway from the substantia nigra to the caudate nucleus is involved in Parkinson's disease. The major input to the basal ganglia comes directly from virtually all regions of the cerebral cortex. The major output of the basal ganglia is to the motor areas of the cerebral cortex by way of the thalamus.

ranging from mild difficulty in moving to serious impairment. Perhaps you have seen elderly people with the disease. They typically have a slow, shuffling walk, are stooped over, and may make repetitive movements such as "pill rolling" with the fingers. The major symptom of Parkinson's is difficulty in starting and sustaining voluntary movements. This is not because the muscles are too relaxed; indeed, the muscle tone may be too high when the muscles are at rest. Affected people often have visible tremors of the limbs. Modern treatments have provided much relief for the symptoms of Parkinson's. Indeed, these treatments are one of the success stories of basic research in neuroscience.

It has been known for some time that Parkinson's disease involves abnormalities of the basal ganglia. At autopsy the brains of people who had suffered from Parkinson's disease had significantly fewer neurons in the substantia nigra than normal. The *substantia nigra*, you will recall, is a midbrain structure, so named because its neurons appear dark due to the presence of the pigment melanin. The major projection site of the substantia nigra is to the *caudate nucleus*, a part of the basal ganglia (Figure 9-14). An advance in understanding the disease came with the development of histofluorescence methods of visualizing neurotransmitters. Examination of the brains of deceased Parkinson's patients revealed a consistent and markedly reduced content of dopamine in the substantia nigra and caudate nucleus (see Chapter 5).

The discovery of low dopamine in the basal ganglia of Parkinson's patients immediately suggested a treatment: give dopamine. This was tried but unfortunately did not help. It turned out that dopamine does not cross the blood–brain barrier. However, L-Dopa, the substance from which dopamine is manufactured in neurons, does cross (see Chapter 5). Administration of L-Dopa produces dramatic and rapid improvement in many Parkinson's patients. The increased amount of L-Dopa is thought to enable the few remaining dopamine cells in the substantia nigra that project to the caudate to produce more dopamine, making possible more normal functions.

Why Parkinson's disease develops in some people and not in others is a mystery. Recent evidence has raised the possibility that the disease may be the result of a form of influenza. A neurologist in Boston was said to have had a case of Chivas Regal waiting for anyone who could demonstrate that a person with Parkinson's disease did not earlier have this form of flu. Direct evidence for the influenza hypothesis, however, is lacking.

No therapy is perfect, and no drug is without side effects. L-Dopa causes loss of appetite and sometimes nausea and vomiting and other unpleasant effects. The side effects can be controlled to some extent with still other drugs. Recently, new forms of L-Dopa emerged from the laboratory that do not cause many of these side effects. In one case dopamine itself was bonded to a lipophilic (attracted to fat) molecule that penetrates the blood-brain barrier and can get to the brain.

One side effect of L-Dopa and other dopamine drugs is much more serious. As we noted in Chapter 5, L-Dopa can induce psychotic symptoms resembling schizophrenia in some Parkinson's patients. The reason for this is that the basal ganglia are not the only dopamine circuit in the brain. Dopamine-containing neurons, as we saw in Chapter 5, also project to the limbic system and cerebral cortex. If this other dopamine system is normal in Parkinson's sufferers, then administration Of L-Dopa will cause it to overproduce dopamine. The excessive dopamine hypothesis is in fact the major current hypothesis of the cause of schizophrenia (see Chapter 5).

A very recent approach to the treatment of Parkinson's disease is brain tissue transplants. In this rather heroic procedure, tissue is actually implanted in the critical dopamine-deficient region of the brain. Like other tissues, brain tissue tries to reject foreign tissue. Hence one procedure involves transplanting tissue taken from the patient's own adrenal gland. Adrenal cells have the necessary catecholamine synthetic enzymes to make dopamine in the brain— if they live. But the most promising approach involves taking living dopamine-system brain tissue from aborted fetuses and implanting it into the critical brain region in Parkinson's patients. Foreign fetal tissues are not as readily rejected as adult foreign tissues.

This work is still in the experimental stage and much more research needs to be done. It is most unfortunate that this has become a major political issue. Many people (but not all) who oppose abortion oppose the use of tissues from aborted fetuses for use in medical research. In my opinion, the two issues should be separated. Regardless of one's opinion on abortion, fetal tissues are available from legal abortions. If they are not used for research that may lead to successful treatment of a devastating and life-threatening disease, they are simply thrown away.

MOTOR CORTEX

The primary motor-sensory cortex was discovered in 1871, when Gustav Fritsch and Edvard Hitzig showed that stimulation of the anterior portion of the cerebral cortex in the dog elicited muscle movements in the opposite side of the body. This cortical region was found to contain giant neurons called Betz cells and to be primarily concerned with the control of movement.

Electrical stimulation of discrete points on the motor cortex in anesthetized animals and humans reveals a very detailed and complete map of the movements of the limbs, face, and body. The diagrams in Figure 9-15 indicate the region of the body that moves following cortical stimulation. As can be seen, the primary motor cortex is in many respects a mirror image of the somatic sensory cortex. The pattern of representation of movement on the motor-sensory cortex of humans shows marked enlargement of the hands, lips, and tongue control areas, as is the case in the somatic sensory cortex. The hand area of the human motor cortex is relatively much larger than in any other species. Each area of the primary motor cortex controls muscles on the opposite side of the body.

The distorted enlargements of the representations of certain parts of the body correspond, as we saw for the somatic sensory cortex, closely to the behavioral use made of that part of the body. Humans use their lips and tongue and their hands much more and with much finer detail of movement than other animals. Hence the motor cortex representing these movements

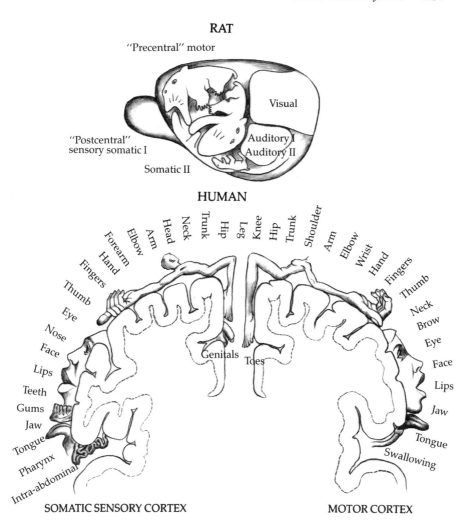

Figure 9-15 Motor and sensory areas of the cerebral cortex (see also Figure 8-13). The muscle movement representation is largely a mirror image of the somatic sensory projections to the primary somatic sensory area (SI). But the motor areas also receive skin and body information, and electrical stimulation of the somatic sensory areas can cause movements.

has become much enlarged to provide fine, delicate control. In the rat, the region representing movements of the head and nose and whiskers is expanded to provide for its mode of exploring the world, just as was true for its somatic sensory cortex.

We have emphasized the movement-control function of the motor cortex, but actually, it could equally well be called a sensory cortex. The detailed representation of the body skin surface on the motor cortex is a virtual mirror image of the representation, just behind it, in the somatic sensory cortex. Further, the mapping of muscles and movements on the motor cortex corresponds closely to the representation in the somatic sensory cortex: movements can also be elicited by stimulation of the somatic sensory cortex. The motor area and somatic sensory area of the cerebral cortex are therefore both sensory and motor in organization and in function. However, one is more sensory and one is more motor in function; hence the distinction.

Our discussion of the motor cortex has so far been concerned primarily with movements elicited by electrical stimulation. This does not necessarily reveal the essential role of the motor cortex in the control of movement. Removal of the primary motor-sensory cortex in humans produces loss of the most delicate and skilled movements, particularly those of the fingers and hand. Early experiments by Karl Lashley showed that although the motor cortex is necessary for delicate or skilled movements, it plays no essential role in the learning or retention of particular sequences of movements. Lashley trained monkeys to perform skilled acts such as opening a puzzle box to obtain food, then removed their motor cortices. After the initial paralysis began to dissipate, the animals could perform the correct sequence of responses necessary to get the reward. Their movements were clumsy and awkward but nonetheless in the correct sequence.

Two major descending systems from the motor cortex mediate cortical control over movement. One, the *pyramidal tract,* has its cell bodies largely in the motor cortex and sends axons down to the cranial motor nuclei and the motor regions of the spinal cord. Many of these pyramidal tract axons do, however, send off collateral (side) branches at many subcortical levels to influence other regions of the brain. The second system descending from the motor cortex is defined by exclusion: it consists of all the other descending motor pathways, arbitrarily grouped together under the label *cortical extrapyramidal system.* The existence of the second system of pathways is demonstrated by the fact that stimulation of the cerebral cortex can induce movements after complete bilateral destruction of the pyramidal tracts. Although the fibers of the descending pathways come in large part from the motor cortex, some come from other regions of the cortex, particularly the somatic sensory cortex and certain association areas.

The pyramidal tract has excited interest because of its late appearance in the course of evolution. It is most developed in mammals and reaches its maximum elaboration in primates. In view of the cortical origin of the pyramidal tract, it is not too surprising that the pyramidal tract is a late evolutionary invention. It is of particular interest that in primates, including humans, but not in other mammals, a significant proportion of the pyramidal tract fibers make monosynaptic connections to or synapse directly with the spinal motor neurons. The motor cortex thereby achieves direct and powerful control of the motor neurons.

The pyramidal tract appears to play an essential role in the performance of highly skilled movements. Sectioning the pyramidal tract bilaterally in monkeys and chimpanzees produces impairment of precision in movements; during the course of executing a movement the animals are not able to modify the movement smoothly. Larger movements of the body are not much impaired. Monkeys with complete section of the pyramidal tract can run, climb, and jump about in a relatively normal fashion.

Understanding of the behavioral functions of the motor cortex and its descending pyramidal tract has been advanced considerably by experiments in which the activity of a single neuron from the motor cortex of the monkey is recorded while the animal is engaged in performing fine movements of the hand and wrist. This work was first done by Edward Evarts. Because damage to the motor cortex or the pyramidal tract severely impairs fine movements of the hand in humans and other primates, Evarts reasoned that the neurons in the motor cortex whose axons descend to form the pyramidal tract must be particularly involved in such movements.

Evarts used an ingenious method for identifying cells from which pyramidal tract fibers originate in the cerebral cortex (Figure 9-16). The vast majority of neurons in the motor cortex are not pyramidal tract neurons; they are interneurons that do not send axons out from the cortex. If a microelectrode were simply inserted in the motor cortex and the activity of a single neuron recorded, there would be no way of telling if it were a pyramidal tract neuron or not. Actually, the chances of finding a pyramidal tract neuron from which to record are a little better than that, because some of these neurons happen to be the largest in the motor cortex and in fact in all of the cerebral cortex. These are the *Betz cells*, named after the Russian neuroanatomist, Vladimir Betz, who first described them.

Although a recording microelectrode implanted at random in the motor cortex is more likely to approach a very large neuron such as a Betz cell and record its activity than to meet with one of the much smaller interneurons, it is less than a certainty. Evarts got around the difficulty by implanting a stimulating electrode permanently in the pyramidal tract of the monkey well below the motor cortex and applying a brief stimulus to it. This initiates action potentials in all of the pyramidal tract axons in the vicinity of the stimulating electrode. The action potentials travel down the pyramidal tract to motor neurons, but such a single volley is not enough to produce a movement. More important, the action potentials travel backward up the pyramidal tract axons to their cell bodies of origin in the motor cortex. We

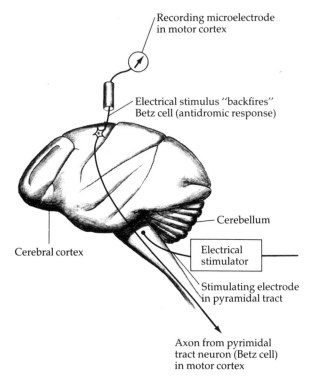

Recording microelectrode
in motor cortex

Electrical stimulus "backfires"
Betz cell (antidromic response)

Cerebellum

Cerebral cortex

Electrical
stimulator

Stimulating electrode
in pyramidal tract

Axon from pyrimidal
tract neuron (Betz cell)
in motor cortex

Figure 9-16 Experimental arrangement for studying the activity of the cells of origin of pyramidal tract fibers in monkey motor cortex (for example, Betz cells) while the monkey is making a skilled movement (see Figure 9-17).

saw in Chapter 3 that when an action potential is initiated at some point on an axon by an electric stimulus, it travels away from that point in both directions: the axon itself is not directional. The action potentials that go backward up the axons from the place of stimulation are called *antidromic* (opposite direction) as opposed to the normal *orthodromic* direction of conduction.

Evarts's microelectrode in the motor cortex could record the antidromic response of the pyramidal tract neuron activated by the electrical stimulation of the pyramidal tract. The antidromic action potential arriving at the cell body of a neuron in the motor cortex can be identified as an antidromic response because it has certain properties that differentiate it from orthodromic potentials. For example, no synapses are crossed, and a high frequency of stimulation, say 100 stimuli per second, will be registered by the corresponding part of the neuron in the motor cortex, which would not be possible for a pathway that had a synapse interposed. A motor cortex neuron that shows an antidromic response to stimulation of the pyramidal tract must be a neuron of origin of a pyramidal tract fiber from the motor cortex.

Having identified pyramidal tract neurons in the motor cortex, Evarts was now in a position to study their role in behavior. He trained monkeys to make small, discrete movements of a handle to get a reward, such as a taste of orange juice. Monkeys enjoy orange juice and will gladly work to get it. Previously the pyramidal-tract-stimulating electrode and a small device for moving electrodes in the motor cortex had been attached by means of surgery, in which anesthetics and all the precautions taken in human surgery were utilized. (Evarts's procedures do not hurt the animals at all. The brain itself has no sense of pain, and so the monkeys cannot even feel the electrodes being inserted into the motor cortex.) The monkey sits in a chair and performs the required movements.

Evarts found that Betz cells in the motor cortex showed a striking increase in activity when the monkeys made even the smallest fine movement. Indeed, the fraction of motor cortex cells that fired during a small, fine movement was far larger than the number of spinal motor neurons involved in controlling the actual wrist movement. Larger movements of the limbs did not engage the pyramidal tract neurons in the motor cortex nearly as much.

An example of the firing pattern of a pyramidal tract cell in the motor cortex during a small movement of a monkey's wrist and finger is shown in Figure 9-17. A monkey had been trained to depress a telegraph key when a light was turned on. After the light went on, the activity of the pyramidal cell rapidly increased; it began firing in the motor cortex after about 150 milliseconds. Actual movement followed the turning on of the light by 250 milliseconds, or about a quarter of a second, so the firing of the cell in the motor cortex preceded the onset of movement by about 100 milliseconds.

The timing of the activity of the motor cortex cell in relation to the behavioral responses came as something of a surprise. The motor cortex, along with the rest of the cerebral cortex, had been traditionally viewed as the highest region of the brain, where the most abstract aspects of behavior and experience are coded and analyzed. For the motor cortex this does not seem to be the case. The responses of the motor cortex cells are very tightly coupled to the actual execution of fine movements. They respond well before the movements begin but long after the monkey has decided to make the movement: the motor cortex is concerned with the actual execution of fine movements and not with the earlier processes that lead the animal to decide to make it.

A very fundamental question about how the cerebral cortex functions concerns "readout." How is the information from the many millions of neurons in the motor cortex put together in the brain to result in a discrete, precise movement? Suppose you trained a monkey to reach out to touch a small light that was placed in any location within reach in front of the

Figure 9-17 The monkey is trained to press a button when a signal light comes on. The cell in the motor cortex begins to fire about 150 milliseconds after the light comes on, about 100 milliseconds before the muscle activity begins.

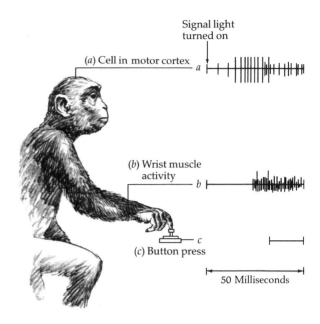

monkey. You now record from single neurons in the motor cortex of the monkey while he is reaching out his hand in a particular direction. If you are recording from a neuron that responds when the animal reaches out, you might expect that this particular neuron would respond only when the monkey reaches in that particular direction. Elegant studies by Apostolos Georgopoulis and associates at Johns Hopkins University showed that this result does not occur. Each neuron they recorded from responded when the monkey reached out in any direction over a wide region. How, then, did the monkey know where to reach? This question is much like the issue of the "grandmother cell" in visual cortex discussed in Chapter 8. (For motor cortex, "grandmother" cells would mean one neuron for each specific direction of reach.)

Georgopoulis's work indicated that there were no "grandmother" neurons in motor cortex. It is not the case that each direction of movement is coded precisely by a group of neurons. However, when the broad range of preferred movements for each neuron was added together for all the neurons a most remarkable result occurred. The summed responses (actually the vector sum) of all the neuron responses for reaching to a particular location predicted that location with great precision (Figure 9-1). The activity of the entire ensemble of neurons together coded the precise direction of movement. Single cells in motor cortex are broadly tuned rather than sharply tuned to the direction of movement, sometimes termed "coarse coding," but the direction of movement is uniquely and precisely coded by a directionally heterogeneous neuronal population.

MOVEMENT CONTROL SYSTEMS IN THE BRAIN

When it became clear from Evarts's work that the motor cortex is much more concerned with the detailed execution of fine voluntary movements than with their initiation, other motor systems of the brain began to be explored using his techniques. The major structures in the brain concerned with movement are diagrammed in Figure 9-18, along with a few of the most important interconnecting pathways.

Neurons in the cerebellum begin to increase their activity well before motor cortex cells when a movement is initiated. Cooling of the appropriate region of the cerebellum in monkeys markedly interferes with and slows down the initiation of voluntary and learned skilled movements. The cerebellum is massively interconnected with the motor cortex, as we noted earlier. Recent work suggests that the actual motor programs, the memory traces that code for complex skilled learned movements, are formed and stored in the cerebellum (see Chapter 11).

Interestingly, neurons in the basal ganglia also show early increases in activity when a voluntary movement is initiated. In fact, they may show the earliest increases in the brain and are at least a candidate for the system that initiates movements. Remember that the major symptom in Parkinson's disease is difficulty in initiating movements and that the major damage in Parkinson's is the destruction of the dopamine pathways from the substantia nigra to the basal ganglia. The basal ganglia are massively connected with cerebral motor cortex.

Important work by Vernon Mountcastle and his associates at Johns Hopkins University indicates that a region of association cortex lying adjacent to the primary somatic sensory cortex may also be of great importance in the initiation of movements in monkeys and by analogy in humans. Neurons in this region become active when a monkey looks at an object and then reaches out for it, but they are not activated if the animal is merely shown the object or if its limbs are passively moved. The animal must see the object and decide to reach for it in order to activate neurons in the association cortex. These "intentional" neurons are organized in columns. One column of cells responds when the arm begins to reach, another when the hand manipulates the object, another when the animal actively moves its eyes to look at the object and so on. There are at least six such functional types of columns and of course many columns of each type. It may be that at least in primates, the decision to make a voluntary movement originates in part in the association cortex.

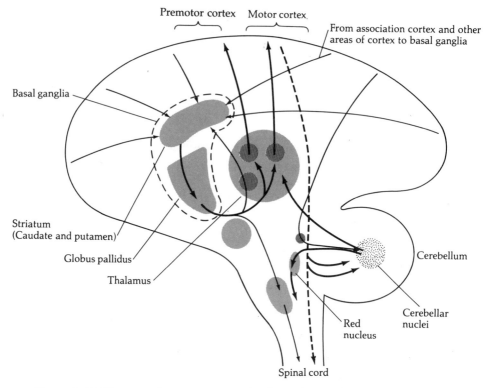

Figure 9-18 The major brain systems involved in voluntary skilled movements. They might work together as follows. Assume that the initial decision to make a movement develops in the association cortex. This can act directly on the basal ganglia and less directly on the cerebellum. The basal ganglia and cerebellum increase their activity and activate the motor area of the cerebral cortex via the thalamus. The motor cortex then acts down on motor neurons in the spinal cord to produce the movement.

Recent work by Mountcastle and his associates focused on the coding of the direction of a visual stimulus by these "visual intention" neurons. Single neurons are broadly tuned to the direction of the visual stimulus—each neuron would respond to stimuli over a wide range of locations. However, when the responses of a population of these neurons were added together, the population vector predicted very accurately the direction of the stimulus. This principle of coarse coding by single neurons but fine tuning by the ensemble of neurons is exactly what we described earlier for neurons in motor cortex coding the direction of a reaching movement.

SUMMARY

It can be argued that the primary purpose of the brain is to produce adaptive behavior—movements. Indeed, a number of brain systems are critically involved in the generation and control of movements. It is helpful to view these motor-control systems as a hierarchy of functions. At the most primitive level are the muscles themselves and the spinal reflexes that exert basic control over them. Skeletal (striated) muscles are activated by motor nerve fibers, and ACh is the neurotransmitter. Activation produces an all-or-none twitch response of muscle fiber. But the total response of the muscle, made up of many fibers, is of course graded. The basic mechanism of contraction involves calcium ion activation of the actin and myosin proteins such that the two bind, sliding the actin and myosin filaments over each other.

Muscles have several types of sense organs; tendon receptors code stretch and spindle receptors code the contraction of the spindle organs in the muscle. Muscles have two types of motor nerve fibers: alpha motor fibers that activate muscles to contract and gamma motor fibers that connect to the spindle organ and cause it to contract, activating the spindle receptors, which in turn activate the alpha motor neurons. Brain motor systems can thus act on alpha motor neurons to produce movements or on the gamma motor neurons, which may not cause movements but can increase the readiness of the muscles to respond. The gamma system is the monosynaptic reflex (for example, knee jerk)—tapping a tendon stretches the spindle organs whose sensory fibers connect directly (one synapse) to the alpha motor neurons. The major function of this system is to maintain and adaptively modulate muscle tone and posture. The flexion reflex is polysynaptic (more then one synapse in series) and is defensive, moving the limbs away from painful and potentially damaging stimuli.

The cerebellum is a very large structure that developed early in vertebrates, probably the first specialized brain structure to evolve for the control and coordination of movement. It is highly fissured, with a layer of cortex many cells thick that rivals that of the cerebral cortex in area. The cerebellar nuclei are buried in the white matter of the cerebellum and (with vestibular nuclei) are the only source of output axons from the cerebellum to other brain systems. There are two major input projection systems: the climbing fibers from the inferior olive that project to the cerebellar cortex (one-to-one on Purkinje neurons) and nuclei and the mossy fibers from the pontine nuclei and other sources. The climbing fibers convey primarily somatic sensory information and appear to function as an error-correcting system; the mossy fibers convey detailed information about the state of muscles and movement of limbs and also auditory and visual information to the nuclei and, via parallel fibers, to the cerebellar cortex. Purkinje neurons are the only output neurons from the cerebellar cortex. They project only to the cerebellar (and vestibular) nuclei and their sole action is to inhibit their target neurons. Computational models of the cerebellum show how it can function as a "learning machine" for the learning and memory storage of skilled movements, and recent evidence strongly supports this view.

The basal ganglia are large neuronal structures in the depths of the forebrain. Like the cerebellum, they are closely interconnected to the cerebral cortex. Damage to the basal ganglia yields severe disorders of movement, the best-known example being Parkinson's disease. The major problem Parkinson's patients have is in the initiation of voluntary movements; they also show disorders in ongoing movements. The cause of the disease is degeneration of dopamine-containing neurons in the substantia nigra that project to the basal ganglia.

The motor area of the cerebral cortex are most evolved in primates and humans, where their output neurons make direct, monosynaptic connection on alpha motor neurons. The primary motor area (and pyramidal tract) seems most involved in direct control of skilled movements, particularly of the mouth, hands, and fingers. Recent work indicates that individual neurons in motor cortex do not code the direction of reach (as when a monkey reaches for an object) very precisely but the vector sum of these neurons' preferred directions of reach predicts with great precision the exact direction of reach (fine-tuning from coarse coding). Although much uncertainty exists, evidence suggests that when primates make voluntary movements (as in reaching for a seen object), the impetus for initiating the movement may originate in parietal association areas of the cerebral cortex.

SUGGESTED READINGS AND REFERENCES

Books

Brooks, V. B. (1986). *The neural basis of motor control.* New York: Oxford University Press.

Evarts, E. V., Wise, S. P., and Bousfield, D. (1985). *The motor system in neurobiology.* Amsterdam: Elsevier Biomedical Press.

Groves, P. M., and Rebec, G. V. (1992). *Introduction to biological psychology* (4th ed.). Dubuque, IA: William C Brown.

Ito, M. (1984). *The cerebellum and neural control.* New York: Raven Press.

Matthews, P. B. C. (1972). *Mammalian muscle receptors and their central action.* London: Edward Arnold.

Rosenbaum, D. A. (1991). *Human motor control.* San Diego: Academic Press.

Schmidt, R. A. (1982). *Motor control and learning: A behavioral emphasis.* Champaign, IL: Human Kinetics Publishers.

Talbott, R. E., and Humphrey, D. R. (1979). *Posture and movement.* New York: Raven Press.

Vander, A. J., Sherman, J. H., and Luciano, D. S. (1990). *Human physiology: The mechanisms of body functions* (5th ed.). New York: McGraw-Hill.

Articles

Evarts, E. V. (1979). Brain mechanisms of movement. *Scientific American, 241,* 98–106.

Georgopoulis, A. P., Schwartz, A. B., and Kettner, R. E. (1986). Neuronal population coding of movement direction. *Science, 233,* 1416–1419.

Grillner, S. (1985). Neurobiological bases of rhythmic motor acts in vertebrates. *Science, 228,* 143–149.

Thach, W. T., Goodkin, H. P., and Keating, J. G. (1992). The cerebellum and the adaptive coordination of movement. *Annual Review of Neuroscience, 15,* 403–442.

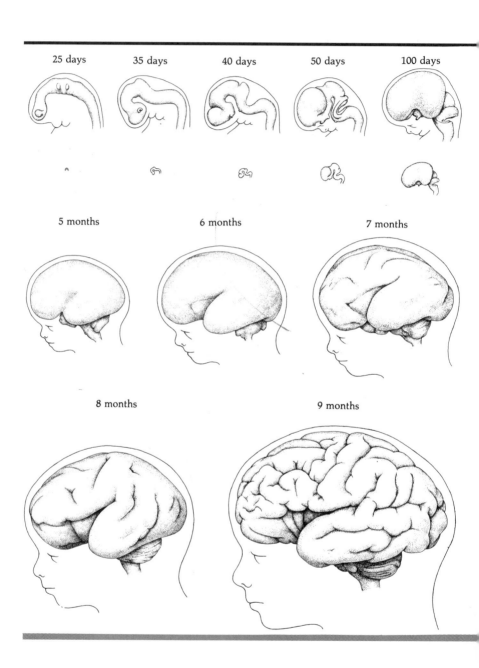

25 days   35 days   40 days   50 days   100 days

5 months   6 months   7 months

8 months   9 months

10

Life Cycle of the Brain: Development, Plasticity, and Aging

The human brain grows and develops from a single fertilized cell into a structure containing billions of neurons that form the myriad of synapses, pathways, and circuits that make up all adult human brains (Figure 10-1). Over the nine months of development, the human embryonic brain gains neurons at the astonishing rate of 250,000 per minute. These billions of neurons develop in what at first seems a chaotic way and then migrate to their preordained destinations. The major circuits in the brain are basically the same in all mammals: there is a high degree of predetermination, or "hard-wiring," in the mammalian brain. The ultimate plan for the hard-wiring comes of course from the genes and their interaction with the cellular environment over the organism's course of development from a single fertilized egg into an adult.

Figure 10-1 *Development of the human brain in stages from 25 days until birth. The drawings from 5 months to 9 months are about one-third life size. Those from 25 days to 100 days are much enlarged—the actual sizes are shown just below (note the little speck at 25 days). The three major parts of the brain—forebrain, midbrain and hindbrain—begin as swellings in the neural tube (see text). As the human brain grows, the cerebral hemispheres (forebrain) expand enormously and cover most of the rest of the brain.*

Current estimates of the total number of genes in the human DNA range up to 100,000. Of these, perhaps 50,000 are functional only in the brain, which suggests the enormous complexity of genetic control over the brain and its development. You might think that the genes determine exactly the diverse connections among the neurons in the brain, but simple arithmetic argues against this. There are literally trillions of synapses in the human brain, far too many connections to be specified in detail by the genes.

To date the most completely characterized nervous system belongs to a rather unglamorous creature, the nematode worm *C. elegans*. It has 302 neurons and about 7,000 synapses, all of which have been identified. In this simple and primitive invertebrate all the synaptic connections do appear to be specified by the genes. Development of the *C. elegans* nervous system proceeds in an extremely rigid, genetically controlled manner. If a cell destined to become neuron 48 is destroyed, the remaining neurons develop but neuron 48 does not.

The humble zebra fish provided a unique opportunity to study the genetic control of brain development in vertebrates. Many of these fish develop as clones from the same fertilized egg. They all have identical genes, as do human identical twins. Anatomical analysis of the fine structure, the detailed synaptic connections, in brains of zebra fish clones at birth showed that the brain of each individual is unique and different from the others. All the major pathways and nuclei are of course the same, as they are in all members of a given species, but the detailed synaptic connections differ. This must mean that the genes alone do not completely determine the fine details of synaptic connections in the vertebrate brain. Developmental processes must play a key role in determining the details of brain development.

We now think that in mammals, in addition to developmental factors, experience from before birth to death continually shapes and reshapes the fine structure of each individual brain. The general plan is the same in all human brains but the detailed organization differs widely from person to person, due to genetic and developmental factors and to each person's lifetime of experience. If we knew how to "read" memories from the synaptic connections we might someday be able to reconstruct the lifetime of memories stored in a brain.

How it is that the human brain grows and develops into a structure of the utmost complexity is a profound mystery. As we noted, a complete "blueprint" of the brain does not exist in the genetic material of the chromosomes. The components of the fertilized cell outside the nucleus, however, are also much involved in organizing development. Norman Wessells, a developmental biologist at the University of Oregon, uses the analogy of a prime contract and subcontracts to describe the role of the DNA and its cellular environment in embryological development. The DNA of the nucleus, the hereditary material, is the prime contract. It specifies the plan for the building blocks (proteins) that constitute the cell's structure and carry out various tasks in the cell, and it also specifies the basic rules for the way the cell's particular job can be done. Outside the nucleus, however, specialized materials in different parts of the fertilized cell provide "subcontracts" that give additional information essential to the form and function the cell and its descendants will take on. Later, as tissues develop, the interactions among them provide still more detailed subcontracts.

A specific example of the interaction of nuclear (DNA) instructions with influences from outside the nucleus is provided by the gray crescent of the fertilized frog egg (Figure 10-2). Normally when the frog egg undergoes its first division, or cleavage, the gray crescent is split so that each of the two new cells has a part of it. If these two cells are separated, they will develop into normal, identical twin tadpoles. However, if a frog egg is made to cleave so that one cell gets all of the gray crescent and the other none, only the cell with the gray crescent will develop into a tadpole, even though both cells have a normal complement of DNA. The gray crescent lies outside the nucleus and has no DNA, yet it carries essential information for development. Ultimately, of course, the DNA was responsible for the development of the gray crescent.

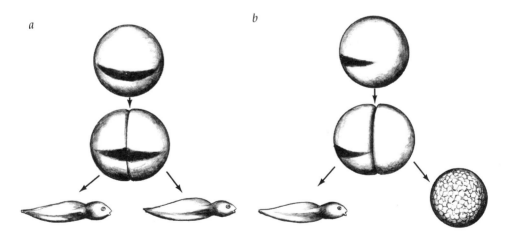

a

b

Figure 10-2 Role of the gray crescent in the development of the frog zygote (fertilized egg). (*a*) Normally, the first cell division splits the gray crescent. Two normal tadpoles develop. (*b*) If the zygote is split so that all the gray crescent is in one cell, only that cell will develop into a tadpole, even though the DNA of the nucleus has replicated and is present and normal in both cells.

The key question about the growth of the human brain is how its precise, detailed, and extremely complicated neuronal circuits develop. The final answers to this question will be found at the level of single neurons and their interactions, their processes of growth and migration, and the physical or chemical events responsible, but very few answers of this sort exist as yet. Let us first look at larger events, the growth of the major components of the human brain, and then return to the question of mechanisms.

Induction is the general principle believed to underlie the development of the nervous system. The mechanisms seem to be more in the nature of sub-contracts than directly derived from the prime contract of the DNA. Neurons are first formed from cells in the outer layer of the embryo, the epidermis, by means of their interaction with cells under them, which will become the backbone and other tissues and will constitute the mesoderm. Before the epidermal cells interact with the mesoderm cells, the epidermal cells can become either nerve cells or skin cells. Presumably the mesodermal cells release a substance or substances that cause certain epidermal cells to turn into neurons.

As the development of the brain proceeds, the fate of the neurons becomes progressively more determined. Initially, the ectodermal cells in the embryo are induced to form a small band of cells called the *neural plate* (Figure 10-3). The head end of the neural plate will later develop into the forebrain and the neural part of the eye, the retina. If a small piece of the developing ectoderm is removed early enough, the cells are replaced and development of the forebrain and eye proceeds normally. If a piece is removed from the neural plate at a slightly later stage, a permanent defect results in either the forebrain or the eye, depending on where the tissue came from.

The neural plate grows, folds in, and forms the *neural tube,* the original tubular nervous system still seen in primitive animals such as the worm. In higher animals, as development proceeds, the fate of each region of the neural tube becomes increasingly determined. Chemical marking substances applied to various regions of the brain of an experimental animal very early in development can be used to reveal the final destinations of the cells from the marked regions in the adult brain.

Neurons initially develop within the neural plate and multiply rapidly at the neural tube stage. Then, at various times, groups of cells stop dividing and

Figure 10-3 (*Right*) Early development of the human nervous system. Drawings at the left are external views; cross sections are shown at the right. Neural cells develop from ectoderm (skin-to-be) cells to form the neural plate, which folds in to form the neural tube. As the developing neurons send out axons, the basic form of the gray matter (cell bodies) and white matter (axons) of the spinal cord develops.

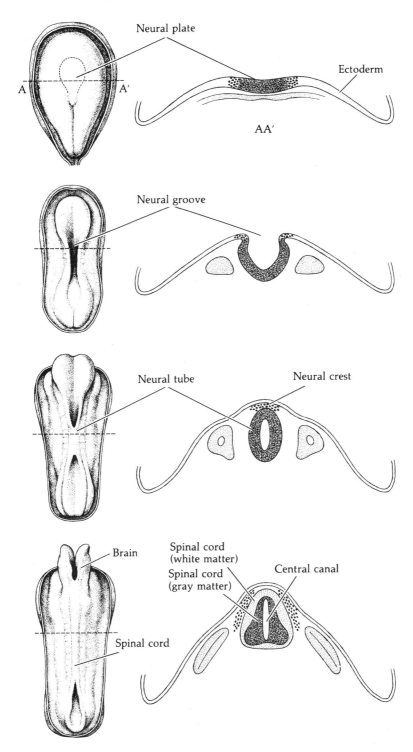

migrate to their ultimate destinations. Migration seems to be triggered by nuclear events in the cell. It begins when a given type of neuron stops dividing and forming new cells. At this point it starts to migrate. For some reason, when neurons lose their capacity to synthesize DNA, they begin to migrate to their final homes in the brain or another part of the nervous system. There are a few exceptions to this rule. The granule cells in cerebellar cortex continue to divide after they have arrived at the granule cell layer.

The stages of development of the human brain are shown in Figure 10-1. The drawings from 5 months on are all to the same scale, about three-fifths life size. The stages in the top row of drawings (25 to 100 days) are enlarged to the same arbitrary size and their actual size is shown below. At 25 days the human embryonic nervous system resembles that of a worm. By 40 to 50 days the brain clearly is that of a vertebrate, but it could be mistaken for the brain of a fish. By 100 days it is clearly recognizable as a mammalian brain, and by five months it has acquired the features of a primate brain. From this point on, however, development—the vast expansion and elaboration of the forebrain, cerebral cortex, and cerebellum—becomes uniquely human. The fact that the early stages of development of the human brain and embryo roughly follow the course of the evolution from lower to higher life forms led to the old notion that "ontogeny recapitulates phylogeny." In an obvious sense this is true, but it has no deeper meaning. At any stage of development, the brain of any one species has unique features (Figure 10-4).

MECHANISMS OF BRAIN DEVELOPMENT

How are the multitude of specific pathways and patterns of connections that are the same in every human brain formed? There are three different principles, really theories, that appear to operate in forming the hard-wiring of the brain: chemical signals, cell and terminal competition, and fiber-guided cell movements.

Chemical Signals

The easiest theory to understand is the idea of chemical signals, or *trophic growth*: growing nerve terminals attach to particular neurons or cells because there is a chemical affinity between them. Chemical gradients of some substances encourage the growth of the axon in a particular direction and to a particular set of target cells.

This general view was developed by Roger Sperry at the California Institute of Technology some years ago. Sperry's classic experiments showing the

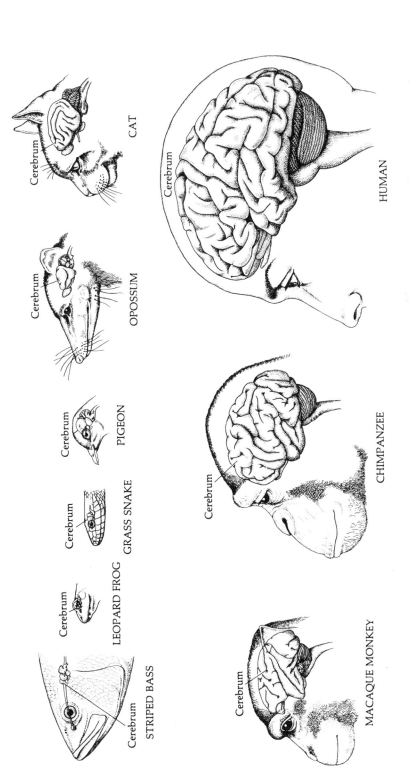

Figure 10-4 Progressive increase in the size of the cerebrum in vertebrates is evident in the drawings, which show a representative selection of vertebrate brains all drawn to the same scale. In vertebrates lower than mammals, the cerebrum is small. In carnivores, and particularly in primates, it increases dramatically in both size and complexity (compare with Figure 10-1).

STRIPED BASS

LEOPARD FROG

GRASS SNAKE

PIGEON

OPOSSUM

CAT

MACAQUE MONKEY

CHIMPANZEE

HUMAN

Cerebrum

action of trophic factors are very simple. He first severed the optic nerve of a frog. Unlike in mammals, the cut optic nerve of a frog regenerates, connecting back to the brain and restoring normal vision in the eye. The test for good frog vision is also simple. Allow the frog to become hungry, cover the eye with the unsevered optic nerve, and present a bug to the frog. It will snap its tongue out and attempt to capture the bug. If the eye is functioning normally, the tongue moves accurately to the bug. These simple observations indicate that the optic nerve terminals grow back to make connections with the same places in the brain to which they were attached before (remember that the cell bodies of the optic nerve fibers are the ganglion cells in the retina).

The optic nerve terminals could, of course, be guided in their regrowth by the remaining cut, degenerating fibers of the optic nerve. Each new fiber could simply grow along the path left by its dying axon. To resolve whether this happens, Sperry cut the optic nerve of another frog and rotated the eye 180 degrees. Now the growing fibers were opposite dying fibers that have very different destinations in the brain. If a fiber followed the path of the dying axon it was now next to, it would reconnect to the wrong part of the visual brain. The results were striking (Figure 10-5). After its optic nerve had regenerated, the frog forever after struck down at a fly that was up, and vice versa. The optic nerve fibers had grown to the parts of the visual brain they had originally connected to, and since the eye was rotated, up now looked down to the frog and down up. The visual brain of the frog is nonplastic, so the frog would never amend its behavior. The mammalian visual brain is much more plastic, as we shall see later in the chapter. Humans can learn to adapt to lenses that invert the visual world and see right side up.

Sperry's experiments proved that cut optic nerve fibers, which went to quite different regions of the visual brain, grew around the dying axons ad-

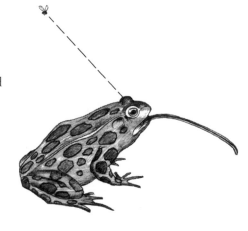

Figure 10-5 Frog with eyeball rotated strikes down at a fly that is up. When the optic nerve is cut and the eyeball rotated 180 degrees, the nerve fibers regrow into the brain and connect to their original locations.

jacent to them to find their proper homes. The easiest way to explain this is that some kind of chemical factor guides the growing axon to its destination. Indeed, it is difficult to think of any other explanation.

If chemical signals somehow guide axons to their correct destinations, as Sperry's experiments strongly indicate, there must be a multitude of them to guide the growth of the literally thousands of different pathways in the brain. The first chemical signal to be discovered was *nerve growth factor* (NGF). In 1951 Rita Levi-Montalcini and Viktor Hamburger discovered this substance in the chick embryo, and subsequently it was found to be present in all vertebrates. Chemically, NGF is a large protein molecule. It is specific to one type of neuron: the neurons of the sympathetic ganglia. Injection of NGF into a chick embryo causes a sixfold increase above normal in the number of neurons in the sympathetic ganglia. It can actually trigger a marked increase in nerve cell division in the developing nervous system.

Perhaps even more striking is the trophic influence of NGF. Levi-Montalcini injected NGF into the brain of newborn rats. (Rats are born at a very early stage of development, and much brain growth occurs after birth.) Normally, nerve axons from the sympathetic ganglia grow only out toward body target organs, never into the brain. But in the rats injected with NGF, a large number of sympathetic axons grew into the brain toward the place where the NGF had been injected. Presumably the NGF diffused from the site of the injection, forming a chemical gradient that was most concentrated at the site of injection and least concentrated at the periphery of the nervous system, where the sympathetic neurons are. The gradient served to guide the growth of the fibers over a very long distance to their new and abnormal home, the site of NGF injection in the brain.

Several other growth factors have now been identified in the mammalian brain. These brain growth factors may someday offer promise of repairing brain damage or even treating degenerative brain disorders like Alzheimer's disease.

Cell Competition and Death

Another general process by which neuronal connections are determined is *cell death*, or at least axon terminal death. This will be treated in more detail in a discussion of how the fibers of the visual system form connections with the visual area of the cerebral cortex. A simple example of cell death is provided by the growth of motor neuron axons out to innervate skeletal muscle fibers (Figure 10-6). In Chapter 9 we saw that a given motor neuron axon connects to one or more muscle fibers, typically several. A given muscle fiber receives input from only one motor axon. In the developing embryo, several motor neurons grow axon terminals that are sent to each muscle fiber. These are

Figure 10-6 Competition in the development of innervation (connection) of motor neuron axons onto striated muscle fibers. At an early stage there is considerable overlap, but as development proceeds, competition results in a given axon winning out over all others until the final pattern of no overlap is established (see also Figure 9-3).

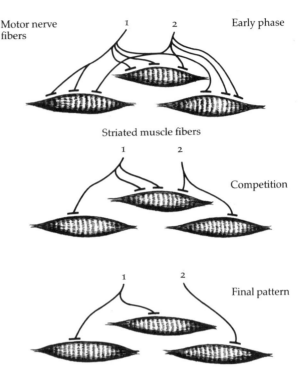

actual functional synaptic connections. As development proceeds, however, the terminal branches of most of the motor neuron axons retract, and one motor neuron comes to dominate a given muscle fiber completely. It is as though the motor neuron axons compete and the one with the strongest innervation wins out. The other synapses die and disappear. Activity at the neuromuscular junction—activation of the muscle fiber by the dominant nerve axon—appears crucial in this competition.

The process of retraction and cell loss appears to be general in the nervous system. To take another example, in certain nuclei in the auditory system there are many more neurons before birth than after. Once again, more neurons and synapses form than are needed, the axons compete, and the numbers of synapses and neurons are reduced. It is easy to see how a process like this can fine-tune the anatomical organization of the embryonic brain, leading to the very precise and detailed organization of synaptic connections in the adult brain. If you are worried about reports that people lose a few neurons and synapses as they grow old, remember that you lost far more by the time you were born.

Fiber-Guided Cell Movement

A third process that helps to account for the growth of hard-wired circuits in the brain might be termed the "bootstrap" process. Briefly, a growing neuron sends out a fiber, that eventually reaches a boundary such as the surface of the brain and cannot grow any farther. The cell body then travels up its fiber to the boundary.

A clear example of the process is provided by the Purkinje cells in the cerebellum (Figure 10-7). These cells are destined to become the principal neurons of the cerebellar cortex, conveying information out from it chiefly to the cerebellar deep nuclei, which in turn send information to other regions of the brain (see Chapter 9). How does a Purkinje neuron come to have its cell body in the cerebellar cortex and its axon projecting out of that region, terminating in a deep nucleus well below the cortex?

The cells that will become Purkinje neurons arise near the cavity of the hollow hindbrain at a very early stage in brain development. Other cells in the general region where the Purkinje neurons originate are destined to become the deep cerebellar nuclei. Some of the newly formed cells send out a process that grows through the developing cells of the hindbrain and then cannot grow any farther. Then the cell body travels up its fiber until it cannot go any farther. This top surface of the hindbrain becomes the cerebellar cortex, and the Purkinje cell body is now in the cerebellar cortex. Its fiber becomes an axon, projecting from the cell body in the cerebellar cortex to the place where the cell started, in the deep cerebellar nucleus. The cell ends up conveying information in the opposite direction to its original direction of growth.

Development of the Cerebral Cortex

Developmental processes can help us understand the unique structural features of particular brain regions. In Chapter 7, we discussed the columnar organization of the visual cortex, the fact that the cortex is organized into vertical columns of neurons having particular functional properties. The anatomical organization of the cerebral cortex into columns is also clear (Figure 1-7). In development, the cerebral cortex begins as a single layer just a few cells thick, the *germinal zone*. As the cells proliferate, some stop dividing and move up to form another layer. From here some cells move up to form the next layer, and so on. The first layer of cortex to develop is thus the bottom layer, layer VI. Layer V forms next and finally the top layer, layer I, forms last (Figure 10-8). Hence a columnar organization is superimposed on the horizontally arranged cellular layers.

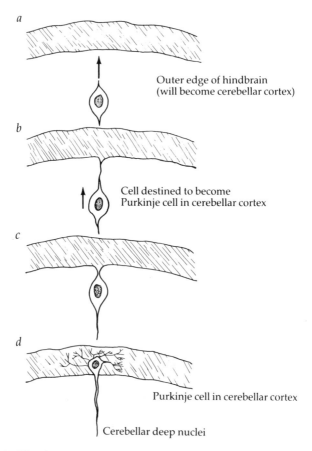

a

Outer edge of hindbrain
(will become cerebellar cortex)

b

Cell destined to become
Purkinje cell in cerebellar cortex

c

d

Purkinje cell in cerebellar cortex

Cerebellar deep nuclei

Figure 10-7 The "bootstrap" process of cell body migration. (*a*) The Purkinje cell of the cerebellum begins in a brain stem region that will become the cerebellar nuclei. (*b*) A fiber grows out from it until it reaches the top edge of the hindbrain and cannot grow any farther. (*c*) The cell body migrates up the axon until it reaches the top of the brain, which is becoming the cerebellar cortex. (*d*) The Purkinje cell body is now in its correct location, in cerebellar cortex, and the fiber becomes its axon connecting down to cells in the cerebellar nuclei, the correct adult pattern of connection.

A type of cell that is particularly important in the development of cerebral cortex is the *subplate neuron*. The cell bodies of subplate neurons lie below the developing cortex in the white matter. They send their axons up into the cortex and they appear to be physiologically active, forming functional synapses on developing neurons in the cortex. Their axons may also serve to guide the growth of cortical neurons and incoming fibers, for example, the projections from thalamic sensory neurons destined to synapse on layer IV neurons in sensory areas

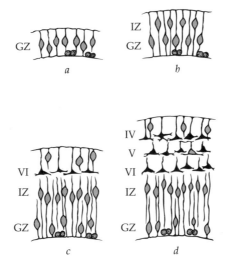

Figure 10-8 Formation of the cerebral cortex. (*a*) Initially the neural tube is just a few cells thick and consists mainly of the germinal zone (GZ). (*b*) As cells proliferate, some stop dividing and move to the intermediate zone (IZ). (*c*) The intermediate zone cells then migrate distally to take up their final positions; the first cells to migrate form the deepest cortical layers (layer VI). (*d*) Cells migrating later form the more superficial layers (here, layers IV and V).

of the cortex. A remarkable fact about subplate neurons is that they die out as the cortex becomes established. We will have more to say about these temporary neurons when we examine the details of development of the visual cortex.

The Growth Cone

A key question in the formation of neural pathways is how an axon grows. At the beginning of development, the axon is called a *neurite* and is destined to become an axon. The growing end of the axon has a special structure called the growth cone (Figure 10-9), which advances as the neurite grows. Axon growth at the junction of the neurite and the cell body could occur by the cell body continually extruding the neurite or by the whole length of the neurite extending or by growth only at the growth cone. A simple experiment showed that the last possibility is the actuality. If particles of an opaque substance are attached to the neurite just behind the growth cone, they remain "on" it at

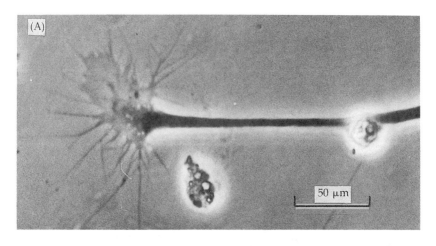

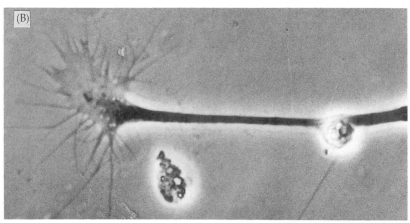

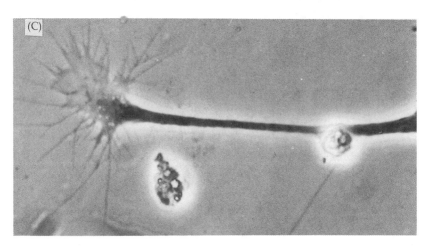

Figure 10-9 Rapid movements of a growth cone (clublike structure at left with many filaments protruding from it) in tissue culture. These three frames (A–C) were taken at 20-second intervals!

exactly that distance from the cell body; hence growth occurs at the growth cone, leaving an increasingly long axon behind.

It is thought that the adding of membrane at the growth cone occurs by membrane vesicles being made in the cell body and transported out the neurite to fuse with the growth cone. Most adult neurons in the brain do not actually move; the growth cone in the developing axon does actually move through space, just as muscle cells move in the adult organism. In order to move, the growth cone must have contractile like mechanisms—and indeed it does. The primary components of the growth cone are actin and myosin, the proteins that make up striated muscle fibers (Chapter 9).

The processes that guide the direction of growth of the growth cone are presumed to include trophic chemical signals and fiber-guided movement. Adhesion is also a factor—a growth cone may adhere to one type of cell or fiber and not to another. Interestingly, electrical fields can also influence the direction of growth. Electrochemical gradients in the developing embryo can be of sufficient strength to control the direction of movement of a growth cone. Whether this is an actual mechanism in controlling the direction of axon growth in normal development is not yet known.

Understanding the mechanisms that are known to function in hard-wiring the developing brain is perhaps only a wedge in opening up to us an ultimate understanding of how the brain comes to be what it is. With increased knowledge of the basic processes of growth and development in the brain, it may someday be possible to regrow damaged parts of brains. Brain damage is one of the most serious modern afflictions of the human race, thanks to the development of the automobile and the motorcycle.

PLASTICITY IN DEVELOPMENT: THE VISUAL SYSTEM

Experience plays a critical role in the ultimate growth and fine-tuning of neural circuits in the brain. Some understanding of this process has been gained from studies of the visual system. David Hubel and Torsten Wiesel and their associates, including Carla Shatz, now at the University of California, Berkeley, made many of the key discoveries. I noted in Chapter 8 that the *lateral geniculate body*, the thalamic nucleus that relays information from the optic nerve to the visual cortex, is separated into six layers in the monkey and the human. These layers are completely segregated in terms of input from the two eyes. All six layers of the left lateral geniculate body project to layer IV of the left visual cortex, and all six layers of the right lateral geniculate project to layer IV of the right visual cortex. The pattern of projection is schematized for just two layers of the lateral geniculate and a given region of visual cortex in Figure 10-10. Layer 1 of the lateral geniculate, with input only from the left

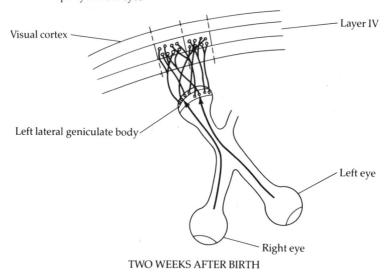

a   No ocular dominance columns; neurons in layer IV connect equally in both eyes

Layer IV

Visual cortex

Left lateral geniculate body

Left eye

Right eye

TWO WEEKS AFTER BIRTH

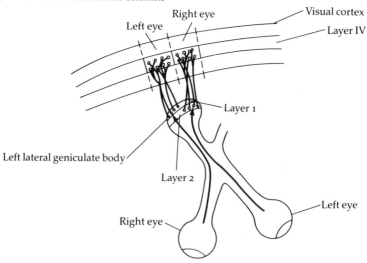

b   Ocular dominance columns

Right eye

Left eye

Visual cortex

Layer IV

Layer 1

Left lateral geniculate body

Layer 2

Left eye

Right eye

ADULT ORGANIZATION

Figure 10-10 Cat visual system. (*a*) Shortly after birth, there is complete overlap of input from the separate layers of the lateral geniculate body (and hence the two eyes) to the columns of cells in layer IV of the visual cortex. (*b*) In the adult pattern of connections from the two eyes to the layers of the lateral geniculate body and to cells in the columns in layer IV in the visual cortex, the inputs from the two eyes are completely separated into alternating columns of cells in layer IV of the cortex (but not in other layers; see Chapter 8).

eye, projects to neurons in alternate columns in layer IV of the left visual cortex. The neurons in layer 2 of the lateral geniculate body, receiving input from the right eye, project to neurons in the remaining columns of layer IV in the left visual cortex.

The lateral geniculate body of the cat, the favored experimental animal for studies of the visual system, consists of only three layers, but the principle of separate layers activated by one of the two eyes is the same. The top and bottom layer receive input from the eye on the opposite side of the body and the middle layer receives input from the eye on the same side. In the cat and the human the topographic projections from the retina to the lateral geniculate body are highly organized. Neighboring regions of the retina make connections with neighboring geniculate cells.

The primary receiving cells in layer IV of the visual cortex are all *monocular*, meaning that they receive input from, say, layer 1 of the lateral geniculate (left eye) or layer 2 of the lateral geniculate (right eye) but never from both. The receptive fields of these primary receiving neurons in cortical layer IV are essentially identical to those in the lateral geniculate, which are identical to those of the ganglion cells in the retina: simple on-center/off-surround or off-center/on-surround. The feature-detecting properties of more complex neurons in the visual cortex are the result of the processing by the neuronal networks of the visual cortex of this simple information conveyed by the layer IV primary receiving cells, as we saw in Chapter 8.

How does this elegant and precise pattern of connections from the two eyes to alternate columns of primary receiving neurons in the visual cortex develop? In cats, monkeys, and humans, if for a certain period of time after birth one eye is kept closed or does not function properly because of some abnormality such as a cataract, that eye will be forever blind. The eye itself is optically normal after opening or cataract removal, or it can easily be made so with a contact lens. Furthermore, the cells in the retina and in the lateral geniculate appear to function normally. Nevertheless, the deprived eye is blind. The changes responsible for this loss of visual function occur in the visual cortex.

The critical period after birth when closing one eye can produce permanent impairment of vision in that eye varies. In cats and monkeys, the critical period extends to several months of age. Over this period the effect of closing the eye becomes progressively less. Closing it for the first two months after birth produces a much greater impairment than closing it for the fifth and sixth months. In humans the critical period seems to last for about the first six years of life. Keeping one eye closed for only a few weeks in the critical period is thought to produce a measurable deficit.

The critical period in visual development corresponds to the period of time when the circuitry in the visual area of the cerebral cortex is still growing and developing. Once the system is completely developed, closing one eye has no effect on vision. An adult can develop a cataract in one eye and wait years for its removal, but once the cataract is removed, vision in that eye is restored (with a contact lens) to complete normality. The fact that the critical period for vision in humans lasts for six years implies that the circuitry is growing and the fine-tuning of its patterns of interconnections is taking place. Normal visual experience has profound effects on the development of circuitry in the visual brain.

If both eyes of a cat or a monkey are kept closed from birth throughout the critical period, and the eyes are then opened, the animals remains functionally blind. In humans, after correction of some malady that prevented sight through the critical period, some vision does seem to be restored, but detail vision is much impaired. However if both eyes are kept closed for relatively brief periods, there is much less impairment of function than if just one eye is closed.

Most of the work on visual system development and deprivation has been done on the cat because its visual cortex is less developed at birth than a monkey's or those of other primates. Presumably the visual processes develop in basically the same ways in cats, monkeys, and humans, although at somewhat different times.

Two techniques have been critical in understanding visual development and the effects of visual deprivation on the brain. One technique is the recording of the activity of single neurons in the visual cortex. The other technique is *anatomical tracing*. A radioactively labeled amino acid is injected into the eye, from which it is taken up by the ganglion cells in the retina and transported to the nerve terminals in the lateral geniculate. Here a process of transneuronal transport occurs. This is a fortunate occurrence in the visual system (and other sensory systems): the labeled amino acid somehow crosses the synapses of the ganglion cells with the lateral geniculate and is taken up by the cells there, which transport it to their axon terminals connecting with layer IV of the visual cortex.

Microelectrode recording studies and anatomical tracing work agree that essentially the following is the pattern of development in the visual system of the cat. During the first two weeks of life there are no *ocular-dominance*, or eye-preferring, *columns* in the visual cortex and, in fact, there is little sign of any ocular dominance at all. Radioactively labeled amino acid transported from either eye forms a uniform band in the visual cortex. The neurons studied at this time with a microelectrode have been shown to be binocular, or to respond equivalently to stimulation of either eye (Figure 10-10).

The pattern of projection to layer IV of the visual cortex in the cat is essentially undifferentiated at birth. This is in striking contrast to the pattern in the young adult cat. At several months of age, labeled amino acid injected into one eye is projected to alternating columns in the cortex, and layer IV cells respond only to input from one eye or the other, which can be determined with a microelectrode.

As development proceeds after birth in the cat, axon terminals from the layers of the lateral geniculate (conveying information from the two eyes) compete. In one small region input from the left eye comes to dominate, and in the next small region input from the right eye dominates. Very recent work provides insights into two processes that appear critical for the development of the ocular-dominance columns. First, electrical activity of the neurons is necessary. In ingenious experiments, Michael Stryker at the University of California at San Francisco showed that if a substance called tetrodotoxin (TTX), the poison in puffer fish that blocks sodium channels and hence stops all action potentials in neurons (see Chapter 3), is infused in the cortex during the time that the fibers from the lateral geniculate body are segregating into the separate columns for the input from the two eyes, the ocular-dominance columns do not develop. Remember that normal visual experience is necessary during this period for normal development of the ocular dominance columns. So if the electrical activity of neurons in the cortex is blocked, visual experience cannot do the job.

The second process involves the subplate neurons. As we learned earlier, these neurons are present only during the development of the cerebral cortex. In visual cortex their axons project to both layer IV and layer I (Figure 10-11).

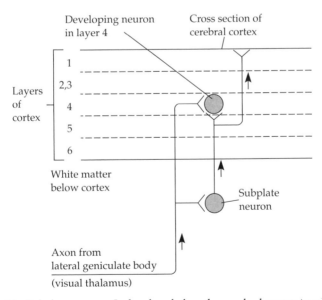

Figure 10-11 Subplate neuron. It develops below the cerebral cortex in white matter and sends its axons up to synapse on developing neurons in layer 4 of the cerebral cortex (sensory-reception layer) and also sends axon branches up to the surface of the cortex. Subplate neurons are physiologically active and are thought to guide the development of sensory-receptive fields in the cerebral cortex. They die out as the cortex matures.

It appears that they synaptically activate the cortical layer IV neurons. Carla Shatz and her colleagues injected a chemical that destroys cell bodies but not fibers in the white matter just below the cortex in the first week after birth in kittens. This killed the subplate neurons but not the neurons in the developing visual cortex. The cortex was examined much later (at more than 7 weeks), after the ocular dominance columns normally would have developed. Dramatically, no ocular dominance columns developed directly over the region where the subplate neurons had been destroyed, but they were present and normal elsewhere in the visual cortex. The subplate neurons somehow guide the growth and segregation of the incoming lateral geniculate neurons to the appropriate small regions of layer 4 to yield the ocular-dominance columns. Again, during this time, after the first postnatal week, the kitten's eyes are open and the visual system is electrically active, which is also necessary for normal development. Shatz speculates that subplate neurons might modulate the interactions between the geniculate fibers and the cortical layer IV neurons by activating glutamate NMDA-type receptors (see Chapter 4).

What happens to the ocular-dominance columns in the visual cortex when one eye is kept closed from birth? The ocular-dominance columns for the deprived eye are much smaller than for the normal eye (Figure 10-12). This is a striking demonstration of the effects of experience on the growth and development of the nervous system. Here the difference in experience is between normal visual stimulation and the dim shades of light that penetrate the closed eyelid. In the absence of normal visual experience, the input to the cortex (via the lateral geniculate) from the open eye comes to dominate and take over a substantial part of the deprived eye's normal dominance column. How this happens is not yet known, but the message is clear: normal sensory experience is critically important for the normal development of the brain. The work with cats has obvious implications for children with visual defects that result in one eye functioning better than the other. Such defects should be corrected as soon after birth as possible.

Norepinephrine may be involved in the development of the ocular-dominance columns in the visual cortex during the critical period. This has been suggested by some recent work. Norepinephrine neurons in the locus ceruleus become functionally mature at the time of the visual critical period. These neurons project from the region of the locus ceruleus in the brain stem widely and diffusely to the cerebral cortex and the limbic system. When activated, they release norepinephrine at their axon terminals in these regions. It is currently believed that this norepinephrine system is not a fast synaptic transmitter system but rather acts more like a local hormone, exerting modulatory influences by way of a second-messenger system (see Chapter 5).

The neurotoxin 6-hydroxydopamine was injected into the region of the locus ceruleus in young kittens at the beginning of the critical visual period;

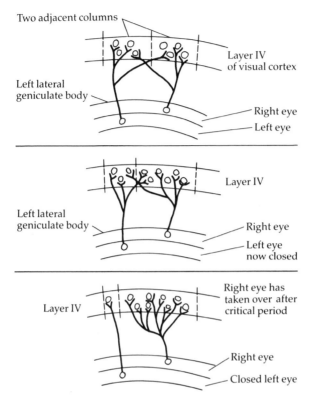

Figure 10-12 Effect of keeping an eye closed over the course of early development, for example, in a cat or monkey from birth until the time the adult pattern is normally formed. Absence of normal visual stimulation from the closed eye results in the input from the normal eye (via the lateral geniculate body) progressively taking over more and more of the cells in layer IV of the visual cortex. The open-eye columns become larger and larger, and the closed-eye columns shrink, ultimately to only about 10 percent of the visual cortex (normally each eye's columns represent about 50 percent of the visual cortex).

the drug permanently destroys norepinephrine neurons. The kittens were then monocularly deprived (one eyelid was kept closed) during the critical period. No changes in ocular dominance developed: the columns in the cortex activated by the open eye did not expand and those that had been activated by the closed eye did not shrink. It is as though norepinephrine is necessary for this neuronal plasticity to occur in the visual cortex.

In other kittens that had one eye closed and had been treated with hydroxydopamine, norepinephrine was perfused directly onto the visual cortex during the critical period. In these animals, the ocular-dominance shift in favor of the open eye developed. Hence adding norepinephrine directly to the visual cortex replaced the normal source of norepinephrine, the locus ceruleus.

The next experiment yielded even more impressive results. One eye was closed in normal adult cats, long after the critical period had passed. By itself, this would have had no effect on the organization of the visual cortex. The experimenters then perfused norepinephrine onto the visual cortex in the cats. Ocular-dominance shifts developed: the columns in the visual cortex activated by the open eye expanded and those from the closed eye shrank. Apparently a new critical period in the visual cortex had been created in adult cats by the addition of norepinephrine directly to the cortex. Such induction of neuronal plasticity could have important applications in the treatment of human conditions such as squint. If a human infant is born with a squint and the condition is not corrected early, the affected eye becomes less functional.

The notion of critical periods in development is very general. A striking example is imprinting in birds. Precocial birds, birds that can walk and feed at birth, such as chickens and geese, for a brief period lasting about two days after birth will become imprinted on, or strongly attached to, almost any object larger than they are that moves. Normally, this object is the mother, but in her absence they will readily attach themselves to substitutes. You may have seen a picture of Konrad Lorenz, who discovered imprinting, being trailed about by a group of young geese who were convinced he was their mother.

Laboratory studies of imprinting in the chicken indicate that a particular region of the forebrain called the *medial hyperstriatum ventrale* seems to be a critical locus for the development of the "memory trace" for the imprinting stimulus. Destruction of this region abolishes the imprinted behavior, and anatomical and chemical changes are reported to occur here that are correlated with the imprinting process. There is some degree of hemispheric asymmetry in the development of imprinting. Imprinting provides a most interesting model of a very specialized form of learning that can occur only in one narrow and early window of time during the development of the nervous system in certain birds.

Suppose that during early stages of development in a mammal a defect of some sort occurs and the embryo does not develop a limb. After the animal is born and matures, will the somatic sensory region of the cerebral cortex have a representation of the missing limb or not? This may seem like a chicken-or-egg question but it is profoundly important for our understanding of the developmental organization of the cerebral cortex. A particularly good model for studying this question is the whisker barrels in rodent somatic sensory cortex we described in Chapter 8 (see Figure 8-17). You will recall that each whisker is represented in the cortex by a ring or barrel of neurons that are exquisitely sensitive to movements of the whisker. Thomas Woolsey and associates, working at Washington University in St. Louis, performed a now classic experiment (Figure 10-13). They removed an entire row of cells from the snout region early in development and allowed the animals to continue developing. When the whisker barrels had developed in the cortex, the entire row of cortical barrels corresponding to the row of removed whiskers was missing.

This experiment demonstrated that the organization of somatic cerebral cortex is extremely plastic early in development and also that cortical organization is dependent on the organization of the peripheral body and, presumably, the normal activity of the corresponding neural pathways during development. But what about adult animals? Michael Merzenich and others at the University of California, San Francisco, showed that if a digit was amputated in monkeys, the receptive field for the digit in the somatic sensory cortex decreased in size. On the other hand if the digit was stimulated by

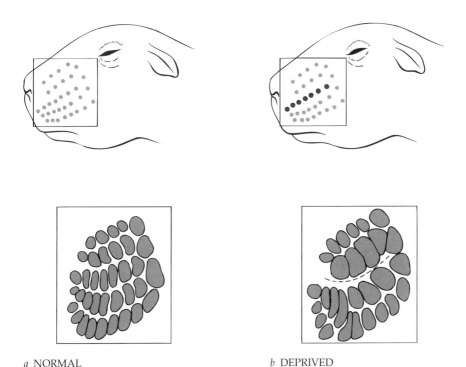

a NORMAL   *b* DEPRIVED

Figure 10-13 Development of the whisker barrel receptive fields in rodent somatic sensory cortex (see Figure 8-17). (*a*) Normal development. (*b*) If one row of whiskers is removed early in development, the corresponding barrels in the cortex do not develop and are completely missing in the adult.

vibration for a long period of time, the cortical receptive field of the digit expanded.

Recently, a very dramatic experiment showed that somatic sensory cortex can undergo massive reorganization in the adult. You may recall the experiment we described in Chapter 9, where monkeys had all sensory input from their forelimbs eliminated by section of the appropriate dorsal roots. They were able to learn to move their arms accurately even without visual guidance. We concluded from this that brain motor systems provide information directly to the brain about where the limbs are supposed to be in space, even without sensory input from the limbs. Ten years later, when the monkeys were elderly, somatic sensory cortex was mapped (see Figure 8-13). An extraordinary reorganization had occurred in the cortex. The forearm representation area was missing. Instead, the region of the cortex representing the face had expanded to occupy the entire region formally occupied by the arm. We might think that this would result in greater sensory sensitivity and discrimination ability of the face. It also raises the possibility that in humans who lose major sensory input, remaining cortical areas representing other sensory input might expand in an attempt to compensate. The acute hearing of people who are blind from a young age might be due in part to reorganization of cerebral cortex as well as to the traditional explanation that they pay more attention to auditory cues. But this is of course only speculation.

The effects of visual experience on the development of the visual cortex provide a specific example of how early experience can influence brain development. Many studies have shown that the richness and variety of early experience can have powerful effects on brain development and behavior in mammals. Pioneering work in this area was done by psychologists Mark Rosenzweig and David Krech together with Marion C. Diamond, a neuroanatomist, and Edward Bennet, a neurochemist, at the University of California at Berkeley. Rosenzweig and Krech devised a rich environment for rats and raised them together in various social groups. (An example of the environment is shown in Figure 10-14). Brothers and sisters of the rich rats (littermate controls) were raised individually in standard laboratory cages (they were the poor rats) and in social groups in large laboratory cages (poor-social rats). Rich rats, poor rats, and poor-social rats were all given sufficient food and water and kept clean.

Rosenzweig and his associates measured a number of properties of the rats' brains, particularly of the cerebral cortex, and also tested their behavioral capabilities. Virtually all of the measures showed increased brain development in the rich rats compared with the poor rats. The poor-social rats generally were intermediate between the two. Indeed, the effects of early experience are evident simply from the weights of brains: rich rats had heavier brains than

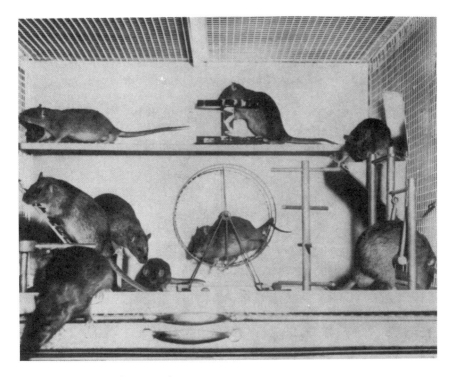

Figure 10-14 A rich rat penthouse environment.

poor ones. The rich rats were also superior at maze learning and other complex behavioral performance tasks.

The two types of measures that have been used most widely in recent work on the effects of experience on the brain are the number and complexity of neuron dendrites and the number of dendritic spines. Much of the work has been done by William Greenough and his associates at the University of Illinois. The dendrites of a neuron, along with its cell body, receive synaptic connections from other neurons, as we saw in Chapter 2. In the cerebral cortex, the dendrites of many neurons are covered with thousands of dendritic spines (see Figure 2-2). Each spine is the postsynaptic part of a synapse formed with the dendrite by an axon terminal from another neuron. The presynaptic axon terminal forms on and around the spine, as we said in Chapter 2, and these dendritic spine synapses are thought to be excitatory.

In the cerebral cortex of a rich rat certain neurons have significantly more complex dendrites and significantly more dendritic spines on them than in the cortex of a poor rat. Since the spines are synapses, presumably excitatory, a rich early environment may result in more excitatory synaptic connections in the brain. Whether the growth of new synaptic connections in the cerebral cortex actually serves to code the memories formed by the rich rats is not known. It could be that more excitatory synapses form as a result of greater stimulation and arousal (and more norepinephrine?) but that they are not directly concerned with memory storage.

An alternative interpretation is that the rich rats are actually normal rats, because rats in the wild live in an environment that is rich in stimuli and stress, if not in food. The poor rats may be abnormally deprived of experience and so develop an abnormally small number of excitatory synaptic connections in the cerebral cortex. Rosenzweig and his associates raised laboratory rats in the seminatural environment of the "wilds" of Berkeley outside Tolman Hall (the psychology building) and found that this may indeed be the case. In these animals the brains were as well or better developed than those of the rich laboratory rats.

The effects of a rich environment on the brain are not completely permanent. If rich rats are later returned to a poor environment, the brain development regresses to some degree. Interestingly, the poor rats show some signs of increased brain development when they are run through mazes and other behavioral tests. The testing and learning experiences can apparently induce some brain development, even in these young adult animals. Stress may also be an important factor. Seymour Levine of Stanford showed that rats that were given electric shock stress experiences as infants performed better on learning tasks after they were adults than did nonstressed controls.

Most of the work on the effects of early environmental experience on brain development has been done on rats and mice. Greenough has also studied the effects of experience on brain development in the monkey. One group of monkeys was housed in individual cages from shortly after birth. Another group lived in similar cages but was allowed to play with other monkeys each day. The third group was raised with other monkeys of all ages in a pair of large, adjoining rooms equipped with play objects and structures. In the rich monkeys the principal neurons of the cerebellum, the Purkinje cells, had significantly greater dendritic complexity than those of the monkeys in the poor and poor–social groups. The cerebellum, as we have seen, is much involved in the control of movement and may also have much to do with the coding of learned responses (see Chapter 11).

In sum, experience can exert powerful effects on the growth of dendrites and the formation of synapses in the brain, particularly during early growth and development. Synapses, the points of functional connections among neurons, are much more plastic than was earlier thought to be the case.

Apparently they can form and disappear in a matter of hours or days. The powerful effects of early experience on brain development in rats and monkeys were among the reasons why programs like Headstart were developed, in the hope that early enriched social and educational experiences prior to the school years would benefit disadvantaged children.

AGING AND THE BRAIN

The average life expectancy is now over 70 years in developed countries such as the United States and has been growing progressively longer. However, the maximum life span has not increased; it remains about 100 years.

The fact that the maximum life span for humans has not increased despite better medicine, including the elimination of many diseases, suggests that there may be built-in aging factors. For a long time it was thought that the organs were primarily responsible for aging: the heart, kidneys, and other organs simply wore out. It is now known that this is not the entire answer. Leonard Hayflick, then at the Children's Hospital Medical Center in Oakland, grew cell cultures of normal human body cells taken from people of different ages. Cells from a human embryo double about 50 times before they die, whereas cells taken from a middle-aged human divide only about 20 times before they die.

Hayflick went on to determine whether this control on cell aging was in the DNA of the cell nucleus, the "prime contract," or if it was in the cell bodies outside the nucleus, the "subcontracts." He exchanged the nuclei in human embryo cells and adult cells and found that whether a cell body was from an embryo cell or from an adult cell, if the nucleus was from an adult, the cell divided only about 20 times. If the nucleus was from the embryo, the cell divided about 50 times. Hayflick's experiments suggested that part of the aging process is genetic, or under the control of the DNA in the nucleus. The only kind of human cell that is immortal is the cancer cell.

A genetic time clock that regulates the number of times a human body cell divides cannot, however, be the whole explanation of the aging process. The most important cells in the human body, the neurons in the brain, never divide after birth. Therefore, resetting of the genetic aging clock in body cells would not solve the problem of possible deterioration of the brain. Aging has become a major area of investigation in biology and neuroscience, perhaps more than coincidentally with the aging of certain influential segments of the population.

Memory and Aging

The mental deterioration that occurs with normal aging in humans has been greatly exaggerated, due in part to confusion between normal aging and a severe type of senility called Alzheimer's disease. Laboratory studies of memory abilities in older people who are not senile indicate that the losses in memory with age are not great. Short-term or recent memory is not impaired, although the ability to divide one's attention between two or more sensory inputs may be, as when one wishes at a party to listen to the person talking to one and to eavesdrop on the conversation of people nearby as well. Long-term memory, the ability to store new information for long periods, does show a significant decline with age but not until the sixth decade or older.

Most of the studies on the effects aging has on human abilities have suffered from a subtle but important defect called the "cohort" problem. As an example of this, if we were to compare the memory abilities of two groups of people, one made up of 20-year-olds and the other of 70-year-olds, they would obviously have had quite different educations and experiences. A 70-year-old who was 10 in 1932 had an education that was quite different from that of a person 20 years old today. Among many other factors, there was no television in 1932. In this context, "cohort" means a group of the same age at the same time followed over their life span. We should really compare Ms. X at age 20 with herself at age 70 to establish accurately changes in memory ability. What data exist on memory ability suggest that people who are 60 today perform significantly better on memory tests than people who were 60 in 1930 (and of course were tested then). Whatever the reason, memory in older people seems to be improving.

Senility and Alzheimer's disease

Senility is a very broad term meaning age-related brain dysfunction and can have many causes, including brain damage, stroke, alcoholism, and Alzheimer's disease. The most striking symptom of senility is memory impairment. An unacceptably high number of people over age 65—10 to 15 percent—suffer from mild to severe symptoms of senility. Alzheimer's disease has traditionally been defined as severe senility that develops before age 65. The symptoms of senility are similar in people under and over 65, however, and so senility that develops after 65 is now generally included as Alzheimer's disease, technically as "senile dementia of the Alzheimer's type" (SDAT). Over 50 percent of people showing symptoms of senility can be included in the Alzheimer's disease category—over a million people in the United States. The incidence of SDAT increases with age and will be an increasingly severe problem in our aging society.

The symptoms of Alzheimer's disease include marked defects in cognitive function, memory, language, and perceptual abilities. In some people the onset is slow and gradual, but in others it is quite rapid. The first and most obvious symptom is the loss of recent memory, particularly the ability to place new information into long-term storage. A clear brain pathology associated with Alzheimer's disease has been known for some time: *senile plaques,* which are clusters of abnormal cell processes surrounding masses of protein; tangles of neurofilaments inside neurons; deterioration of neuron dendrites; and loss of neurons (Figure 10-15). These changes are particularly evident in the hippocampus and certain regions of the cerebral cortex, regions much concerned with complex cognitive processes and memory. Regrettably, the disease is

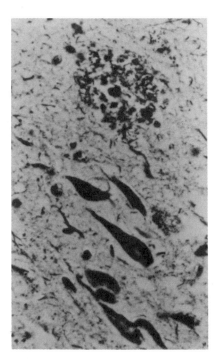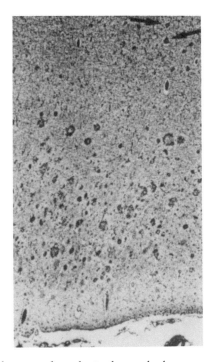

Figure 10-15 Photomicrographs of senile plaques and tangles in the cerebral cortex from a patient who died from Alzheimer's disease (*a*) High-power magnification showing one plaque above and several neurofibrillary tangles below. (*b*) Lower-power magnification of cross section through cerebral cortex showing numerous plaques, and tangles in neurons below (arrows).

progressive—people gradually lose their permanent memories and ultimately die as the brain degenerates.

The neurotransmitter ACh may have some involvement in Alzheimer's disease. To quickly review (see Chapters 4 and 5, particularly Figure 5-2), ACh is the neurotransmitter chemical at the neuromuscular junctions between motor neurons and skeletal muscle fibers and in some brain systems. ACh activates target cell receptors and is in turn broken down by an enzyme, acetylcholinesterase (AChE), back into its two simple chemical constituents, acetyl and choline. A form of acetyl is present in all cells, and choline is present in many normal food substances. The nucleus basalis at the base of the forebrain, which projects to the cerebral cortex and hippocampus, utilizes ACh as a neurotransmitter. Studies of the brains of a number of patients who had died from Alzheimer's disease indicated a marked loss of cells in the nucleus basalis, which contains ACh neurons projecting to the cerebral cortex, and much lower levels of certain chemicals associated with the ACh system.

It has been known for some time that anticholinergic drugs, which counter the effects of ACh, impair memory in rats and monkeys but that anticholinesterase drugs, which block AChE, facilitate memory. If AChE is blocked, there will be more ACh. Thus it seems that more ACh is good for memory and less ACh is bad for it, at least in rats. But the same is true for a number of other substances, for example, NE (see Chapter 11).

It is not yet known whether the loss of ACh neurons is the sole or even a major cause of Alzheimer's disease, nor whether there is any causal relation between the appearance of the senile plaques, neuron loss in the cerebral cortex and hippocampus, and the marked loss of ACh neurons in the nucleus basalis. However, now that a correlation between the disease and the loss of ACh neurons has been established, these questions are more approachable.

Drugs acting to increase ACh in the brain ought to improve memory in humans. This has indeed been found to be true for normal young adults. However, many of these drugs have rather serious side-effects. Such drugs have been used to treat Alzheimer individuals, with some reports of success with people who are only mildly senile. Feeding choline to very aged mice, who also show deficits in placing new information into long-term memory, is reported to result in improvements in maze-learning performance. Choline is a safe treatment, but clinical studies in which choline was fed to senile patients did not report that the patients improved. However, when choline and the drug physostigmine, which antagonizes the action of the breakdown enzyme AChE, are jointly administered, the memories of Alzheimer individuals are helped somewhat according to some studies but not according to other studies. Even if these treatments were to help, they would at best be very temporary.

We still do not know the actual causes or precipitating factors in Alzheimer's disease. In at least some cases there appears to be a genetic predisposition—the disease can run in families. The general notion prevalent today is that certain genes may suddenly begin expressing proteins that lead to plaques and tangles or may cease producing proteins that prevent these abnormal phenomena or both. If this proves to be the case, then chemical therapies may be possible. Thus, if genes start expressing abnormal proteins, drugs might be developed that will prevent the expression of these proteins. Perhaps the ultimate preventive treatment will involve some form of genetic engineering. Study of the causes and possible treatments of Alzheimer's disease is one of the most active areas of research in neuroscience today.

SUMMARY

The number of neurons of the human embryo increases by an average of 250,000 every minute from conception to birth. How this multitude of neurons migrates, grows, and develops into the human brain is one of the major mysteries in neuroscience. The blueprint for the development of the structural organization of the human brain is found in the genes, and developmental processes, for example, induction, are critical. Further, the fine structure of synaptic connections in the brain is not under direct genetic control but rather is shaped and reshaped throughout development and life from conception to death by experience.

Mechanisms of neural growth and development include chemical signals, cell and terminal competition, and fiber-guided cell movements. Certain types of cells release chemical signals (for example, NGF) that guide the growth of nerve fiber terminals to them. At a relatively late stage of prenatal development there are many more neurons and many more competing synapses on neurons than there are in the adult. Only some win out. Many neurons and synapses die as a result of this competition, leading to the fine-tuning of connections in the adult brain. Finally, neurons send out growing axons, at the end of which are growth cones that produce the actual growth. In many cases these growing axons continue to grow until they reach a barrier, for example, the edge of the brain. The cell body then moves up the axon to take its final position, as in a Purkinje neuron in the cerebellar cortex.

Development of the visual brain system has provided much of our understanding of how the cerebral cortex forms and develops. Early in development, neurons in layer IV of visual cortex receive input from both eyes (via the visual thalamus). However, ultimately cells receive input from only one eye or the other. It turns out that normal neuronal activity due to visual experience after birth is necessary for this process of synapse selection. Another key process involves subplate neurons that develop, guide the growth of axons into the correct critical locations in the cerebral cortex, and then die out.

Organization and reorganization of the cerebral cortex is not limited to development; it appears to occur throughout the lifetime of each individual. Studies on monkeys show that altered input, for example from the fingers, can cause rapid increases or decreases in size of receptive fields in the somatic sensory cortex. Experiences during postnatal growth and development and in adulthood has profound effects on the growth and development of the cerebral cortex. Enriched experience can increase the thickness of the cortex and the numbers and organization of synaptic connections in both the cerebral and cerebellar cortices.

The deleterious effects of normal aging on brain organization and memory processes have often been exaggerated. There are no age-related impairments in short-term memory, and impairment in ability to place new information in long-term storage begins to appear only in the sixth decade or later. Alzheimer's disease, on the other hand, is a devastating disorder that causes massive changes in the brain (plaques, tangles, neuron loss) and corresponding impairment in memory abilities and memories. As yet there is no effective treatment for this terrible disorder that afflicts some 15 percent of people over the age of 65.

SUGGESTED READINGS AND REFERENCES

Books

Diamond, M. C. (1988). *Enriching heredity: The impact of the environment on the anatomy of the brain.* New York: Free Press.

Fidia Research Foundation (1991). *Proceedings of the course on developmental neurobiology.* New York: Thieme Medical Publishers.

Finch, C. E. (1990). *Longevity, senescence, and the genome.* Chicago: The University of Chicago Press.

Gilbert, S. F. (1988). *Developmental biology* (2nd ed.). Sunderland, MA: Sinauer Associates.

Greenough, W. T., & Juraska, J. M. (1986). *Developmental neuropsychobiology.* Orlando: Academic Press.

Heston, L. L., & White, J. A. (1991). *The vanishing mind: A practical guide to Alzheimer's disease and other dementias.* New York: W. H. Freeman.

Purves, D. (1988). *Body and brain: A trophic theory of neural connections.* Cambridge, MA: Harvard University Press.

Purves, D., & Lichtman, J. W. (1985). *Principles of neural development.* Sunderland, MA: Sinauer Associates.

Articles

Brun, A. (1983). An overview of light and electron microscope changes in Alzheimer's disease. In Reisberg, B. (Ed.), *Alzheimer's disease.* New York: Free Press, pp. 37–47.

Cowan, W. M. (1979). The development of the brain. *Scientific American*, *241*, 112–133.

Ghosh, A., & Shatz, C. J. (1992). Involvement of subplate neurons in the formation of ocular dominance columns. *Science*, *255*, 1441–1443.

Gorski, R. A. (1988). Sexual differentiation of the brain: Mechanisms and implications for neuroscience. In Easter, S. S., Jr., Barald, K. F., & Carlson, B. M. (Eds.), *From message to mind: Directions in developmental neurobiology*. Sunderland, MA: Sinauer Associates, pp. 256–271.

Hamburger, V. (1988). Ontogeny of neuroembryology. *Journal of Neuroscience*, *8*, 3535–3540.

Levi-Montalcini, R. (1982). Developmental neurobiology and the natural history of nerve growth factor. *Annual Review of Neuroscience*, *5*, 341–362.

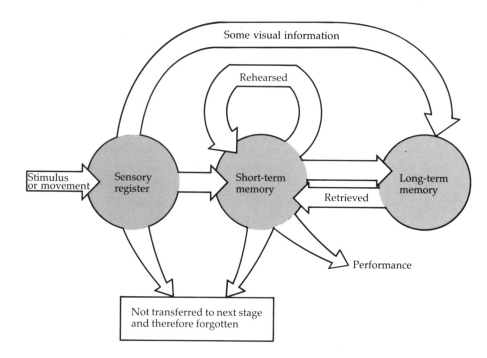

Some visual information

Rehearsed

Stimulus or movement

Sensory register

Short-term memory

Long-term memory

Retrieved

Performance

Not transferred to next stage and therefore forgotten

11

Learning, Memory, and the Brain

Memory is the most extraordinary phenomenon in the natural world. You who are reading this book have literally millions of bits of information stored in your long-term or permanent memory. Your memory store includes your vocabulary and knowledge of language, all the facts you have learned, your memories of your own life experiences and people you have known, all the skills you have learned, from walking and talking to swimming and tennis, and much more. Somehow the brain stores all this diverse information so that it

Figure 11-1 *Hypothetical scheme of the human memory system. Sensory information, including information about movements being learned (as in tennis) enters a sensory register or "iconic" memory where it is held in detail for a brief period. Some of this information is transferred to a short-term memory store (for example, memory of a new telephone number). Some visual information is also transferred directly from iconic to long-term memory. Some of the information from short-term memory can be transferred to long-term memory, usually by rehearsal or practice. But some aspects of our ongoing experience (episodic memory) appear to be transferred from short-term to long-term memory automatically, without practice. But much information from iconic and short-term memory is not stored and is simply lost. When you remember something, it is called up into short-term or working memory from long-term memory storage. Performance, as in reporting memories or showing improvement on skilled motor tasks, is the net outcome of all these processes. Short-term memory is roughly equivalent to consciousness or awareness (see Chapter 12).*

can easily be accessed and used. It may be that each well-educated adult has as many bits of information stored in memory as he or she has neurons in the brain. But this is not to say that individual memories are stored in individual nerve cells. Instead, we think that memories are coded and stored by alterations in the patterns and excitability of the myriads of synaptic connections among the neurons in the brain. Different brain systems play particular roles in different aspects of learning and memory, as will become clear in this chapter. *Learning,* incidentally, refers to the acquisition of information or skills, and *memory* refers to the expression of information or skills.

ASPECTS OF MEMORY

Much of the learning we do is learning to make movements. Reaching is a simple example. At one month of age an infant shows erratic and inaccurate movements of the arms when reaching for an object; by five months of age the reaching movement is smooth and accurate. Interestingly, patients with damage to certain regions of the cerebellum show impairments in reaching movements much like the one-month-old infant. Learning to walk is a long and sometimes painful process; learning to talk, to speak language, requires years. The act of speaking clearly requires the learning of complex sequences of skilled and precise movements of the lips, tongue, and mouth. Some scientists have argued further that learning to understand spoken language involves internal representations of the act of speaking. In any event, the learning of skilled movements is a major part of the learning we do.

There is of course much more to memory than learning movements. Do you have a photographic memory? Can you look briefly at a page of text or a list of numbers, then look away, see the material with your "mind's eye" and repeat it accurately? Most of us do not have this ability but a few people who do have been found and studied. A famous case was documented in a book by the Russian neuropsychologist Alexander Luria entitled *The Mind of a Mnemonist*. The person, identified by Luria only as "S," could remember long lists of digits dictated to him, long lists of objects shown to him, and even lists of complex mathematical formulas (he did not know mathematics). He was even able to recall accurately a matrix of random numbers that had been presented to him 16 years earlier! Interestingly, S was not above average in intelligence and in fact complained that his memories kept getting in his way when he was trying to solve problems. Past images and lists of numbers would intrude and disrupt his thought processes.

Actually, all of us have visual photographic memories. This is the good news. The bad news is that they last for only about a tenth of a second. This surprising fact was discovered in ingenious experiments by the psychologist

George Sperling. He used a device termed a tachistoscope that can present visual stimuli for very brief periods—a few milliseconds. He showed people an array of random individual letters, say a five-by-five array containing 25 letters that did not spell any words. The array was flashed for a few milliseconds and the person asked to recall the letters. People could correctly recall only four or five letters, typically those in the corners of the array. But of course it took the person a second or more after seeing the array to begin reporting letters.

Sperling then added a cue; a dot of light would appear in the place in the empty array where a letter had been. He presented this cue at various times shortly after the array of letters had been turned off. If the dot was presented within 100 milliseconds after the array, people would almost always recall correctly the letter that had been in the space where the dot was located, regardless of which position it was in. In other words, people were able to hold the entire array of letters in memory for about 100 milliseconds. Sperling systematically increased the delay time from turning off the array of letters to presenting the dot and found that the photographic memory had decayed in about 200 milliseconds (Figure 11-2). This very short-term photographic memory is termed *iconic memory* from the Greek word icon, meaning image. Surprisingly, the brain systems that store iconic visual memories are not yet known. The retina and visual pathways, including the visual areas of the cerebral cortex, are a reasonable guess, but evidence is lacking.

Studies with children suggest that they may have photographic-like visual memory abilities until about 6 years of age, about the time they begin to learn to read. Interestingly, studies by anthropologists of peoples living in remote corners of the world who do not have written language suggest that even the

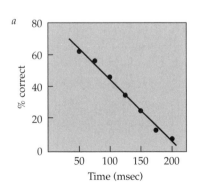

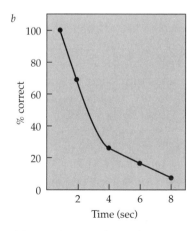

Figure 11-2 Decay of memory. (*a*) Time course of decay of sensory (iconic) memory following very brief (a few milliseconds) exposure to an array of visual information. (*b*) Time course of decay of short-term memory.

adults may have photographic-like visual memory abilities. Walking on a well-traveled jungle trail that has thousands of leaves along the path, they notice when just a few leaves have been moved.

These observations probably have implications for brain substrates of visual memory and language. So far as we know, the human brain evolved to its fully modern form well over 100,000 years ago; no changes in brain structure or organization have occurred for a very long time. Yet written language and hence reading were invented only about 10,000 years ago. Reading is after all an unnatural act. There was no evolutionary pressure to develop reading ability in the brain. It is tempting to speculate that the human species evolved very special photographic-like visual memory abilities. Such abilities would clearly have adaptive value. Learning to read is a slow and difficult task for children and particularly so for those who learn to read as adults. Perhaps the regions of the brain (in the cerebral cortex?) that evolved for photographic visual memory are the regions used to learn to read. Our cultural evolution has forced us to use certain areas of our brain on tasks for which nature never intended them to be used. Spoken language, on the other hand, must have evolved along with the evolution of our species and is clearly adaptive. Brain substrates of language will be treated in Chapter 12.

Short-term memory and its annoying lack of persistence is familiar to all of us. You look up a new number in the telephone book and remember it for the few seconds it takes to dial it, and then it is gone from memory. To remember it, you have to repeat it to yourself a number of times, to rehearse it, just as you have to rehearse the lines in a play or a poem to place the text in long-term memory. Careful studies of short-term memory where people were prevented from rehearsal, for example, by counting backward, indicate that short-term memory decays to virtually zero in about 10 seconds. (Figure 11-1). It is also the case that short-term memory has a very limited capacity—about seven items of completely new information, like a telephone number. But in real life, as opposed to the psychology laboratory, short-term memory generally involves things that are at least partly familiar to you, as in having a conversation with someone. Short-term memory merges with longer-term memory and experience. This more natural shorter-term memory is continuous and persists much longer than 10 seconds and is often called *working memory*.

Remarkable experiments by the psychologist Saul Sternberg give us a glimpse of the machinery of the brain in short-term memory. He presented people with a list of random digits, one at a time, to form a short-term memory set. The number of digits in the memory set varied from one to six. A few seconds after the memory set was presented, a test digit was shown. If it had been presented in the set, the person pulled a "yes" lever and if not, a "no" lever. Sternberg simply measured how long the subject took to make his or her response; that is, he measured the subject's reaction time or *response latency*. Results were striking. Response latency was a virtually perfect straight vector,

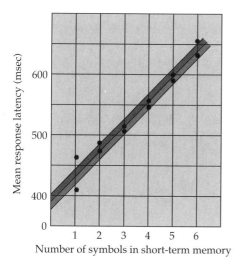

Figure 11-3 Relationship between the number of items in short-term store and the response latency as people search through their memory store.

increasing as a function of the number of symbols in memory (Figure 11-3). This indicated that the memory search was accomplished in a serial fashion (from the first to the last symbol presented in the memory set) and was very fast, averaging about 25 or 30 symbols per second. One has the sense of a computerlike machine functioning in a rigid manner searching through a memory bank.

With practice, new information and skills are stored in long-term or permanent memory. Actually, visual long-term memory may be a special case in humans. This was shown in a dramatic experiment by the psychologist Ralph Haber at the University of Rochester. He collected thousands of home slides, pictures of persons and places, from people in his community. In an introductory college psychology lecture he showed the students more than 1000 slides, one after the other, at the rate of 1 per second. Two days later, at the next lecture, he showed all of the same slides, but each one now shown side-by-side with a new slide. The position of the previously seen slide was randomly on the left or right. After each slide pair the students simply had to score which slide, left or right, they had seen before. They scored an amazing 90% correct. It is as though some aspects of the visual scene in each slide had somehow been stored directly in visual long-term memory without any practice or rehearsal. Consider all the faces you have seen in your life. If you see one again you are likely to recognize it, even if you only saw it briefly years ago and couldn't possibly remember the name that goes with the face. The visual memory ability to remember and recognize faces may be unique to people and perhaps other primates. Primates are animals with visual abilities well-suited to living in social groups.

There appear to be several different kinds of long-term memory. One type is time-tagged, or *episodic*, characterized by Endel Tulving at the University of Toronto. You remember what you had for breakfast, a conversation you had with a friend last week, and what you did on your last birthday. Every person has a vast memory store of his or her own past experiences. You remember roughly when these experiences happened in the past and their appropriate sequence in time. Another type of memory is *semantic* knowledge. You remember the meanings of words and the multiplication table, but not when you learned them. Semantic knowledge is not time-tagged.

Motor skill memory is very similar to semantic memory. In learning a foreign language (semantic memory) you associate the foreign words and phrases with English equivalents and concentrate on rehearsing these associations many times. As you become fluent in the language and the meanings become well-learned, they are stored in long-term memory. You are not normally aware that the new language is in your memory, but when you need to use it, it is there. By the same token, when you learn any new motor skill, from playing tennis to playing the piano, you learn to associate particular stimuli with particular precise sequences of movements, an activity that requires considerable effort and concentration. You must practice these stimulus-associated movements many times. As the skill becomes well-learned, you cease concentrating on it—it becomes stored in long-term memory. You are not normally aware that this skill is in your memory, but when you use it, it is there. Semantic and motor skill learning have many of the same basic properties. For example, distributed practice—an hour a day for seven days—is much more effective for both types of memory than seven hours in a row of massed practice.

Another way of classifying long-term memory is as *declarative*—learning what—and *procedural*—learning how. Declarative memory includes both episodic and semantic memory and procedural memory includes motor skills and Pavlovian conditioning (discussed later). These various ways of classifying different types or aspects of memory have arisen because different brain systems seem to be involved, as we will learn later in the chapter.

A general scheme for the mammalian memory system is shown in Figure 11-1. To recapitulate, sensory information, received through the eyes, ears, and other senses, is registered very briefly in iconic memory. If it is a face or a visual scene, at least part of the information may be transferred directly into long-term memory. Some residue of the information from iconic memory persists for a few seconds in short-term memory. If it is new information or a new motor skill and you do not practice it, some of it may be stored in long-term memory but most will fade away. If you practice enough you can store it in long-term memory, where it may remain essentially forever. Some small part of your ongoing experience, however, is continuously stored in permanent memory.

BASIC PROCESSES OF LEARNING AND MEMORY

The behavioral phenomena of learning and memory can be grouped into a few general categories that apply equally to humans and other animals. The simplest and most primitive forms of learning, habituation and sensitization, are *nonassociative*. *Habituation* is simply a decrease in a response elicited by a stimulus as a result of repeated stimulation. *Sensitization* is an increase in a response elicited by a stimulus as a result of (usually strong) stimulation. If a rat (or human) is presented with a sudden loud sound, it will jump or start. If the same sound is given repeatedly with no other consequence, the rat (or human) will gradually cease jumping at the sound (habituation). On the other hand, if the rat (or human) has been given a painful shock just before the loud sound, it will jump more at the sound than it did before the shock (sensitization).

Habituation can easily be viewed within the general scheme of mammalian memory (Figure 11-1). The first one or few presentations of the stimulus enter short-term memory and are lost. But with repetition, a memory of the stimulus and the fact that it has no meaningful consequence—it is not followed by reward or punishment—is formed and stored in long-term memory. This is essentially the theory of habituation proposed by the Russian neuroscientist Eugene Sokolov. He further suggested that when the stimulus continues to be presented, it is compared (in short-term memory) with the long-term memory of the stimulus. If the two are the same, the animal or human does not respond. But if a very different stimulus is suddenly presented, there will be a large discrepancy between the representation of the new stimulus in short-term memory and the representation of the habituated stimulus from long-term memory and sensitization may occur.

Associative is a very broad category that includes much of the learning we do, from learning to be afraid to learning to talk to learning a foreign language to learning to play the piano. In essence, associative learning involves the formation of associations among stimuli and/or responses or movement sequences. It is generally subdivided into classical and instrumental conditioning or learning. *Classical* or *Pavlovian conditioning* refers to the procedure where a neutral stimulus, termed a *conditioned stimulus* (CS), typically a sound or light, is paired together with some stimulus that elicits a response, termed an *unconditioned stimulus* (US), for example, food that elicits salivation or a shock to the foot that elicits limb withdrawal. Ivan Pavlov, a Russian physiologist who had been studying digestion in dogs, discovered classical conditioning by accident, a celebrated case of serendipity. Pavlov received the Nobel prize, incidentally, for his work on digestion. He noticed that the mere sight of the food dish caused the dogs to salivate and decided to continue the experiment to see if dogs would also salivate in response to a bell heralding feeding time. Pavlov trained dogs to stand in a harness and, after the sound of a bell, fed them meat powder. He recorded the salivary responses of the dogs. At first, the

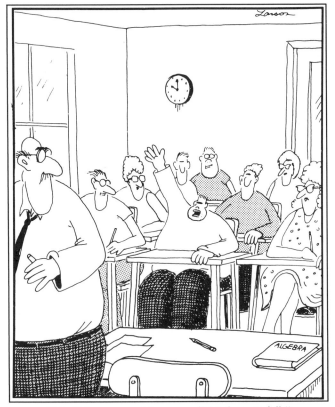

"Mr. Osborne, may I be excused? My brain is full."

bell did not elicit any response; the meat powder of course elicited reflex salivation, termed the *unconditioned response* (UR). He noted that after a few experiences they began to salivate when the bell rang, before they received the meat powder. This is termed the *conditioned response* (CR). This type of conditioning came to be called reward or appetitive conditioning (Figure 11-4). If

Figure 11-4 (Right) Pavlovian conditioning. (*a,b*) A conditioned stimulus (CS) such as a light or a bell is given, followed by an unconditioned stimulus (US), food. (*c*) At first the food elicits salivation, an unconditioned response (UR), but the light (CS) does not. After repeated pairings, the CS elicits salivation. An association has been formed between the CS and the US. This Pavlovian, or classical, conditioning works best if the CS precedes the US by a brief period of time (200 msec to a few seconds, depending on the kind of response to be learned), that is, if the CS predicts the occurrence of the UC (*b*). (*d*) The conditioned response (salivation in response to the light) is learned rapidly. Then, if the food is omitted and the light presented repeatedly, the conditioned response of salivation disappears, or is extinguished.

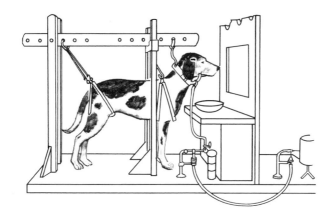

a

b **Delayed conditioning**

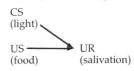

CS
(light)

US
(food)   Time ⟶

c **Before conditioning**

CS ⟶ No response or
(light)   irrelevant response

US ⟶ UR
(food)   (salivation)

During conditioning

CS
(light)

US ⟶ UR
(food)   (salivation)

After conditioning

CS ⟶ CR
(light)   (salivation)

d

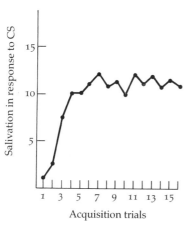

Salivation in response to CS

Acquisition trials

Extinction trials

the bell or another stimulus was followed by an unpleasant event, such as a strong electric shock, then a variety of autonomic responses became conditioned. This type of conditioning is often termed aversive or *fear conditioning*. A key aspect of Pavlovian conditioning is that the animal or human subject cannot control the occurrence of the CS and the US; they are determined by the experimenter. *Instrumental learning* describes a situation in which the animal or person must perform some response in order to obtain reward or avoid punishment. That is, the subject can control the occurrence of the US.

All aspects of learning and memory can be included within these broad categories. But as we noted, long-term associative memory can be categorized in several different ways, for example, episodic, semantic, procedural. Some authorities would argue that some aspects of declarative memory, particularly episodic memory, differ fundamentally from other aspects of associative memory and should not even be considered associative in nature.

Contiguity and Contingency

The concept of associative learning is ancient; the classical Greek philosophers observed it and the British school of "associationist" philosophers in the eighteenth and nineteenth centuries elaborated it. The basic notion is very simple: events that tend to occur together in time become associated with one another in the brain. If you place your finger in a flame the immediate consequence is pain and finger withdrawal. Association of events in time is termed *contiguity* and is an essential requirement for associative learning.

Important studies by the psychologist Robert Rescorla, now at the University of Pennsylvania, showed that in many associative learning situations, contiguity by itself is not sufficient to yield good learning. Suppose you are studying learned fear in a group of rats. The animals are given several trials of a tone followed by a mild shock, a shock that is aversive or unpleasant but not necessarily painful. If you then measure a fear response in the rats, you will find that the tone now elicits a vigorous fear response. Contiguity was enough to establish learning. But suppose that you give another group of rats a number of experiences of the shock without the tone, as well as the same number of paired tone–shock trials as in the previous group of animals. You will find that in this group of rats the tone elicits much less fear response than in the original group. This seems counterintuitive; animals in the second group received *more* shocks than animals in the first group, yet they developed much *less* learned fear. In extensive and ingenious studies, Rescorla showed that the degree of learning in this sort of situation depended on the proportion of trials where the tone and shock were paired (Figure 11-5). Indeed, if enough shock-alone trials are given, animals that are also given the same number of paired tone–

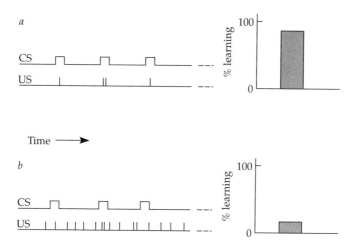

Figure 11-5 Role of contingency in associative learning. (*a*) Rats are given a CS (a tone) that is always paired with a US (footshock) for a number of trials, and the degree of fear they learn to the tone is measured—they learn very well. (*b*) The *same number* of paired tone CS/shock US trials are given, but a number of shock-alone presentations are also given unrelated to the tone CS. Under these conditions, where the contingency between tone and shock (the probability that tone and shock will occur together) is much lower, animals (including humans) learn poorly.

shock trials as the original group will not learn any fear at all. Rescorla stressed that the key underlying requirement for associative learning is *contingency*. The degree of learning that occurs depends on the probability or contingency that two events will occur together—it is contingent on the proportion of times they are associated. Simple contiguity, although necessary, is not sufficient to account for learning.

The psychologist Richard Herrnstein at Harvard University found similar results in situations that involve different rates of response for differential rewards. Human subjects were given two levers to press; the probability of reward (money) was less than 1 for each lever and different for each lever, for example, 35% for lever one, 65% for lever two. The number of times the subjects pressed each of the two levers was in exact proportion to the percent of times each lever was rewarded, even though the subjects were not consciously aware of this fact. Herrnstein termed this the *matching law*: mammals (and birds) respond in exact proportion to the probability that reward will occur. The contingency between the response, the lever pressed, and the reward determined the behavior very precisely. Note that in this situation the subjects would have won more money if they had pressed only the lever that was rewarded 65% of the time.

Temporal Law of Associative Learning

The exact times of occurrence of two events that are associated is critically important in associative learning. This is obvious when sticking one's finger in a flame—placing the finger in the flame always occurs just before pain and finger withdrawal. The pain doesn't occur before the finger is placed in the flame. This kind of inevitable temporal sequence of events led the British associationists to their definition of causality, cause and effect, which is generally accepted in science to this day: if event A is always followed by event B, A can be said to cause B.

It appears that the nervous system evolved to detect cause and effect from its early beginnings in relatively primitive animals like certain mollusks. Associative learning requires that the neutral warning stimulus (CS) must occur before the stimulus that has biological consequences (US) in order for learning to occur. Further, the degree of learning that develops depends on the time between the onsets of the two stimuli. Even more remarkable, the form of the functional relationship between the onset times of the two stimuli is essentially the same for all kinds of associative learning. This is illustrated in Figure 11-6, showing degree of learning for animals trained at various CS-US onset intervals in several different learning situations: rabbits learning to blink their eye to a tone, rats learning to lick for a reward, rats learning a fear response and learning a taste aversion. Humans show essentially identical functions.

We consider some of these learning situations in more detail later. The key point here is that there is a critical range of time intervals between CS onset and US onset that yield best learning. The actual values of this range differ greatly in different kinds of learning. They are around 200 to 500 milliseconds for eyeblink conditioning, 2 to 4 seconds for licking conditioning, 10 to 20 seconds for fear learning, and 1 to 2 hours for taste-aversion learning. But the form of the relationship is the same in all cases. If the CS onset and the US onset occur at the same time, or even if the CS onset occurs before the US onset for some brief period of time, no learning occurs. As the critical range of intervals is reached, the learning function increases rapidly and then gradually dies away as the interval is made increasingly long. The universal nature of this function suggests that it reflects some basic property of plasticity of the nervous system. One of the major unsolved challenges in the study of brain mechanisms of learning and memory is accounting for the form and properties of the temporal law of associative learning.

Pavlovian conditioning is perhaps the most basic aspect of associative learning (Figure 11-4). In general terms it is a process by which an organism benefits from experience so that its future behavior is better adapted to its environment. In more specific terms, it is the way organisms, including humans, learn about causal relationships in the world. It results from exposure

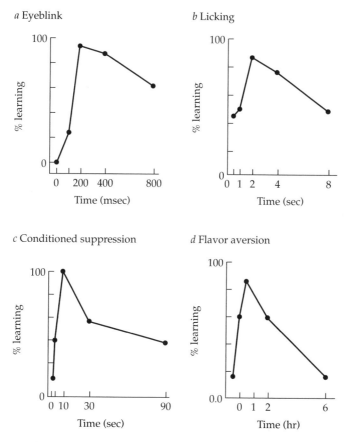

a Eyeblink

b Licking

c Conditioned suppression

d Flavor aversion

Figure 11-6 The temporal law of associative learning. Four quite different kinds of associative learning tasks are shown in terms of how well animals (humans, too!) learn as a function of the time between the onset of the CS and the onset of the US. (*a*) Rabbits are trained in eyeblink conditioning with a tone CS and a puff of air to the eye as the US. (*b*) Rats are trained to lick a spout for a reward (US). (*c*) Rats are first trained to lick and then separately given fear training to a tone CS paired with a shock US. When the tone is then presented while they are licking, it causes suppression of licking, a measure of learned fear. (*d*) Rats are given a good-tasting solution CS (saccharin, for example) followed by an injection of lithium chloride (US) that makes them sick. They learn to avoid the taste of the CS. The time range between CS and US onsets for best learning varies from a few hundred milliseconds to an hour, depending on the situation, but the *form* of the function relating amount of learning to time between CS and US onsets is the same in all cases.

to relations among events in the environment. To quote Rescorla, "Such learning is a primary means by which the organism represents the structure of its world" (1988, p. 152). Viewed in this way, Pavlovian conditioning is a basic aspect of complex, cognitive learning. For both modern Pavlovian and cognitive views of learning and memory, the individual learns a representation of the causal structure of the world and adjusts this representation through experience to bring it into tune with the real causal structure of the world, striving to reduce any discrepancies or errors between its internal representation and external reality.

BRAIN SUBSTRATES OF LEARNING AND MEMORY

Karl Lashley, then working at Johns Hopkins University, began the search for long-term memory traces in the mammalian brain (he termed them "engrams") about 75 years ago. He stressed the now obvious point that it will not be possible to analyze the neuronal mechanisms underlying memory storage until the locations of the memory traces in the brain are known. Near the end of his career, in 1950, no memory traces had yet been localized, leading him to the following rather pessimistic conclusion:

> This series of experiments [as of 1950] has yielded a good bit of information about what and where memory is not. It has discovered nothing directly of the real nature of the engram. I sometimes feel, in reviewing the evidence on the localization of the memory trace, that the necessary conclusion is that learning just is not possible. It is difficult to conceive of a mechanism which can satisfy the conditions set for it. Nevertheless, in spite of such evidences against it, learning does sometimes occur. (Lashley, K. S. (1950). *In search of the engram.* Soc. Exp. Biol. Symp. 4, 454-482, pp. 477–478.)

Following Lashley's original dictum, most research on brain substrates of memory in vertebrates in the past 40 years has focused on identifying the brain systems critical for various aspects of learning and memory, with the goal of localizing the sites of long-term or permanent memory storage in the brain. If critical memory systems can be identified, it ought to be possible to localize the memories themselves within these critical circuits and hence to analyze the biological mechanisms of memory formation and storage.

Habituation and Sensitization

Habituation, as we noted, is simply a decrease in response to repeated stimulation under normal behavioral conditions. It is a process that occurs in the central nervous system and is distinguished from receptor adaptation or muscle fatigue. Sensitization is the other side of the coin: it is an increase in response, usually as a result of some other (strong) stimulus.

Habituation and sensitization of behavioral responses are ubiquitous in animals with nervous systems. The sea anemone, belonging to the lowest phylum of animals to have a nervous system, shows habituation clearly: if it is touched, it contracts, but if it is touched again soon after, it contracts less. (Try this some time when you are at the seashore.) Hence even a nerve net, the most primitive type of nervous system, can produce habituation.

Because habituation is common to a wide range of animals, from anemones to humans, it is possible that a common neuronal mechanism may subserve it. Comparison of habituation in different animals can also serve to define the behavior and to distinguish it from such processes as muscle fatigue. The common properties of habituation in higher and lower animals make it possible to use simpler systems, such as spinal reflexes and the reflexes of simple animals, as model systems in which to analyze the mechanisms through which it occurs.

Work on both mammals and invertebrates has shown that habituation and sensitization are two quite different processes, both behaviorally and neuronally. Habituation seems to be due to a process of *synaptic depression*, a decrease in the efficacy of transmission at certain synapses as a result of repeated activation. The basic process is presynaptic, a decrease in the probability of release of neurotransmitter at the synapse. The process of sensitization, where it has been analyzed at the synaptic level, appears to be a superimposed facilitation, either presynaptic or postsynaptic.

A favored animal used in studying nonassociative learning is the *Aplysia*, also called the sea hare or sea slug (Figure 11-7). It is a mollusk with a rather simple nervous system containing only about 5,000 neurons. The neurons are grouped into several ganglia, which control different aspects of the animal's behavior. Eric Kandel and his many associates at Columbia University have made good use of this little beast to study basic processes of neuronal plasticity. If the head of the animal is touched, it withdraws its gill; with repeated touches, the gill-withdrawal reflex habituates. If the tail of the animal is shocked, the gill now withdraws vigorously to head touch—sensitization.

Habituation could be shown to occur across one synapse (Figure 11-8). The mechanism, as we said, is a decrease in the probability of transmitter release. But the transmitter is not used up. Instead, it appears that the entry of Ca^{++} ions into the terminal decreases (you will recall that Ca^{++} entry is the key event for transmitter release at neuron terminals). The decrease in Ca^{++} entry, in turn, seems to occur by the action of a second-messenger system that alters the Ca^{++} channels as a result of repeated activation.

Sensitization occurs at the same synapse but by the actions of another neuron terminal, activated via interneurons by the tail shock, that acts on the synaptic terminal (Figure 11-8). The tail-shock-activated terminal releases a neurotransmitter, perhaps serotonin, that activates second-messenger systems within the target terminal that result in increased Ca^{++} entry into the terminal. Habituation and sensitization both alter Ca^{++} entry into the terminal but do so by different mechanisms, so both can occur together. The sensitization process we have described is short term. If repeated sensitization training is given, a long-term sensitization process develops that seems to result in

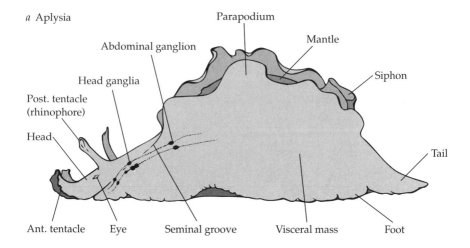

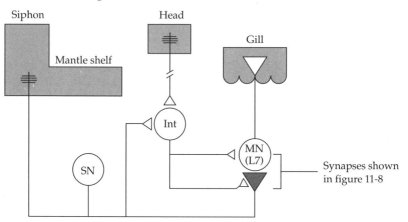

Figure 11-7 (*a*) Marine mollusk *Aplysia*, showing the major body structures and the locations of the major neural ganglia. The gill is inside the parapodium and cannot be seen in this drawing. (*b*) A simplified schematic of the basic circuit controlling the gill reflex, used to study habituation and sensitization.

actual structural changes in the synapse. We return to the long-term sensitization process later; it is also used as a model for associative learning.

Habituation usually occurs to stimuli given in a time range from about one per second to one per hour or more. Stimuli given at faster rates than about one per second may produce fatigue effects. Not all synapses habituate. Synapses in the auditory system faithfully follow up to several hundred impulses per second. In general, sensory systems show little habituation. Instead,

HABITUATION

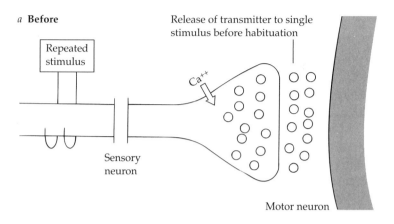

a **Before**

Repeated stimulus

Release of transmitter to single stimulus before habituation

Ca^{++}

Sensory neuron

Motor neuron

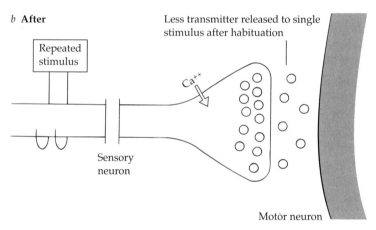

b **After**

Repeated stimulus

Less transmitter released to single stimulus after habituation

Ca^{++}

Sensory neuron

Motor neuron

Figure 11-8 Basic mechanisms of habituation and sensitization for the key synapses shown in the circuit in Figure 11-7. Sensory synapse on the motor neuron before and after habituation (*a, b*). Repeated stimulation of the sensory axon results in a persisting decreased Ca^{++} influx into the terminal, which results in decreased transmitter release at the synapse. Sensory synapse on the motor neuron before and after sensitization (*c, d*). A sensitizing stimulus to the head activates an interneuron that synapses on the sensory neuron terminal. This results in a persisting increase in Ca^{++} influx into the terminal when it is activated by stimulation of its axon. This in turn results in increased transmitter release. The two processes of habituation and sensitization can both occur at the same synapse and appear to involve different intracellular mechanisms.

habituation develops mostly at places in the nervous system where sensory information connects to motor pathways. It makes good adaptive sense to see, hear, and feel the world accurately but to be able to "decide" whether or not to respond to a given stimulus.

SENSITIZATION

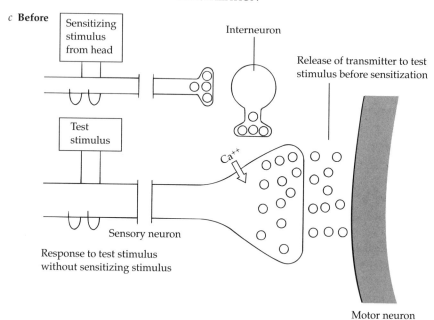

c **Before**

Sensitizing stimulus from head

Interneuron

Release of transmitter to test stimulus before sensitization

Test stimulus

Ca^{++}

Sensory neuron

Response to test stimulus without sensitizing stimulus

Motor neuron

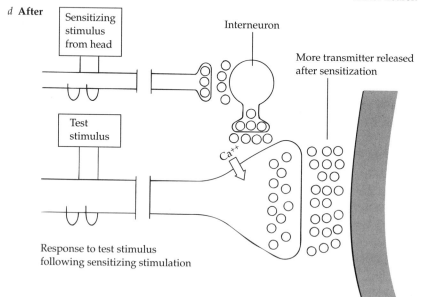

d **After**

Sensitizing stimulus from head

Interneuron

More transmitter released after sensitization

Test stimulus

Ca^{++}

Response to test stimulus following sensitizing stimulation

Animals respond to a novel stimulus or event. If the stimulus or event occurs repeatedly and has no interesting consequences, the animal stops responding to it. In this sense habituation is a very adaptive aspect of behavior. Without it, animals would spend most of their time responding to all kinds of irrelevant stimuli. However, as we said, it is useful that the higher regions of the brain continue to receive accurate sensory information about the habituated event—it may become important some time. A person walking along a street in his or her neighborhood has not stopped seeing the familiar sights; he or she just doesn't respond to them anymore.

Sensitization is also a very adaptive aspect of behavior. A sudden or painful stimulus arouses an animal and increases the likelihood and strength of a variety of responses. If you hear a loud and unexpected sound (or in Southern California, when you feel the floor begin to sway), you immediately become alert and aroused, your autonomic system becomes more active (you feel a tickling under your arms and your heart pounds), and you look about for the source of the sound, which might signify danger. When you have satisfied yourself that the sound does not mean danger, you stop being sensitized to it. In the laboratory, when a strong sensitizing stimulus is given repeatedly to an animal and does not actually cause harm, the animal ceases being sensitized. The process of sensitization also habituates.

Associative Learning and Memory

Much of the learning that birds and mammals do is associative, which, as I have said, is learning to associate a stimulus with a response or event. Learning occurs most readily when it has adaptive consequences, such as obtaining food or avoiding injury. There are clear biological constraints on what can be learned. In the wild, a rat's world resembles mazes, and rats learn a maze very well in the laboratory, especially if it leads to food or away from punishment. Pigeons readily learn to peck a key to obtain grain, a behavior very much like pecking grain itself. Rats cannot learn to peck and pigeons are poor maze learners. Humans learn language naturally but no other species does.

Birds in particular can learn in some interesting and rather specialized ways. We saw in Chapter 2 that the "song" region of the brain in male canaries doubles in size as the bird learns its new seasonal song and then shrinks after the mating season as the bird forgets the song.

Pavlovian Conditioning of Fear Fear learning or conditioning is basic in birds and mammals and can have most important consequences for the human condition. It is likely that many aspects of fear and anxiety, in particular neurotic fears and even phobias, are the result of fear conditioning. Change in heart rate is a simple measure of an autonomic response that is believed by many scientists to reflect learned fear. In a typical laboratory study of fear conditioning, an animal or human volunteer is given a tone or light stimulus followed by an unpleasant shock that cannot be avoided. The shock itself causes a large increase in heart rate. After a few trials when the tone or light has been followed by a shock, the tone or light comes to elicit a change in the heart rate.

Studies of several species, pigeons, rabbits, and baboons, have shown that a region of the hypothalamus is critical for the learned change in heart rate in response to the tone. Orville A. Smith, Jr., at the University of Washington in Seattle, studied the learned heart rate response in the baboon. He also measured heart rate and blood pressure changes when the animals exercised. Finally, he trained the animals to "tell" him when they were afraid. The baboons were equipped with a system that would deliver a squirt of orange juice if they pressed a lever. Shock and fear would cause the animals to stop pressing the food reward lever for a while. Initially the tone had no effect on the lever pressing, but after the tone had been paired with a shock a few times the animal would stop pressing the lever when the tone came on. This is a behavioral indication of fear that is termed *response suppression.*

After the animals were well-trained and showed both a conditioned heart rate response and a suppression of lever pressing after the tone, a tiny lesion was made in a region of the hypothalamus believed to be involved in the control of the cardiovascular system. The lesion completely abolished the learned heart rate response to the tone. However, the heart rate response to the shock was not altered, nor were the heart rate changes associated with exercise. Thus there was no change in the reflex regulation of the heart rate; only the learned heart rate response was abolished. Interestingly, the animals still showed suppression of lever pressing in response to the tone; they stopped pressing the lever for juice when the tone came on. The learned heart rate measure of fear was abolished by the brain lesion, but the learned lever-pressing measure was not (Figure 11-9).

This result seems paradoxical. The baboon was no longer afraid of the tone insofar as its heart rate was concerned but was still very much afraid of the tone as indicated by its lever-pressing behavior. Smith interpreted this to mean that the hypothalamic region is critical for the expression of the learned (but not reflex) heart rate response. Another way of saying this is that the hypothalamic region was on the efferent or output side of the fear memory-trace circuit. If this is true, then the fear memory trace itself must exist in a structure that projects to the hypothalamus. One such candidate structure is the amygdala (see Chapter 1).

There is now converging evidence from several species of mammals and also pigeons that lesions of the amygdala markedly impair or prevent fear learning of heart rate and blood pressure. Lesions of the amygdala also markedly impair or abolish behavioral signs of learned fear. We use the elegant studies of Michael Davis and associates at Yale University as an example. Davis made use of a classical study of learned fear done by Judson Brown and associates at the University of Iowa many years ago. They first measured the startle response of rats to a sudden loud sound in a stabilometer cage that

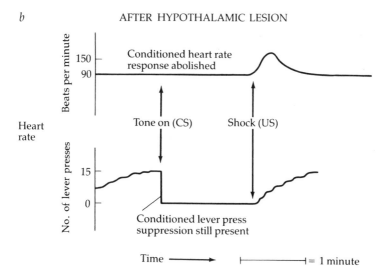

Figure 11-9 Effect of a small hypothalamic lesion on two measures of conditioned fear: heart rate (autonomic) and lever press suppression (behavioral). The animal had learned to press a lever repeatedly to obtain food. A tone was then paired with shock a few times and a Pavlovian conditioned response of increased heart rate developed in response to the tone. At the same time the animal learned to stop pressing the lever when the tone came on (a behavioral sign of fear?). After the hypothalamic lesion, the tone no longer caused a learned increase in heart rate (although the heart rate still increased reflexively to shock). However, the animal still stopped pressing the lever when the tone came on. The autonomic and behavioral signs of fear were apparently dissociated by the hypothalamic lesion.

would record the force of the rat's startle jump. They then placed the rats in another cage and gave them a series of light–shock trials—classical conditioning of fear to the light stimulus. The rats were then put back in the startle device, and the strength of the startle response to the loud sound was compared to the strength of the startle response when the light just preceded the loud startle sound. As you might expect, the light, which elicited learned fear, resulted in a much larger startle response to the sound. They termed this effect *fear potentiation of startle* (Figure 11-10).

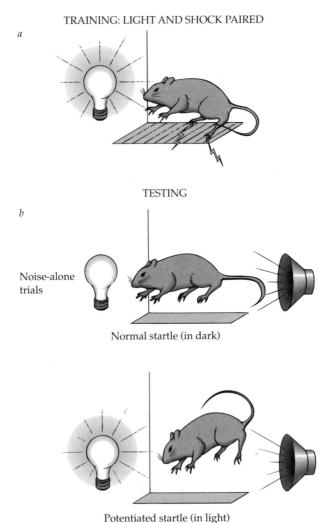

TRAINING: LIGHT AND SHOCK PAIRED

a

TESTING

b

Noise-alone trials

Normal startle (in dark)

Potentiated startle (in light)

Figure 11-10 Conditioned potentiation of startle. (*a*) The rat is first given fear conditioning: a light (CS) and footshock (US) are paired in a distinctive environment (chamber). (*b*) Next, the rat is tested for the startle response to a loud sound. Then the light CS is presented and the same loud sound now yields a much larger startle response than occurred to the sound alone.

Davis made use of this procedure to localize the fear circuit in the brain. But first he had to identify the auditory startle circuit in the brain, which took several years. As indicated in Figure 11-11, the auditory startle stimulus activates auditory nuclei in the brain stem that relay to a nucleus in the reticular formation that acts down ultimately on motor nuclei to yield the startle response. Davis and his colleagues then gave animals fear training (light–shock), which yielded marked fear potentiation of the startle response, and explored the brain circuitry necessary for this learned fear potentiation. They made use of a number of techniques—lesioning structures and pathways, stimulating the circuit electrically, tracing the key pathways anatomically, and succeeded in identifying most of the CS circuit for the learned fear to the light CS.

Joseph LeDoux and his associates at New York University used an auditory CS—for example, a tone—in fear conditioning and a simple measure of learned fear—changes in blood pressure. That is, they paired tone and shock and showed a learned change in blood pressure to the tone. They found that for the auditory CS there were both direct connections from the auditory

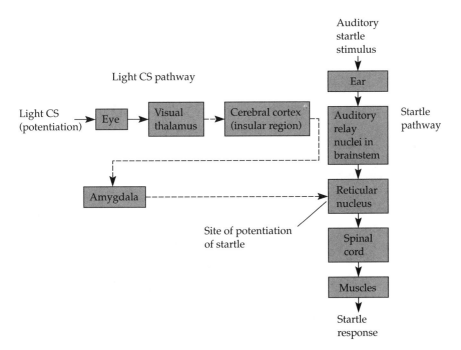

Figure 11-11 Brain circuitry for conditioned potentiation of startle. The startle pathway to the loud sound relays from auditory nuclei to a nucleus in the reticular formation to brain stem and spinal cord motor nuclei that generate the startle response. The conditioned fear potentiation from the light CS relays from the visual pathways to regions of the cerebral cortex to the amygdala and from here to the reticular nucleus to act to potentiate the startle response.

thalamus (medial geniculate body) to the amygdala and also connections from the auditory area of the cerebral cortex to the amygdala. The auditory cortex of course receives direct projections from the auditory thalamus. Either pathway can serve to convey information about the occurrence of the auditory CS to the amygdala.

The amygdala appears to be the key structure for the learning of fear. Both the Davis and LeDoux groups (and other laboratories as well) showed that lesions of the amygdala prevent learning of fear and abolish fear that has been learned. The lesions also impair unlearned or reflex fear responses—to shock, for example—suggesting that information about the shock US also reaches the amygdala.

We now return to the question we asked about Smith's experiment (Figure 11-9): Is the amygdala the locus of the fear memory trace or merely on the input or output side of the trace? Evidence to date supports the view that at least the initial fear memory trace is formed in the amygdala. Lesions of the auditory thalamus, for example, prevent fear learning to a tone but not to a light, whereas amygdala lesions prevent learning to both, arguing that the amygdala is not on the input side of the trace. Lesions of the hypothalamus, on the other hand, can selectively interfere with different fear responses: destruction of lateral hypothalamus (LH) prevents learned blood pressure change (the same result Smith found in his studies on the baboon), but lesions of the periaqueductal gray (a part of the slow pain system; see Figure 6-3) abolish another behavioral measure of fear—freezing (discussed later). But the LH lesion has no effect on fear-learned freezing and the periaqueductal gray lesion has no effect on blood pressure. These results confirm Smith's suggestion that the hypothalamus is on the output side of the fear memory trace and support the view that the trace is formed in the amygdala.

The most direct evidence that the fear memory trace is formed in the amygdala comes from Davis's laboratory. He and his coworkers infused APV, a substance that blocks the NMDA-type glutamate receptors (see Chapter 4), into the amygdala during fear training, using their fear-potentiated startle response procedure. They found that APV completely prevented fear learning to either a tone or light CS. You will recall from Chapter 4 that blocking the NMDA receptors in the hippocampus prevents the induction of long-term potentiation (LTP).

But learned fear is a long-term or permanent memory. Is the permanent fear memory stored in the amygdala? Work from James McGaugh's laboratory at the University of California at Irvine suggests that it is not. They trained animals in an instrumental fear task and then made lesions of the amygdala either immediately after training or several days after training. Lesions made immediately after training abolished the fear memory but lesions made several days after training had little effect on the fear memory! So the permanent fear memory trace may reside elsewhere in the brain.

Nonetheless, the initial fear memory formed to light and tone stimuli seems to develop in the amygdala. As you will see later in the chapter, the hippocampus plays a key role in memory—in rodents it is particularly important for spatial memory, memory for places. Jeansok Kim and Robert Fanselow, at the University of California at Los Angeles, made use of the freezing response in rats as an index of learned fear. When rats are very fearful, they freeze and remain motionless for some period of time. Kim and Fanselow trained rats to be afraid of a particular place or context—a special cage with distinctive features where they were given shocks. When placed in this cage without shock the day after training, the animals immediately froze—an index of learned fear to the context (cage). Lesions of the hippocampus were made either one day after fear training or one, two, or four weeks later. Context fear (freezing) was abolished in the animals who had lesions one day after training but not in the animals with lesions made later. So here too a brain structure is critical for the initial fear memory, in this case the hippocampus rather than the amygdala, but the permanent fear memory seems to be stored elsewhere in the brain. Context, incidentally, seems a very natural stimulus for fear, as you will know if you have ever found yourself alone in a run-down section of a strange city at night.

In summary, the memory trace for initial learning of fear associated with tones or lights appears to develop in the amygdala and for fear associated with context in the hippocampus, but the permanent memory traces seem to be formed elsewhere. As of this writing, it is not known where that elsewhere is. Another loose end in this story is the US pathway: the circuit activating the amygdala and hippocampus by the shock US is not yet known.

Fear is a very nonspecific kind of learning; it involves many different kinds of responses, particularly of the sympathetic nervous system and hypothalamus–pituitary–adrenal system, as well as behaviors like freezing or fleeing. Indeed, it closely resembles the initial syndrome (set of responses) to a sudden stress (Chapter 7). There is a well-developed theory in psychology that characterizes learning to deal with unpleasant events as occurring in two phases or processes: an initial and nonspecific learning of fear and subsequent learning of specific behavioral responses to deal with aversive stimuli or situations. Examples of specific learned response would be leg flexion to deal with paw shock and closing the eyelid to deal with an aversive puff of air to the eye. Specific response sequences can of course be much more complex; leg flexion and eyeblink are elementary movements widely used in the laboratory.

Pavlovian Conditioning of Discrete Responses   A vast amount of research has been done using Pavlovian conditioning of the eyeblink response in humans and other mammals. The eyeblink response exhibits all the basic laws of Pavlovian conditioning equally in humans and other mammals. The basic procedure is to present a neutral CS like a tone or a light followed a quarter of a second or so later by a puff of air to the eye (US). Initially there is no response to the CS and a reflex eyeblink to the air puff US. After a number of such trials, the eyelid begins to close in response to the CS before the US occurs, and in a well-trained subject, the eyelid closure CR becomes very precisely timed so that it is maximally closed at the exact time that the air puff US strikes the eye. This very adaptive timing of the eyeblink CR develops over the range of CS–US onset intervals where learning occurs, about 100 milliseconds to 1 second (see Figure 11-5). So the conditioned eyeblink response is a very precisely timed elementary learned motor skill.

More than 20 years ago some colleagues and I decided to make use of the vast amount of behavioral information available on eyeblink conditioning and use it as a model system to localize memory traces in the brain. Isidore Gormezano at the University of Iowa and his many students had published extensive behavioral data on eyeblink conditioning in rabbits—all the properties of the learned response and control procedures had been worked out in detail—so we selected the rabbit as our experimental subject.

How does one go about finding a memory trace? We had no idea what brain structures or systems might be involved when we began this work. We decided to record the activity of nerve cells in various brain systems as the animal learned the conditioned response in the hope of finding regions where the activity of the neurons increased before the onset of the behavioral CR and predicted the form—the amplitude and time course—of the actual eyeblink CR. An example of such a response—a neural activity reflection of a memory trace—is shown in Figure 11-12. We developed a miniature microdrive system that allowed us to advance microelectrodes through brain tissue without bothering the animal. Our microdrive was similar to but much smaller than those developed earlier for study of neuron activity in the monkey by Evarts and others (see Figure 9-16).

Two brain systems showed dramatic examples of possible neural memory traces: the hippocampus and the cerebellum. The example shown in Figure 11-12 is from the interpositus nucleus in the cerebellum. Lesions of the hippocampus did not abolish the learned eyeblink response but lesions of the cerebellum did. Subsequent work in our lab and other laboratories replicated these findings. The hippocampus does play an important role in eyeblink conditioning when the learning situation is made much more difficult. Several lines of evidence suggest that a memory trace may be established in the hippocampus and that it involves changes in the AMPA-type glutamate receptor (see Chapter 4).

But this higher-order memory trace in the hippocampus is not necessary for basic learning and memory of the CR, whereas a region of the cerebellum is (Figure 11-13). The critical region of the cerebellum is very small—lesions no larger than a cubic millimeter completely and permanently prevent learning if made before training and completely and permanently abolish the memory if made after training. Importantly, the lesion that abolishes learning

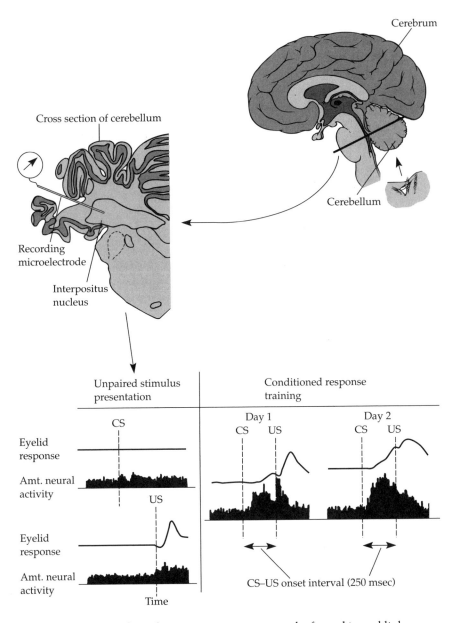

Figure 11-12 Site where the memory trace appears to be formed in eyeblink conditioning. The electrode is recording the action potentials from nerve cells in the interpositus nucleus in the cerebellum. By themselves, the tone CS and airpuff to the eye US do not elicit very much increase in the nerve cell discharges (below left). However, when the stimuli are paired and the animal learns, neural activity in the CS period increases to form a neural response that predicts the occurrence and form of the behavioral conditioned eyeblink response (below right). Upward movement of the eyelid response line indicates eyelid closure. Conditioned responses are eyelid closures (upward movement of line after CS onset and before US onset). The neural activity is shown as histograms. A number of trials are added and the height of each little bar indicates the number of nerve cell discharges in that little time period.

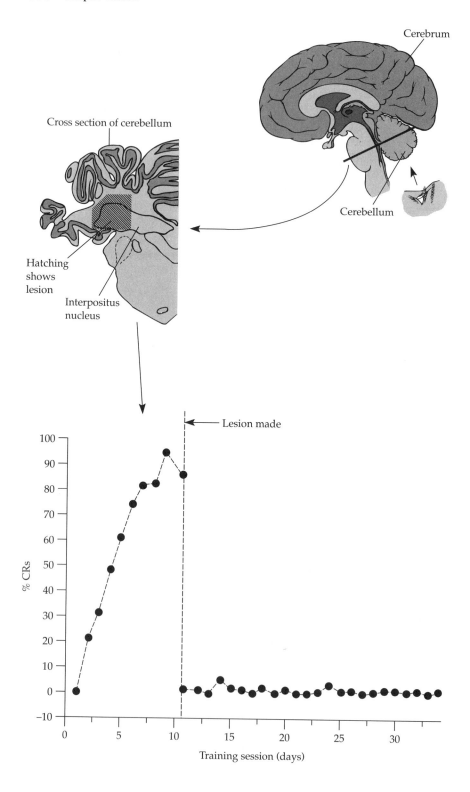

Cerebrum

Cross section of cerebellum

Cerebellum

Hatching
shows
lesion

Interpositus
nucleus

Lesion made

% CRs

Training session (days)

Figure 11-13 (*Left*) Effect of lesion of the region of the interpositus nucleus shown in Figure 11-12. The lesion is made on the same side of the brain as the eye being trained. It completely and permanently abolishes the conditioned eyeblink CR but has no effect at all on the reflex blink to the airpuff. The other eye can be trained normally after the lesion. In contrast to the cerebral cortex, sensory and motor representations in the cerebellum are on the same side of the body: left cerebellum, left eyeblink; right cerebellum, right eyeblink.

and memory of the CR has no effect on the animal's ability to perform the reflex response—to blink to the air puff. Recently, the very same lesion results we found in rabbits have also been obtained in humans with cerebellar damage. So all the results we have obtained on rabbits are likely to hold true for humans as well.

But the fact that a small lesion in the cerebellum abolishes the learning and memory of the conditioned response does not prove that the region destroyed is the locus of the memory trace. In order to prove this it is necessary to identify the entire essential brain circuitry, from the tone CS and the corneal (eye) air puff US to the eyeblink CR. This was the next step in our work. We used lesions, electrical stimulation, recording of nerve cell activity, and anatomical tracing of pathways and succeeded in identifying the circuitry, schematized in Figure 11-14. In brief, information about the tone CS is relayed from auditory nuclei to the pontine nuclei and from there to the cerebellum as mossy fibers. Information about the corneal air-puff US is relayed from somatic sensory nuclei (trigeminal nucleus for air puff to the eye) to the inferior olive and from there to the cerebellum as climbing fibers (see Chapter 9, particularly Figure 9-13, and Figure 11-14). The conditioned response pathway exits from the interpositus nucleus of the cerebellum to the red nucleus and from there descends to the motor nuclei in the brain stem to generate the learned eyeblink CR.

Having identified the entire circuit necessary and sufficient for the learning and memory of the conditioned response, we next focused on where the memory trace was localized in the circuit. We reasoned that it must be in regions of convergence where information from the CS and US come together in activating neurons. This does not happen in the inferior olive and does not appear to happen in the pontine nuclei; it does happen in the cerebellum, in both cerebellar cortex and the interpositus nucleus. We developed a number of lines of evidence arguing against the memory trace being in any structures in the circuit except the cerebellum. But this evidence was indirect.

Recently, direct evidence has been obtained that we feel proves that the memory trace is formed in the cerebellum. Our colleague at the University of Southern California, David Lavond, developed a cold-probe system for revers-

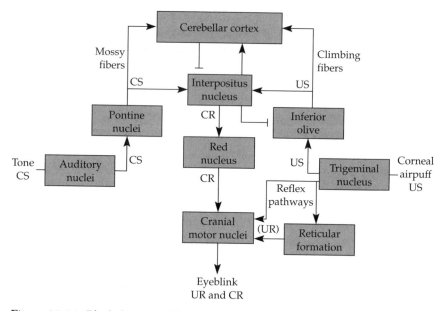

Figure 11-14 Block diagram of the brain circuitry essential for classical conditioning of the eyeblink response. The memory trace is formed and stored in the cerebellum (we think in both the interpositus nucleus and the cerebellar cortex).

ibly inactivating but not damaging local regions of the brain by cooling them. We accomplished the same thing, reversible inactivation, by infusing drugs, for example, lidocaine, a local anesthetic, and muscimol, a GABA agonist that activates GABA$_A$ receptors on neurons and temporarily inactivates them by hyperpolarization (see Chapter 4). The basic idea is to reversibly inactivate a brain region during training. If it is a part of the circuit essential for memory-trace formation then no CRs will be expressed during training with inactivation. If it is the site of memory-trace formation, then after the inactivation has been discontinued, the animal will show no signs of having learned and will have to be trained from scratch. If, on the other hand, the region inactivated during training is beyond the site of the memory trace in the essential circuit, then no CRs will be expressed during training with inactivation. However, after the inactivation has been discontinued, the animal will immediately show that it has learned: it will show well-developed conditioned responses.

Results from both Lavond's laboratory using reversible cooling and our lab using pharmacological inactivation are clear and consistent. Inactivating the critical region of the cerebellum completely prevents expression of CRs during training and after inactivation the animals show no signs of learning—they must be trained from scratch. Reversible inactivation of the output from the interpositus and its target, the red nucleus (see Figure 11-14), also completely prevent expression of CRs during inactivation training. However, after inactivation is discontinued, the animals show that they have fully learned the CR during inactivation training. The conclusion is clear: the essential long-term memory trace is formed and stored in a very localized region of the cerebellum To our knowledge, this is the first conclusive evidence for the localization of a long-term memory trace in the mammalian brain.

It is important to note that our results do not apply just to the conditioned eyeblink response; they hold for the associative learning of any discrete movement. By appropriate activation of the cerebellar circuit we can elicit any movement: limb flexion, head turn, and so on. These movements can all be trained to any arbitrary neutral stimulus, like tone or light. As we noted earlier, precisely timed movements such as these are examples of the learning of elementary skills. Hence our results strongly support the classical theories of the cerebellum as a machine for the learning and memory storage of motor skills (see Chapter 9, pp. 282-283).

Instrumental Learning: Consolidation and Modulation of Memory   The field concerned with possible brain substrates of instrumental learning is vast; there have been many thousands of studies over the 75 years since Karl Lashley began his search for the engram. A wide variety of different tasks has been used, varying from one-trial passive avoidance to the operant procedures developed by B. F. Skinner at Harvard to maze learning and puzzle boxes. To simplify our discussion we will treat studies of monkeys and humans separately from the enormous amount of work that has been done on the rat or mouse. The brain circuits essential for any instrumental learning memory task have not yet been worked out, although considerable progress is being made. Rather than trying to cover this vast and somewhat inconclusive literature, we select memory consolidation and modulation as an example of some of the most interesting work in the field.

The consolidation story has two origins. In the 1940s Carl Duncan, working at Northwestern University, first made use of electroconvulsive shock (ECS) to impair memory. He trained rats in an instrumental avoidance task. The animals were on one side of a shuttle box, a box with a grid floor, two compartments and a connecting alley. When a light came on they had 10 seconds to cross to the other compartment or receive a foot shock from the grid floor. They were given one trial a day for 18 days. Control rats quickly learned the task, avoiding the shock on all but the first few days. Duncan ran a number of groups of experimental rats that received ECS (delivered through ear clips) at intervals ranging from 20 seconds to 14 hours after each day's trial. The results were striking. Animals receiving ECS 20 seconds after each learning trial learned nothing at all. As the time between learning trials and ECS increased, the animals learned better and better, showing no memory impairment if the ECS came an hour or more after the training trial.

Duncan's result paralleled work in the field of psychiatry where patients with various forms of mental illness were given ECS treatments. The basic notion was that there is some period of time when recent memories are fragile and can be obliterated by inducing brain seizures. In the case of mental patients, the rationale was that recent memories and anxieties would be more impaired than well-established memories. With one exception ECS turned out to be of little help for the patients. The exception is severe depression. Even today some severely depressed patients do not respond to the many antidepressant drugs now available (see Chapter 5). For these few people, ECS does help and is still used.

ECS induces *retrograde amnesia*: events just prior to the ECS are forgotten. It has a gradient—the older the memory the better it is retained. But the gradient can be long. After a series of ECS treatments, patients may not be able to remember any of their experiences for a period of a year or more. Fortunately, most of these memories usually return, although the events immediately surrounding the ECS are usually not remembered. As with humans, so with rats.

Duncan's experiment began a large field of research. A number of possible explanations for the memory impairment were explored. Among the possibilities that were ruled out were that the ECS was strongly aversive (conditioned fear); that the ECS became conditioned to the apparatus (context conditioned fear); that the body seizures were necessary. The fact that the ECS memory impairment also occurred when the ECS was given to anesthetized animals and humans seemed to rule out these possibilities. James McGaugh and his coworkers at the University of California at Irvine showed that the critical memory impairment could be obtained by disruptive electrical stimulation of the amygdala; seizures of the entire brain are not necessary. We return to the amygdala later.

The other origin of the memory consolidation story occurred early in the century in independent studies by Karl Lashley and Clark Hull, who showed that administration of strychnine or caffeine markedly improved maze learning performance. Since they gave these substances before training, the effects could be more on the animals' performance than on memory. But McGaugh and others showed that the same memory facilitation occurred if the drugs were given shortly after training rather than before training. Possible rewarding effects of the drugs were also ruled out. Most recent work on memory facilitation has used simple one-trial learning procedures. Passive avoidance is a favorite. The animal is placed in a lighted compartment and allowed to step into a dark compartment (rats like the dark). But the grid in the dark compartment is electrified. After the animal receives a shock, it is removed. The next day it is placed in the lighted compartment and the time before it goes into the dark is measured—the longer the time, the better memory is presumed to be.

This test by itself can be misinterpreted. For example, a sedative drug like a barbiturate that makes the animal inactive would produce a spurious memory. But other tests are also used, for example, active avoidance, the test Duncan used in his ECS study. Tasks involving food reward have also been used.

The bottom line in this work is that a wide range of drugs given after the learning experience can facilitate or impair subsequent memory performance in all these tasks, depending on the type of drug and the dose used (Figure 11-15). Earlier, it was thought that both ECS impairment and drug facilitation or impairment of memory acted on a specific brain process of consolidation, for example, circulating electrical activity in the brain that gradually stamped in memories. If this is so, then there ought to be a gradient of consolidation, a relatively fixed time period. However, there is no gradient, or rather there are many gradients, depending very much on the details of the procedure used in a particular experiment. This and other problems with the simple consolidation notion have led scientists to stress *modulation* rather than consolidation. Most workers in the field believe that ECS or drug administration modulates how well recent memories are stored in long-term memory.

Epinephrine (E) is among the most effective substances for memory facilitation, and it is of course an autonomic neurotransmitter and a critical hormone, released along with norepinephrine by the adrenal medulla in response to stress. In other words, in the real world we and other mammals tend to remember best those experiences that occur at times of arousal and moderate stress. Memory-facilitating drugs like E show the same inverted U effect on memory as a function of drug dose that holds in general between performance and arousal (compare Figures 11-15 and 7-6). This has been termed the "flashbulb" phenomenon—older readers will remember where they were and what they were doing when they learned that President Kennedy had been assassinated; younger readers will remember where they were when they learned that the space shuttle had blown up. We remember best those events associated with a state of moderate arousal and stress—the top of the inverted U.

This satisfactory state of affairs for the notion of memory modulation seemed in danger of falling apart when it was found that E does not readily cross the blood–brain barrier. Systemic (bloodstream) doses of E that yield maximal memory facilitation are much too low to enter the brain to any appreciable degree. So how could they act on memory storage? There are at least two alternative possibilities. One is that memory-enhancing drugs act via a structure such as the subfornical organ. You may recall from Chapter 7 that the subfornical organ lies outside the blood–brain barrier, can be acted on by substances in the blood (angiotension II for thirst), and sends nerve fibers to the hypothalamus. The other possibility is that E activates autonomic sensory fibers—the vagus nerve, you will recall, contains sensory nerve fibers that convey extensive information to the brain about the state of the heart,

a Peripheral injection

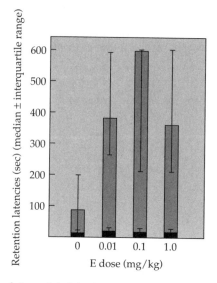

b Amygdala injection

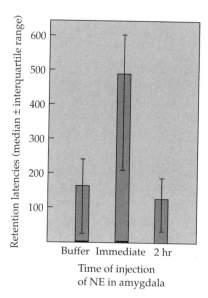

Figure 11-15 (*a*) Effect of increasing concentrations of E injected into the blood stream in rats following training on memory performance in the passive avoidance task (the better they remember the longer the latency). Note that memory is best at an intermediate dose (0.1 mg/kg) and the overall function is an inverted U, just like the relation between arousal and performance (see Figure 7-6). (*b*) Same facilitation of memory performance when NE is injected directly into the amygdala. (the same form of dose-effectiveness function holds as in *a*). Here, we show also the time course of memory facilitation. Amygdala injection immediately after training is much more effective than two hours after training.

stomach, and other internal organs. This is the favored hypothesis at present, but as of this writing the issue is unresolved.

Given that systemically injected drugs act indirectly on the brain to produce memory facilitation, where might they act? Recent work in McGaugh's laboratory suggests that the amygdala is critical. Very small doses of drugs infused directly into the amygdala also produce memory facilitation (and impairment), and destruction of the amygdala prevents the memory facilitation by systemically (in the bloodstream) injected drugs. McGaugh's current working hypothesis about the role of the amygdala in memory facilitation and impairment is shown in Figure 11-16. This notion can account for the effects of diverse types of drugs such as E, NE, naloxone (opiate antagonist), and picrotoxin (GABA antagonist).

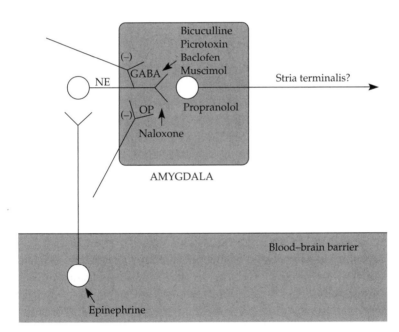

Figure 11-16 McGaugh's amygdala hypothesis for memory modulation. Both peripheral epinephrine (E) and central norepinephrine (NE) act on neurons in the amygdala, as do related drugs (propranolol). GABA and its agonists (muscimol, baclofen) impair memory and its antagonists (bicuculline, picrotoxin) facilitate memory, presumably acting at a GABA synapse. Opiates (OP) and brain endorphins also impair memory, and their antagonist (naloxone) facilitates memory, acting at an opioid synapse. Drugs that influence NE synapses also are believed to act here to influence memory.

The amygdala hypothesis can account for both the facilitating and impairing effects of hormones and drugs on memory storage. However, it does not tell us where the memories themselves are actually stored. In our discussion of conditioned fear we noted the experiment by McGaugh showing that amygdala lesions impaired instrumentally learned fear (passive avoidance task) if made shortly after the learning experience but had no effect on the memory for the learned fear if made several days after learning. This suggests that the long-term memory of the experience is not stored in the amygdala. As of this writing, we do not know where in the brain these memories are stored.

Is there a memory pill? Most of the drugs that facilitate memory in rats are extremely dangerous—either very poisonous or producing serious side effects—and are not recommended for humans. In spite of rumors to the contrary, as of this writing there are no effective memory pills or drugs. However, there is one readily available substance that does enhance memory performance—sugar. Extensive research by Paul Gold and his associates at the University of Virginia showed that glucose injections are as memory enhancing in rats as E. Glucose also enhances memory performance in young adult humans and can have beneficial effects on aged people experiencing problems with memory. You can try the experiment yourself: eat a candy bar after each lecture in a course and then another an hour before the exam.

Memory and the Brain in Humans and Other Primates

The basic processes of associative learning and memory we have considered so far, Pavlovian conditioning and instrumental learning, have the same properties in all mammals, including humans. Furthermore, the brain systems that appear to subserve these phenomena—hypothalamus, amygdala, cerebellum—have the same basic circuitry in all mammals. In those instances where brain substrates have been studied in humans, they appear to be the same as in other mammals. Electroconvulsive shock causes retrograde amnesia in humans just as it does in rats. Lesion of the appropriate region of the cerebellum prevents learning of discrete movements in humans just as it does in rabbits. It therefore seems likely that as we come to understand more fully how memories are formed in the brain in these basic aspects of associative learning in studies on animal models, this knowledge will apply directly to humans.

With the critically important exception of language, it is not at all clear that any aspects of learning and memory are unique to humans. The flow diagram of memory shown in Figure 11-3 applies to all mammals, so far as we know. But we suspect that the storage capacity of the human brain is much greater than that of other animals. This seems likely to be due at least in part to specialized visual memory capacities as well as language abilities in humans.

Visual Learning   It appears that the visual system in the cerebral cortex of primates has been much elaborated over the visual regions in lower mammals. You may recall from Chapter 8 that at least 20 different visual areas have been identified in the monkey and that humans presumably have even more visual areas. These areas seem specialized for different aspects of visual function, for example, area V4 for color and area V5 for movement (Figure 8-11). As we noted in Chapter 8, humans with localized damage to one or another of these areas can show specific kinds of defects in visual function, for example, inability to see color with all other aspects of visual perception normal or inability to see movement with all other aspects of vision normal.

Are these areas the places in the brain where "memories" for color and movement are stored? The answer is probably no. They are necessary for normal perception of color and movement, but this probably results from hard-wired circuits. They are needed for seeing but not remembering. On the other hand, if you can't see different colors you can't remember that you have seen them before in a memory test. This question is very difficult to answer in evaluating effects of damage to visual areas on memory. Are the memories stored in the area or do the stimulus codings or "perceptions" necessary to form memories occur there but the memories are stored elsewhere?

There appear to be two visual memory systems in the monkey brain. The details of these systems have been worked out mostly by Mortimer Mishkin and his many associates at the National Institute of Mental Health in Bethesda, Maryland. They used the lesion method and tested the monkeys in a variety of different visual tasks. One of these systems extends along the temporal lobe from the primary visual cortex (OC in Figure 11-17) through visual association areas to area TEO and finally to area VTE. The other system projects from the primary visual cortex to the parietal cortex. Monkeys are trained on visual discriminations where they must remember which of two objects seen over and over again is correct ("what"), and in other tests they must learn the locations of objects in space ("where"). Lesions of the temporal area TEO markedly impair discrimination performance ("what" task) but not location performance ("where" task). Lesions in the parietal area have just the opposite effect, impairing performance on "where" tasks but not "what" tasks. Neurons in area TEO have very complex receptive fields for visual objects and neurons in the parietal association region seem to code the direction of intended reaching (described in Chapter 9, pp. 293–294). So these two regions of cortex are necessary for these two types of visual memory tasks. Are the memories formed and stored there? It is reasonable to propose that they might be but conclusive evidence is lacking.

The final cortical destination of the temporal visual system is area VTE, the region where Charles Gross first found "hand" cells (Chapter 8, p. 248). Lesions here have quite different effects than do lesions of TEO. Animals are not much impaired on visual discrimination but they are impaired in visual recognition.

Figure 11-17 Mishkin's hypothetical flow diagram for the storage of visual memory in the monkey. The key events involve the transfer of information from the visual area (OC) to the visual association areas (OA, OB, and TEO). For long-term storage of spatial visual memory, information is transferred to areas PG (inferior parietal cortex). For recent visual memory, information is transferred from area TEO to a region of the temporal lobe (VTE) and into the hippocampus (and possibly the amygdala).

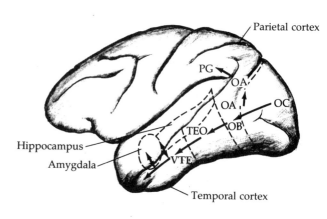

Mishkin trained monkeys to perform a simple short-term visual recognition memory task. A monkey is first presented with a single small block or toy covering a food well that contains a peanut. The monkey reaches out and displaces the object and gets the peanut. After a delay period with a screen in front of the monkey so that it cannot see the objects, another tray is presented to the monkey with the old object and a new object each covering a food well. But only the well under the new object has a peanut. In the following trials with different objects, the monkey must learn the principle of always selecting the new object; of course the monkey must remember which was the old object. Monkeys learn this task well. It is called the *delayed nonmatching to sample task* (see Figure 11-18). (Interestingly, the *delayed matching to sample task*, where the animals are required each time to choose the old object, is more difficult.) Delayed nonmatching to sample was much impaired, particularly with long delays, by lesions of area VTE.

Memory and the Hippocampus   Studies on humans have identified at least three different types of long-term memory formation: declarative (learning what), procedural (skill or learning how), and implicit. The distinction between declarative and procedural memory grew out of studies on patients with damage to structures in the medial temporal lobe of the brain, particularly the hippocampus.

The hippocampus has loomed large as a structure specialized for memory in mammals. The initial impetus for interest in the memorial functions of the hippocampus came as a result of brain surgery done on a now famous patient named H. M. (in the clinical literature patients are never identified by name; initials are used, and generally not the correct initials, to preserve privacy). H. M. underwent extensive neurosurgery many years ago to treat severe and life-threatening epilepsy. The surgery was relatively successful in treating his epilepsy but it had severe side-effects on his memory abilities. To this day, H. M. has an above-average I.Q. and seems perfectly normal and capable in ordinary conversation. However, he is severely impaired in his ability to store new information and experience in long-term memory, an instance of *anterograde amnesia.* Suppose you were introduced to H. M. and talked with him for a while, then left and returned a few minutes later. He would have no memory of having met and talked with you before. H.M.'s loss of the ability to learn new things, particularly to remember his own experiences, dates to about the time of his surgery, actually to a period beginning a few months before the surgery.

Other aspects of H. M.'s current memory are not impaired. His earlier memories of his life before the surgery are intact and normal. He has a normal memory for motor skills. He can learn a complex new motor skill such as playing tennis about as well as other people can. H. M. also has normal short-term memory and therefore can remember a new telephone number long enough to dial it as well as you can. However, if you were asked to memorize the number, you could do so by repeating it to yourself over and over or perhaps developing a trick association—a mnemonic device—to remind you of it. H. M. cannot. He is very good at developing trick associations to help him to remember things, but this works only so long as he can keep repeating the information to himself. As soon as he is distracted, he forgets both the number and the trick association. They never get stored in long-term memory.

It is difficult to imagine what it would be like to live forever in the present. As H. M. once expressed it in an interview:

> Right now, I'm wondering. Have I done or said anything amiss? You see, at this moment everything looks clear to me, but what happened just before? That's what worries me. It's like waking from a dream. I just don't remember. (Milner, B. (1966). Amnesia following operation on the temporal lobes. In Whitty, C. W. M. and Zangwill, O. L. (Eds.) *Amnesia.* London: Butterworths, pp. 112-115.)

The brain surgery that was done on H. M. removed the hippocampus. Like almost all other structures in the brain, there is a hippocampus on each side, one in each temporal lobe. Removal of just one hippocampus—either one—does not seem to cause much impairment of memory ability. However, in H. M.'s case both were removed. Actually, portions of both temporal lobes

a Delayed nonmatching to sample Visual discrimination

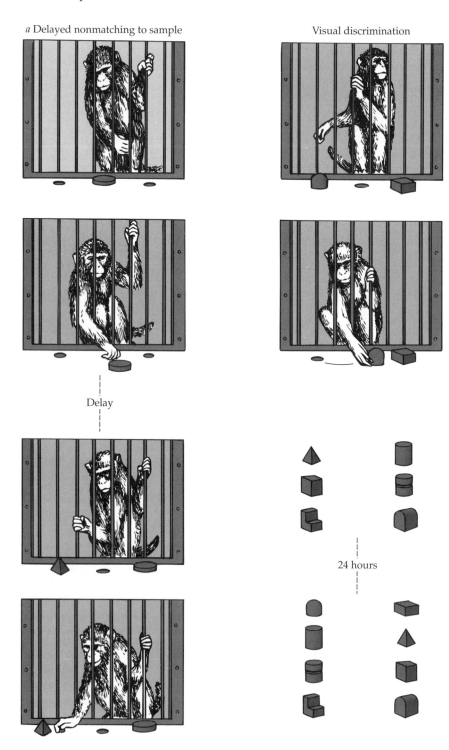

Delay

24 hours

b Delayed nonmatching to sample

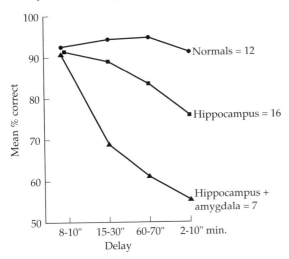

c Delayed nonmatching to sample

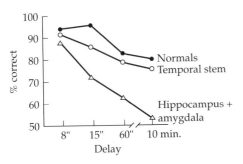

d Visual discrimination

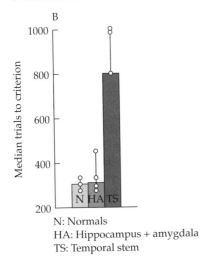

N: Normals
HA: Hippocampus + amygdala
TS: Temporal stem

Figure 11-18 (*a*) Short-term and long-term memory tasks in the monkey. Delayed nonmatching to sample is shown in the left column. One object is presented and the animal rewarded. A screen is lowered, the old object and new object are placed on the tray, and only the new object is baited with reward. The animal must choose the new object to be rewarded and scored correct. Different pairs of objects are then used, and so on. The animal must learn the rule (pick new object) but only need remember the specific object for the brief period of the delay. In visual discrimination learning, shown in the right column, the animal is repeatedly tested on the same two objects until it always chooses the correct one, then it is trained on another pair, and so on. The animal must then remember which objects are correct for 24 hours or longer— long-term visual memory. (*b*) Performance of normal, hippo-campal-lesioned, and combined hippocampus- and amygdala-lesioned animals on delayed non-matching to sample as a function of delay time. (*c*) Same as *b* with the inclusion of a group of "tem-poral stem"-lesioned animals. This lesion destroys fibers con-necting to visual association areas, particularly area TEO (see Figure 11-17). This lesion does not impair performance on delayed nonmatching to sample. (*d*) Performance of normal, hip-pocampus-plus amygdala-lesioned, and temporal stem-lesioned animals on the visual discrimination task (right column in *a*). The temporal stem lesion (area TEO fibers) marked-ly impairs visual long-term memory but the hippocampus plus amygdala lesion does not.

were removed, including the hippocampus and portions of the amygdala and adjacent cerebral cortex.

The hippocampus is a part of the limbic brain, an ancient system that formed the highest region of the brain in primitive vertebrates such as the crocodile. In mammals the cerebral cortex expanded and surrounded the hippocampus and eventually came to dominate enormously in terms of relative size. In a rat, the hippocampus is almost as large as the cerebral cortex, but in monkeys and humans the cerebral cortex is very much larger. Nonetheless, the hippocampus plays critically important roles in learning and memory in all mammals, including humans; H. M. is proof of that. The hippocampus and limbic system are diagrammed in Figures 11-19 and 11-20.

Removing H. M.'s hippocampus did not abolish his memories of his life, his vocabulary, and the facts he had learned before his surgery; it prevented him from storing new memories after the operation. Hence the hippocampus is not where long-term experiential (episodic) and factual (semantic) memories are stored, but it seems to play a critical role in placing these types of new memories in storage. We have stressed H. M.'s difficulty in remembering new experiences and new facts. He is impaired in declarative memory. As we noted, his procedural memory for learning new motor skills is normal. In fact he can learn very complex new skills. A dramatic example is mirror reading. Hold a page of text to a mirror and try to read it—it is very difficult. With extensive practice normal people can succeed in learning to read mirror text. H. M. was trained on this task and learned to read mirror text as well as did normal people. The only difference was that after a training session he had no memory of what he had read, whereas normal people of course did.

Since H. M., a number of other patients with damage to the medial temporal lobe and anterograde amnesia have been studied. Larry Weiskrantz and Elizabeth Warrington, at Oxford University, showed that these patients can learn the conditioned eyeblink task (procedural memory) normally, even though they have no recollection of the experience. Patients with cerebellar damage, on the other hand, cannot learn this task but do remember the experience of hearing tones and feeling puffs of air to the eye.

Recent work, particularly by Daniel Schacter, now at Harvard University, shows that a type of experiential memory ability is preserved in temporal lobe patients: *implicit memory*. To oversimplify, the kind of declarative memory impaired in H. M. involves awareness—we are normally aware of memories when we remember them (*explicit memory*). Implicit memory need not involve awareness. As an example, if people are trained to memorize a list of words, we can test their explicit memory by asking them to repeat the words or to identify them from a larger list. We could test their implicit memory by giving them a list that has just the first two letters of each word; if a word were "tomato," we would give them "to-" and ask them to say the first word that occurs to them. This task is called *priming*. Patients with anterograde amnesia,

RABBIT

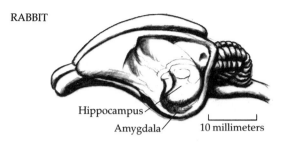

Hippocampus

Amygdala

10 millimeters

Figure 11-19 Hippocampus and amygdala buried in the depths of the temporal lobe in the rabbit, the monkey, and the human.

MONKEY

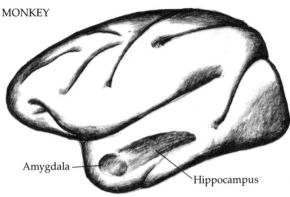

Amygdala

Hippocampus

HUMAN

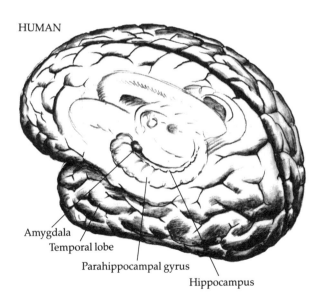

Amygdala

Temporal lobe

Parahippocampal gyrus

Hippocampus

like H. M., perform the implicit task virtually normally, even though they cannot perform the explicit task—they cannot remember the words if asked. They seem to "know" the correct words without being aware of them.

Figure 11-20 Major structures of the limbic system with the surrounding cerebrum dissected away; compare with Figure 11-19 (c).

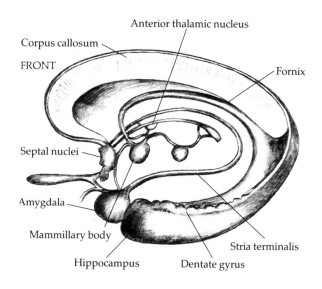

Anterior thalamic nucleus

Corpus callosum

FRONT

Fornix

Septal nuclei

Amygdala

Mammillary body

Stria terminalis

Hippocampus

Dentate gyrus

There is even some evidence that if lists of words are presented verbally to patients undergoing surgery who are unconscious—at the surgical depth of anesthesia—they later demonstrate that they do have some implicit memory for the words, even though they are completely unaware of it. The bottom line here is that the brain system necessary for explicit (declarative) memory, involving the hippocampus and medial temporal lobe, does not seem necessary for implicit memory. We do not yet know the brain circuits for implicit memory.

The fact that amnestic patients have normal implicit memory suggests that categories like "declarative" and "procedural" are much too broad. Semantic (factual), episodic (experiential), and implicit memory are declarative. Some authorities argue that the necessary brain circuits for these aspects of declarative memory differ. This seems clearly so for implicit memory. Others argue that semantic memory is simply extremely overlearned episodic memory. You can't remember the first time you learned the meaning of "tomato" because you have used the word so often. "Procedural" is even more of a grab-bag category. Pavlovian conditioning of discrete responses is procedural and requires the cerebellum. A rat learning to press a lever for food is showing procedural learning, yet this may not require the cerebellum. Much work remains to be done.

The memory impairment shown by H. M. led to much research attempting to develop animal models of H. M.'s deficit, but the work has proved very difficult. Neurons in the hippocampus do seem to be particularly "interested" in behaviors that involve learning. They increase their discharge rates in a learning-dependent manner in many different kinds of learning situations in all mammals that have been studied: rats learning a task for a food reward or to avoid shock, rats learning a maze, rabbits learning the conditioned eyeblink task, cats learning a limb flexion task, and so on. In rats, the hippocampus appears to play a critically important role in spatial learning and memory. Ingenious studies by John O'Keefe at the University of London, James Ranck at New York University, and others demonstrated "place" neurons in the hippocampus. If an animal is running a maze, a given neuron might respond only when the animal is in one particular place in the maze—it is a "place-recognition" neuron. By the same token lesions of the hippocampus markedly impair spatial learning performance in the rat. We might say that learning "where" for rats is like learning "what" for humans.

Working Memory and the Brain   Mishkin explored the effects of limbic lesions in monkeys, using his delayed nonmatching to sample task. He found that removal of both the hippocampus and the amygdala on both sides massively impaired this recent visual memory task, particularly with longer delay times, a result very much like lesions of cortical area VTE (see Figure 11-18 and corresponding text). The monkey still remembered the principle that it was to choose the new object, but it could not remember which was the old object. These monkeys can still see the difference between objects—they can be trained to choose one and not the other—and so it appears that their perceptions of objects are still normal. What has been lost is the ability to remember briefly what they have seen. Another scientist working on the same problem, Larry Squire of the University of California at San Diego, has recently reported that monkeys with lesions only to the hippocampus have this memory deficit, so the importance of the amygdala is at present not entirely clear. Current work suggests that cerebral cortex adjacent to the hippocampus and amygdala may also play a critical role.

The task Mishkin used for his effective limbic and visual area VTE lesions, delayed nonmatching to sample, is really a test of short-term or working visual memory. A localized region of the frontal lobe anterior to the motor areas also seems to be critically involved in short-term memory. The task used is delayed response. The monkey is shown two food wells; one is baited with a preferred food, and both are covered with identical objects. An opaque screen is placed between the animal and the objects for a short period of time. The screen is lifted and the animal must reach out and displace the object over the food to obtain it. Note that this is not a visual discrimination as such but rather memory of a location, a *spatial* kind of short-term memory. Destruction of a very localized region of frontal cortex (sulcus principalis) severely disrupts the animal's ability to perform this task, even at relatively short delays (Figure 11-21). Interestingly, animals with these lesions are able to perform normally on the delayed nonmatching to sample test for *visual* short-term memory.

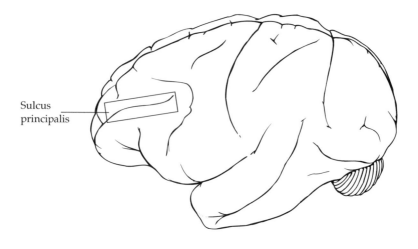

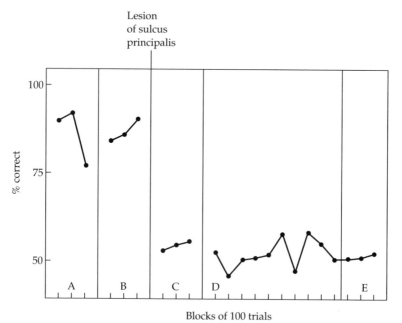

Figure 11-21 Location of the region of the frontal lobe critical for the delayed response task—it is a small region in the banks of the sulcus principalus. Bottom: Delayed response test showing the devastating effect of the sulcus principalus lesion, with a moderate delay of 5 seconds (opaque screen down during delay) between baiting one of two identical objects and the choice period. A: Performance at the end of training. B: Performance six months later showing excellent retention. After B, the lesion is made bilaterally and the animal is given a very long period of post operative training. C, D, E: The animal could never relearn the delayed response task.

The devastating effect of this frontal lesion on delay memory in monkeys was first reported by a scientist named C. F. Jacobsen in 1935. In addition, Jacobsen's lesions, which were large, also produced marked "taming" of the animals. A neurosurgeon heard this report and immediately began removing frontal lobe tissue in humans—the frontal lobotomy procedure—to treat psychiatric problems. Many thousands of operations later it was realized that this damaging procedure was of little help in the treatment of mental illness. A most unfortunate chapter in the history of psychiatry, the procedure is no longer used today.

To summarize, lesions of area VTE and the hippocampus (and amygdala?) impair short-term or working visual memory in monkeys. Frontal cortex lesions impair short-term spatial memory in monkeys. Recently, Charles Gross and his associates at Princeton University identified an area of auditory association cortex necessary for short-term auditory memory in monkeys. Studies by Weiszkrantz and Warrington on patients with localized damage to certain association areas of the cerebral cortex have identified perhaps analogous areas in human cerebral cortex that appear to be specialized for short-term visual and short-term auditory memory (Figure 11-22).

I, at least, am impressed with the extent to which lesions in various association areas of the cerebral cortex in both monkeys and humans impair short-term or working memory processes. Short-term or working memory seems the special province of the cerebral cortex. The evidence for long-term memory storage in the cerebral cortex is less compelling.

Long-Term Memory and the Brain Impairment of visual discriminations with TEO lesions is among the very few examples where lesions of the cerebral cortex impair long-term memories in monkeys. Or do they? Remember that a lesion deficit in memory performance per se can show only that the damaged structure plays a necessary or important role in the expression of the memory

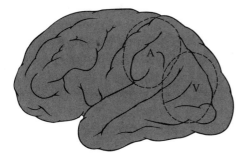

Figure 11-22 General location on the human cerebral cortex where brain damage markedly impairs short-term auditory (A) and visual (V) memory. Such damage does not impair the ability to form long-term memories.

or in the perception necessary for the memory; it does not demonstrate that the memory is stored in the damaged structure.

The short-term visual memory deficit Mishkin found in monkeys with hippocampus plus amygdala lesions seems rather different from H. M.'s inability to place new experiences and facts into long-term memory. Larry Squire and Stuart Zola-Morgan, at the University of California at San Diego, devised a task that does seem to mimic some aspects of H. M.'s impairment. They trained monkeys on a long series of visual discriminations where the animal had to learn which of two objects was correct for each pair. This would seem to involve long-term memory storage. Hippocampal lesions were made at the end of training. Discriminations learned shortly before lesion were much impaired. However, when the training was given a month or more before lesion, the animals remembered as well as trained but not lesioned control animals. Recall that H. M.'s memories for events prior to several months before his surgery were normal. This study on monkeys also provides further evidence that long-term memories are not stored in the hippocampus.

PET–Scanning the Brain for Memories   The recently developed techniques of brain imaging offer promise of identifying memory circuits in the human brain. In one procedure, radiolabeled water (H_2 ^{15}O) is injected into the bloodstream in volunteer subjects. This is a safe procedure because the half-life of ^{15}O is only about 120 seconds. A procedure that involves scanning the brain for radioactivity—*positron emission tomography*, or PET—is used and the subjects engage in a task for about 40 seconds. Increased radioactivity in a given brain area means increased blood flow to that area, which is what is actually measured. There is a relationship between increased neural activity and increased blood flow in brain areas, as shown many years ago in classic studies by Seymore Kety at the National Institute of Mental Health.

We give one example of current work, a study by Larry Squire, in collaboration with Marcus Raichle at Washington University in St. Louis, and their colleagues. Before the PET scan, the subjects had learned a list of words. In one condition they had to remember the words during the 40-second scan (declarative explicit memory). In another condition the priming test was used, where the subjects simply said the first words that came to mind upon seeing the first two letters of the words (implicit memory). Results suggested that in the explicit or declarative task, blood flow increased in the right hippocampus, but in the implicit memory task blood flow increased primarily in the occipital or visual areas of the right cerebral cortex. These results support the notion we mentioned earlier that the brain substrates for explicit and implicit memory may be different.

Mechanisms of Long-term Memory Storage

Long-term, well-learned memories are permanent. This must mean a permanent change of some kind in neurons. Everything we know about how neurons function says that the changes must occur at synapses, the points of interconnections among neurons. There are two broad classes of possibilities, structural changes and functional changes.

Overwhelming evidence shows that experience results in structural changes at synapses. This is particularly true for experience early in life. William Greenough and his associates at the University of Illinois have developed strong evidence in many experiments that a wide variety of early experiences causes an increase in the extent of dendritic branding in principal (output) neurons, particularly in cortical structures. In addition, the number of spine synapses on the dendrites (excitatory) appears to increase dramatically (see Chapter 10). Possible structural change in neurons due to specific learning experiences have been a much more difficult problem, as yet unsolved.

In our discussion of elementary learning processes in a ganglion of the *Aplysia* (pp. 347–348) we noted that long-term sensitization has been used as a model of associative learning. Eric Kandel and his many associates found that long-term sensitization at the modifiable synapse of the sensory neuron to the motor neuron in the gill-withdrawal reflex resulted in clear structural changes at the synapse. We might note that the shorter-term processes of sensitization and classical conditioning appear to involve similar mechanisms at this synapse, hence the use of long-term sensitization as a model of memory formation. The degree to which structural changes of the sort seen in the sensitized *Aplysia* synapse occur in the mammalian brain is unknown at present.

Are gene actions required to produce structural changes? That is, does memory involve changes in gene expression in neurons? You may recall from Chapter 10 that in humans something like 50,000 genes are active—express proteins—only in neurons in the brain. Proteins are of course the building blocks of all cells, including neuron synapses. Some substances can inhibit (block) protein synthesis; the antibiotic puromycin is an example. Some years ago in a number of studies mammals, mostly rats, were trained in long-term memory tasks either with or without injections of protein-synthesis inhibitors. The bottom line was that if protein synthesis was inhibited within a short time after training, memory was markedly impaired. Most of these studies used systemic (in the blood or body tissue) injections of the inhibitors, which act everywhere in the body and make animals very sick. In careful studies, Bernard Agranoff at the University of Michigan trained goldfish in a simple task and injected puromycin directly into the brain. Results were striking. If the substance was injected up to 30 minutes after training, memory was abolished.

If puromycin was injected just before training, initial learning occurred but the subsequent memory was abolished, implying that short-term memory did not require protein synthesis but long-term memory did. Kandel and associates showed that local infusions of protein-synthesis inhibitors blocked the development of long-term sensitization at the *Aplysia* synapse.

All this evidence seems to argue that protein synthesis, and hence gene expression, is necessary to form permanent memories. But is protein synthesis, and hence gene actions, absolutely necessary for structural changes at synapses? The answer is no. In an important theoretical article, Gary Lynch and Michel Baudry, both then at the University of California at Irvine, showed how processes occurring at the synapse and not requiring new or additional proteins can result in structural changes that could markedly increase synaptic excitability. Certain proteins can actually change their shape when activated —the actin and myosin in muscle are obvious examples. Lynch and Baudry argue that certain structural proteins at the synapse can be activated by a cascade of intracellular processes triggered by Ca^{++} entry and can act on synapse proteins to change their shapes, thus altering the properties of the synapse. This process does not require gene expression.

Structural changes, whether due to gene expression or other mechanisms, are a straightforward way of changing synapses. But how can nonstructural, or functional, changes store long-term memories? We actually gave an example of a functional change without a structural change in Chapter 7: Larry Swanson's biochemical switching hypothesis (Figure 7-5). This, however, does involve changes in gene expression. The two most prominent functional mechanisms suggested for memory storage are long-term potentiation (LTP) and long-term depression (LTD).

We considered the mechanisms of LTP at some length in Chapter 4. You will recall that it is a long-lasting increase in synaptic excitability as a result of associative activation of the NMDA Ca^{++} channels.

As we saw earlier, several lines of research support the view that memory storage for at least some period of time occurs in the hippocampus. This storage seems likely to involve a process like long-term potentiation (LTP). Richard Morris at Edinburgh University in Scotland, in collaboration with Gary Lynch and Michel Baudry, explored the role of the glutamate NMDA-type receptors in the hippocampus in spatial memory in the rat. As we noted, activation of NMDA receptors is the critical event for the initiation of hippocampal LTP. They infused the NMDA antagonist APV into the hippocampus and tested the effect on the animal's memory in a water maze. In this task the animal has to swim to find a platform hidden under the water. The water is opaque and the only cues the animal has are the distinctive spatial cues in the room. Rats learn this task well. However, blocking the hippocampal NMDA receptors markedly impaired memory for the task. Another line of evidence favoring LTP that we noted earlier is Michael Davis's finding that

APV infused in the amygdala prevents fear conditioning (LTP can also be induced in the amygdala). Yet another line of evidence comes from work by George Tocco and others in my laboratory in collaboration with Michel Baudry at the University of Southern California. When rabbits learn the conditioned eyeblink task, there is a massive learning-dependent engagement of hippocampal neuron activity, as we noted earlier. This is accompanied by a marked increase in binding to the AMPA-type glutamate receptor in the hippocampus. In current work in Gary Lynch's lab at the University of California at Irvine and in our labs at the University of Southern California, it appears that increased activation or binding affinity of the AMPA receptors may be a mechanism underlying expression of LTP (see Chapter 4).

Tim Bliss and T. Lomo discovered long-term potentiation in the hippocampus and it has since been found in other structures as well, for example, the amygdala and the cerebral cortex. It could well prove the mechanism for permanent memory storage in the cerebral cortex, if some types of permanent memories, for example, visual memories and declarative memories, are indeed stored there. By the same token, long-term depression (LTD) was first discovered by Ito in the cerebellum, and it has now also been seen in the hippocampus and cerebral cortex. You may recall (Chapters 4 and 9) that if parallel fibers and climbing fibers in the cerebellar cortex are activated together repeatedly, there is a long-lasting decrease in excitability of the parallel fibers to Purkinje neuron synapse, thought to be mediated by the AMPA-type glutamate receptors. In studies in my laboratory at the University of Southern California, eyeblink conditioning resulted in a decrease in the Purkinje neuron response to the tone CS-activated parallel fibers. Further, appropriate pairing of stimulation of mossy parallel fibers and climbing fibers can produce normal learning of the behavioral response evoked by the climbing fiber stimulus. This would seem to argue that a process of LTD in cerebellar cortex may be a key mechanism of memory storage in classical conditioning of discrete responses (motor skill learning).

It is of interest that the mechanism of expression of LTD appears to be a decrease in AMPA receptor function and the mechanism for LTP is thought, at least by some workers, to be an increase in AMPA receptor function. The AMPA receptor (there are actually several subtypes) may hold the key to permanent memory storage in the mammalian brain. Whether or not LTP and LTD involve changes in gene expression is unresolved at this writing.

SUMMARY

The ability of the human brain to store and retrieve memories is perhaps the most extraordinary phenomenon in the natural world. Each of us has literally millions of bits of information stored in long-term memory.

There are several different time-dependent processes in memory: very short-term sensory or iconic memory, lasting about 100 milliseconds; short-term memory lasting a few seconds, working memory bridging recent experiences, and long-term or permanent memory. New stimuli or events are stored in detail very briefly in iconic memory, some fraction of them are held in short-term memory, and some, if rehearsed (for verbal material) or practiced (for motor skills), are gradually placed in long-term memory.

Memory can be described in several categories. Nonassociative memory includes habituation, a decreased response to repeated stimulation, and sensitization, an increase in response following a strong or arousing stimulus. Associative learning entails forming associations among stimuli and/or responses or movement sequences. A basic form of associative learning is classical or Pavlovian conditioning, where neutral stimuli are paired with reinforcing stimuli (reward or punishment). In instrumental learning, the organism must perform some response in order to obtain reward or avoid punishment. Long-term associative learning and memory can be categorized in several ways: episodic (experience coded), semantic (knowledge), declarative (experience dependent), procedural (motor skills, Pavlovian conditioning).

Most of the learning we and other mammals do is associative. Key processes are contiguity (close temporal association among stimuli and events) and contingency (the likelihood that the stimuli and events will occur in close temporal association). Basic associative learning (Pavlovian conditioning) is the way that organisms, including humans, learn about the causal structure of the world. The temporal law of associative learning indicates that in a wide range of learning situations the signal or CS must precede the reinforcement or US by some period of time. Although this CS–US interval for best learning varies widely for different tasks, it has the same functional form in all tasks.

Habituation, where it has been analyzed, appears to be due to a decrease in the probability of transmitter release at synaptic terminals as a result of repeated activation, due in turn to a decreased entry of calcium ions into the presynaptic terminals when the action potential arrives, due in turn to repeated activation of second messenger systems within the terminal. Sensitization (short-term), on the other hand, appears to be due to increased probability of transmitter release, due to an increase in calcium entry at presynaptic terminals as a result of sensitization-pathway terminal neurotransmitter actions on second-messenger systems at the terminal. Changes in excitability of the postsynaptic neuron membrane can also occur in sensitization.

Fear conditioning (pairing a neutral stimulus with an aversive stimulus like an electric shock) appears to critically involve the amygdala, as does fear-potentiated startle. Lesions of the amygdala attenuate learned fear to all modalities of neutral stimuli (tone or light) and all aspects of expression of fear (freezing, heart-rate changes), whereas lesions in the hippocampus can selectively abolish specific aspects of fear. Infusion of NMDA antagonists in the amygdala prevents learning but not expression of learned fear, suggesting that a process like long-term potentiation in the amygdala may be involved.

Classical conditioning of discrete skilled movements (eyeblink, leg flexion) critically involves the cerebellum. The neutral CS (tone, light) pathway activates mossy fiber projections to the cerebellum and the aversive US (corneal air puff, paw shock) activates the inferior olive and its climbing fiber projections to the cerebellum. Small lesions of the cerebellar interpositus nucleus completely abolish all components of the conditioned response to all modalities of CS and have no effect on the reflex US. Reversible inactivation studies suggest that the memory trace is formed and stored in the cerebellum.

Memory consolidation is a powerful and pervasive phenomenon—memories are remembered best if learned in a state of arousal. Posttraining injection of a wide range of drugs can substantially improve or impair subsequent memory performance on instrumental learning tasks. As with Pavlovian fear learning, the amygdala is critical. Interestingly, amygdala lesions abolish both memory-enhancing and memory-impairing drug effects. Lesions of the amygdala made shortly after instrumental tasks are learned (typically passive or active avoidance) abolish subsequent memory, but if the same amygdala lesion is made a week after the learning experience, the memory is not impaired. This suggests that the amygdala is essential for the initial formation of the memory but that the long-term memory is stored elsewhere.

Visual learning and memory in primates involves two different systems in the cerebral cortex. One system relays from V I through visual association areas to area TEO on the temporal lobe. Lesion of this area impairs the animal's ability to learn visual discrimination tasks (long-term memory). Another system projects from V I and visual association areas to parietal association cortex. Lesions there impair the animal's ability to learn the location of objects in space but not its ability to discriminate objects (vice versa for TEO lesions).

Area TEO projects a temporal association area termed VTE (where "hand" cells were found in the monkey) and area VTE projects to the hippocampus. Lesions of VTE or the hippocampus markedly impair short-term or working memory—the delayed nonmatching to sample task. (Lesions in a region of prefrontal cortex permanently impair short-term memory for locations of objects—the delayed response task.) Lesions of a temporal lobe area of cerebral cortex in the monkey impair short-term auditory memory tasks. Analogous cortical lesions in humans selectively impair short-term auditory and visual memory performance. If monkeys are trained on a long series of visual discrimination tasks (long-term memory), hippocampal lesions shortly after training massively impair memory for the discriminations learned just before the lesion but not for those learned earlier. The hippocampus is not the site of long-term memory storage. Studies with human amnesiac patients, most notably H. M., indicate that extensive bilateral hippocampal damage causes severe anterograde amnesia. New experience and information cannot be stored in long-term memory, but memories of experiences prior to a few months before the lesions are retained. Interestingly, one type of experience-dependent memory ability, implicit memory, revealed by the priming procedure, is present in these amnesiac patients.

As yet, the mechanisms that form long-term memories in the brain are not known. Long-term potentiation, first discovered in the hippocampus, and long-term depression, first discovered in the cerebellar cortex, both occur in hippocampus and cerebral cortex and are the leading candidate mechanisms of memory storage at present.

Impairment in protein synthesis markedly impairs or prevents memory formation in invertebrate systems and in certain types of learning situations in fish and mammals. This implies that changes in gene expression are involved in long-term memory formation. Study of this molecular biology of memory is a promising new area of research.

SUGGESTED READINGS AND REFERENCES

Books

Bryne, J. H. , and Berry, W. O. (1989). *Neural models of plasticity: Experimental and theoretical approaches*. San Diego, CA: Academic Press.

Changeux, J.-P., and Konishi, M. (1987). *The neural and molecular bases of learning.* Chichester, England: John Wiley & Sons.

Davis, J. L., Newburgh, R. W., and Wegman, E. J. (1988). *Brain structure, learning, and memory.* AAAS Selected Symposium.

Dudai, Y. (1989). *The neurobiology of memory: Concepts, findings, trends.* Oxford: Oxford University Press.

Groves, P. M., and Rebec, G. V. (1992). *Introduction to biological psychology* (4th ed.). Dubuque, IA: William C Brown.

Kandel, E. R. (1976). *Cellular basis of behavior.* San Francisco: W. H. Freeman.

Lynch, G. (1987). *Synapses, circuits, and the beginnings of memory.* Cambridge, MA: MIT Press.

Martinez, J. L., Jr., and Kesner, R. P. (1991). *Learning and memory: A biological view* (2nd ed.). San Diego, CA: Academic Press.

Squire, L. R. (1987). *Memory and brain.* New York: Oxford University Press.

Articles

Bailey, C. H., and Chen, M. (1983). Morphological basis of long-term habituation and sensitization in *Aplysia. Science, 220,* 91–93.

Carew, T. J., and Sahley, C. L. (1986). Invertebrate learning and memory: From behavior to molecules. *Annual Review of Neuroscience, 9,* 435–487.

Davis, M. (1992). The role of the amygdala in fear and anxiety. *Annual Review of Neuroscience, 15,* 353–376.

McGaugh, J. L. (1989). Involvement of hormonal and neuromodulatory systems in the regulation of memory storage. *Annual Review of Neuroscience, 12,* 255–288.

McGaugh, J. L., and Liang, K. C. (1985). Hormonal influences on memory: Interaction of central and peripheral systems. In Will, B. E., Schmitt, P., and Dalrymple-Alford, J. C. (Eds.), *Brain plasticity, learning, and memory*. New York: Plenum.

Rescorla, R. A. (1988). Pavlovian conditioning: It's not what you think it is. *American Psychologist, 43*, 151–160.

Squire, L. R., and Zola-Morgan, S. (1991). The medial temporal lobe memory system. *Science, 253*, 1380–1386.

Thompson, R. F. (1986). The neurobiology of learning and memory. *Science, 233*, 941–947.

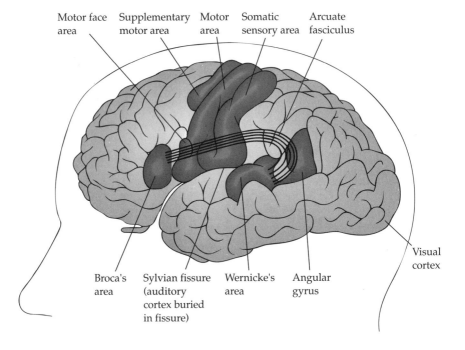

Motor face area   Supplementary motor area   Motor area   Somatic sensory area   Arcuate fasciculus

Broca's area   Sylvian fissure (auditory cortex buried in fissure)   Wernicke's area   Angular gyrus   Visual cortex

12

Language, Consciousness, and the Brain

Language is the most astonishing behavior in the animal kingdom. It is the one species-typical behavior that sets humans completely apart from all other animals. We use our native language so naturally and fluently that we are completely unaware of the extraordinary complexity of the process. Before examining brain substrates of language a few words are in order about the nature of language.

Figure 12-1 Primary language areas of the human brain are thought to be located in the left hemisphere, because only rarely does damage to the right hemisphere cause language disorders. Also shown are motor and supplementary motor areas, the somatic sensory area, and the auditory and visual areas. Broca's area, which is adjacent to the region of the motor cortex that controls the movement of the muscles of the lips, the jaw, the tongue, the soft palate, and the vocal cords, apparently incorporates programs for the coordination of these muscles in speech. Damage to Broca's area results in slow and labored speech, but comprehension of language remains intact. Wernicke's area lies between Heschl's gyrus, which is the primary receiver of auditory stimuli, and the angular gyrus, which acts as a way station between the auditory and the visual regions. When Wernicke's area is damaged, speech is fluent but has little content, and comprehension is usually lost. Wernicke and Broca areas are joined but a nerve bundle called the arcuate fasciculus. When it is damaged, speech is fluent but abnormal, and the patient can comprehend words but cannot repeat them.

SPEECH AND LANGUAGE

Language is of course a means of communication. But many animals can communicate information (the "honey dance" of the bee, for example). Human language permits communication about *anything*, even about things like unicorns that have never existed. The key lies in the fact that the units of meaning (morphemes or words) can be strung together in different ways, according to rules, to communicate different meanings.

The most elemental component of language is the *phoneme*, the smallest possible sound distinguishing one word from another. The word "pin" has three phonemes, p, i, and n. Change any one and a different word emerges: sin, pen, pit, and so on. Languages have rules for combing phonemes. In English, we cannot begin a word with a t followed by an l, as in "tlip." But another non-word, "glip," is perfectly all right. It just has not yet been given a meaning. As Eric Warner, at the Russell Sage Foundation, puts it, if a new concept comes along and it needs a name, "glip" is ready, willing, and able. All languages are based on various combinations of about 90 phonemes. English uses 40 and other languages have from 15 to 40 of these basic phonemes or sounds.

Morphemes are combinations of phonemes into elementary units of meaning, usually words. "Boats" has two morphemes, "boat" and "s," the plural morpheme meaning more than one boat. Morphemes follow rules too. Consider "glip" as a verb that we wish to use to indicate that you can't glip someone. Clearly, that person is "unglippable." We know that this is the correct form, even though "glip" does not exist.

English has more than 100,000 morphemes, which arranged in various ways yield the million-word English vocabulary. A typical educated adult has a vocabulary of about 40,000 words; an exceptional individual might have a 100,000-word vocabulary.

Finally, words can be combined into sentences according to rules called *syntax*. The rules for a language like English were not spelled out in advance of developing the language; they exist in us the speakers. Many rules have been spelled out—the rules of grammar we learned in school—but the rules existed long before the first grammar was written. Finally, the most complex aspect of language is *semantics*, the way language expresses meaning.

Consider what has to happen when one person is speaking to another. The speaker has to translate thoughts into spoken language, using syntax and semantics to construct sentence patterns that convey the desired meanings, using the sounds of speech to pronounce the sentences correctly. The listener must use the sounds of speech to figure out the words being spoken, syntax to figure out the pattern of words, and semantics to interpret the meaning. Amazingly, this complex process from thought to speech and from speech back to meaning occurs virtually without awareness.

The modern field of psycholinguistics has done much to clarify the essential properties of language. Noam Chomsky at the Massachusetts Institute of Technology has been particularly influential in developing the field. Chomsky hypothesized that languages have two kinds of structures: surface structures that relate to the particular forms and sequences of words in a given language and "deep" structures, a more fundamental kind of organization or syntax that may be common to all languages.

To oversimplify greatly, all but the last of the following sentences have differing surface appearances but the same "deep" meaning; the last sentence has a very different "deep" meaning:

Matthew eats the cookie.

The cookie was eaten by Matthew.

Matthew ate the cookie.

The cookie ate Matthew.

Roger Brown at Harvard University completed an extensive analysis of the acquisition of language by children. In his view there is a common semantic and grammatical order of progression for children learning any language, which he terms natural language acquisition. He was able to characterize a series of stages in language learning that all children go through, regardless of their native language. The rate of language learning in young children is quite amazing. Somewhere between 10 and 15 months the first word is spoken. By age 2, children know about 50 words; by age 8 the average vocabulary is 18,000 words. Between the ages of 1 and 8, the child is learning at the rate of 8 new words a day!

Apparently the deep structure of all languages is similar. At an early stage an infant "babbles" essentially all the sounds (phonemes) used in all languages. Children are thought by some linguists to develop a similar initial universal deep grammar, as Brown's work implies. Perhaps most surprising is the fact that languages show little sign of evolution or development. All languages, from English to obscure dialects of isolated aborigines, have the same degree of complexity and similar general properties. It is as though humans came into the world equipped with a well-elaborated, complex, and biologically determined language system. In short, it would seem that we may have speech and language centers in the brain that are in some ways predetermined or preprogrammed.

Language is a motor activity: speech; an auditory activity: hearing words; and a complex linkage to thought processes. Reading and writing, as we noted in Chapter 11, are unnatural activities that developed only a few thousand years ago, long after the brain had evolved to its present form and long after languages and their implicit rules had developed.

Large areas of the human cerebral cortex are specialized for language, and in very special ways. As we will see later, damage to one or another of these areas can cause loss of ability to understand written but not spoken language, but not vice versa; loss of ability to write but not speak; loss of ability to speak but not understand language, and vice versa; and so on. If ever there was a clear case for detailed localization of function in the cerebral cortex, it would seem to be language.

LANGUAGE IN ANIMALS?

Language as we have characterized it is generally said not to occur in animals in the natural state. But there are some interesting examples that come very close to language in monkeys. Most monkeys are social animals, living in groups that make sounds that clearly convey various meanings to the members of the group. Squirrel monkeys, a small South American species, have a variety of such communication sounds. One study reported that some neurons in the auditory cortex of this monkey responded selectively to certain of these species-typical sounds but not to any pure tones—they respond like feature-detector neurons to sounds that convey meaning.

An extraordinary example of learned speech in monkeys was recently described by Pete Marler and his associates at Rockefeller University. They were studying vervet monkeys living freely in their natural state in Amboseli National Park in Kenya, Africa. Vervet monkeys make alarm calls to warn the group of an approaching predator. All the adult animals make the same three different sounds to identify three common enemies: leopards, eagles, and pythons. The leopard alarm is a short tonal call, the eagle alarm is low-pitched staccato grunts, and the python alarm is high-pitched "chutters." Other alarm calls could also be distinguished, including one given to baboons and one to unfamiliar humans but not to humans they recognized.

The Rockefeller group focused on the leopard, eagle, and snake alarms. When the monkeys were on the ground and one monkey made the leopard alarm sound, all would at once rush up into the trees, where they appeared to be safest from the ambush style of attack typical of leopards. If one monkey made the eagle alarm, they would all immediately look up to the sky and run into the dense bush. When a python alarm was made, they would all look down at the ground around them. The investigators recorded these sounds and played them back to individual monkeys, with the same results.

Perhaps most interesting were the alarm calls of the infant monkeys. The adults were very specific. The three alarm sounds were not made to the 100 or so other species of mammals, birds, and reptiles seen regularly by the monkeys. The infants, on the other hand, gave the alarm calls to a much wider range of species and objects—for example, to things that posed no danger, such as wart hogs, pigeons, and falling leaves. Even the infants, however, understood the categories: they gave leopard alarms to terrestrial mammals, eagle alarms to birds, and python alarms to snakes or other long, thin objects. As the infants grew up, they learned to be more and more selective in the use of alarm calls. This is clearly an example of learned communication, perhaps even a very primitive forerunner of basic language.

Can apes learn language? For many years, attempts to teach chimpanzees spoken language failed completely. Chimpanzees are simply not predisposed to talk. However, more recent attempts to teach language to chimps have used sign language with considerable success. Beatrice and Allen Gardner at the University of Nevada trained a chimp named Washoe in the American Sign Language.

There is good reason to use the chimp as an animal model of language learning. The chimp is the closest living relative of the human species—99% of the DNA in chimps and humans is identical. The Gardners' approached teaching young Washoe sign language just as one would teach spoken language to a child. They lived with her, constantly talked to her in signs, and rewarded her for appropriate signs. Washoe learned over 100 signs and could string them together in phrases as long as five signs. Examples are given in the following passage from the Gardners:

> A listing of Washoe's phrases, together with the contexts in which they occurred, is striking because the phrases seem so apt. For play with her companions, she would sign "Roger you tickle, you Greg peekaboo," or simply "catch me" or "tickle me." She indicated destinations with phrases such as "go in," "go out," or "down in bed." Other phrases produced descriptions: "drink red" for her red cup, "my baby" for her dolls, "listen food" or "listen drink" for the supper bell, and "dirty good" for the toilet chair. Asking for access to the many objects that were kept out of sight and out of reach by the various locked doors in her quarters, Washoe signed, "key open food" at the refrigerator, "open key clean" at the soap cupboard and "key open please blanket" at the bedding cupboard. Combinations with "sorry" were frequent, and these were appropriate for apology and irresistible as appeasements: "please sorry, sorry dirty, sorry hurt, please sorry, good," and "come hug-love sorry, sorry."
>
> These examples of apt phrases are by no means exceptional; there were hundreds of other such phrases, and particular phrases were observed repeatedly, as their appropriate situation recurred. Any participant in this project saw and responded to "go out" and "tickle me" far more often than he would care to remember. (Gardner, B. T. and Gardner, R. A., Two-way communication with an infant chimpanzee. *Behavior of Non-human primates*, 4, 166–167, 1971.)

In more recent work, the Gardners compared Washoe's sign language learning to children's learning of sign language and found them to be very similar, with the chimp apparently going through stages of natural language acquisition.

A major debate in the field of language is not whether chimps can learn a large vocabulary of signs and communicate very effectively with them. The

Gardners' work and studies by other groups show quite clearly that they can. The debate is whether this is "really" language—a system of communication with syntax and deep structure. David Premack, then working at the University of California at Santa Barbara, trained a chimp named Sarah to communicate using differently shaped objects as symbols for words. Sarah learned to use several hundred such symbols and did so very effectively. Premack carried out a number of studies with Sarah to determine the extent to which her use of the symbols had the properties of language. The answer seemed to be that it did not. However, one major difference between Sarah and Washoe, who learned sign language, was that Sarah used her symbols only in the test situation, not spontaneously, whereas Washoe used signing spontaneously all the time.

A discovery that may prove to be extremely important was recently made by Sue Savage-Rumbaugh and Duane Rumbaugh working at the Yerkes Primate Center in Atlanta, Georgia. Researchers there used a simple language (called Yerkish) made up of symbols; the chimps can communicate by pressing the symbols on a large keyboard. As in other studies, the chimps learned to do this very well—they could communicate their wants and feelings, and they pushed the correct symbols showing pictures of objects. As in other chimp studies, the Rumbaughs' chimps did not learn to respond to spoken language.

The Rumbaughs' previous work had all been done with the common chimp (*Pan troglodytes*). The pygmy chimp (*Pan paniscus*), is a different species found only in one region of Africa. The pygmies are not actually much smaller than the common chimp but have longer and more slender bones, tend to walk upright on their feet more of the time, and have a much wider range of natural vocalizations. They seem more humanlike. Indeed, they differ so much from common chimps that a separate genus has been proposed—*Bonobo*.

Matata was one of the first pygmy chimps the Rumbaughs studied. She was caught wild and her son, Kanzi, was born at Yerkes. In contrast to common chimps, at 6 months of age Kanzi engaged in much vocal babbling and seemed to be trying to imitate human speech. From this time until he was 2 ½, Kanzi accompanied Matata to her Yerkish training sessions. He was then separated from his mother for several months while she was being bred and was cared for by humans. The Rumbaughs decided to try to teach Kanzi Yerkish in a manner more like that of natural language learning by humans (no food reward for correct responses, no discrete trial training). He began using the keyboard correctly and spontaneously, which no common chimp had ever done. And quite by accident, it was discovered that Kanzi was learning English! Two of the experimenters were talking together. One of them spoke a word to the other and Kanzi ran to the machine and pressed the correct symbol for that word. Upon testing, Kanzi proved to have a vocabulary of about 35 English words at that time.

The issue of "true" language in chimps may seem a bit academic—they learn to communicate very well, particularly with symbols and sign language.

In the natural state, they and many other primates have primitive vocal communication systems, as we noted. But this is a surface reflection of a much deeper issue, namely, the extent to which human language is determined by the structure of the human brain. A particular language is obviously learned. Perhaps all aspects of language, including syntax and deep structure, are learned. Some years ago the eminent psychologist B. F. Skinner made a heroic effort to show that this is the case, that language is learned by infants as a result of rewards and reinforcements. There are many counterarguments for the more deterministic biological view, as we noted earlier. An interesting example has to do with the way in which young children learn the past tense of verbs. They learn the rule for forming the past tense of regular verbs and go through a period when they erroneously use this form for irregular verbs, as in "I digged a hole." They never hear the word "digged" from their parents and are not instructed at age 3 or 4 in the rules of grammar; they come up with the general rule on their own. It is difficult to see how this could be learned by rewards. On the other hand, it is possible to construct an artificial associative learning network in a computer that will learn and use such incorrect general rules at one stage in its learning of language, as we will see later.

BRAIN SUBSTRATES OF LANGUAGE

In normal adults, language has a very clear set of biological substrates in the brain, especially in the cerebral cortex. The language areas of the cortex are localized and usually on the left hemisphere (Figure 12-1). Indeed, there are clear structural asymmetries between certain of the speech areas on the left hemisphere and the corresponding regions on the right hemisphere. Particularly striking is the enlarged posterior speech area, called Wernicke's area, of the left hemisphere. This area lies around the end of the Sylvian fissure, the large fissure that separates the temporal and frontal lobes of the brain. In most humans, this cortical area is much larger in the left hemisphere than in the right hemisphere.

Language and Asymmetries of the Hemispheres

Work by Marianne LeMay and Norman Geschwind at Harvard Medical School, and others, has extended this analysis to our ancestors. The temporal lobe and Sylvian fissure leave a clear identification and ridge on the inner surface of the skull, which is different on the two sides because of the enlarged speech area on the left in modern humans. The same enlarged left temporal area was found in the skull of our brutish-looking cousin, the Neanderthal.

Neanderthals, incidentally, may have looked brutish, but they had brains as large as those of modern humans, apparently with larger posterior regions and smaller frontal regions than our own. (In *The Clan of the Cave Bear* the novelist Jean Auel develops some interesting speculations about possible differences in the "minds" of Neanderthals and modern humans). The Neanderthal skull that was studied is more than 30,000 years old and was found in France. Even more remarkable is the same enlarged speech area seen on the left hemisphere of a skull of Peking man in Asia, our much more remote ancestor *Homo erectus*. The skull examined is thought to be 300,000 years old. Other evidence indicates that Neanderthals possessed language. They buried their dead ceremoniously, along with objects indicating a religion, which seems unlikely to have existed without a language. Although we have no such extra evidence for language in *Homo erectus*, the enlarged speech area alone strongly points to language capability.

The astonishing quadrupling in size of the human brain over the past three million years must have been molded powerfully by natural selection. Language is the major difference between humans and apes, and much of the human cerebral cortex is involved in language. It seems evident that improving communication with developing language gave a competitive edge in survival to big-brained social animals. Some great apes, chimps, and orangutans also have an enlarged area of the left hemisphere in a region analogous to the human language area, although it is nothing like the human asymmetry. Monkeys, however, do not have this type of cerebral asymmetry.

The existence of speech areas in the left hemisphere of the human brain has been known for nearly 100 years from the study of patients with brain damage. The discovery of anatomical differences between the hemispheres is quite new. The posterior speech area is not only larger in extent in the left hemisphere in the majority of people, it is also larger in terms of tissue at the microscopic level: as much as 700% more tissue occurs in the left speech area than in the corresponding area in the right hemisphere. The difference in the two hemispheres develops in the human embryo at about 31 weeks after fertilization.

The original sign of hemispheric dominance was handedness. About 90 percent of humans in all societies and throughout history have been right-handed. Even our most remote ancestors that could be called humanlike, the Australopithecines, who lived in Africa several million years ago, may have been mostly right-handed. Australopithecines walked upright and apparently used crudely chipped stone tools, although their brain was only about the size of a modern chimp's. Judging by how they bashed in the skulls of the animals they ate, they were right-handed.

Both sensory input from the hand to the brain and motor control of the hand from the brain are crossed—left hemisphere for right hand and vice versa. Why the left hemisphere should come to dominate for both handedness and speech is not clear, although one can make guesses. Handedness is involved in motor tasks and learning of motor skills. Speech itself is a very complex motor skill. If the left hemisphere is specialized for motor skills, including speech, then it makes sense to localize the comprehension of language to the same hemisphere. As we will see, there are two major speech areas on the left hemisphere: the "motor" speech area (Broca's area) and the "comprehension" speech area (Wernicke's area). The right hemisphere is more important than the left hemisphere for certain kinds of spatial functions, such as figuring out three-dimensional patterns, and for certain aspects of music, emotional behavior, and attention.

Although the speech areas are in the left hemisphere in the vast majority of humans, there are exceptions. The speech areas are in the right hemisphere in about 5% of right-handers and in about 30% of left-handers. Location of the speech areas becomes a key question when brain surgery is necessary. Damage to the speech areas can be devastating to the life of the patient; comparable damage to the other hemisphere is much less debilitating—typically an impairment in spatial abilities like map reading and finding one's way about, abilities that many of us are relatively deficient in anyway. A very simple test was developed by the neurologist Juhn Wada at the University of British Columbia to determine which hemisphere has speech. A barbiturate is injected in, say, the left carotid artery in the neck—this artery supplies blood to the left hemisphere. If speech is in the left hemisphere, it is lost in a few seconds. By the time the barbiturate circulates through the right hemisphere, it is diluted and has less effect. So if speech is in the right hemisphere, it is not lost immediately.

Cortical Speech Areas

Virtually all of the information scientists possess about the brain mechanisms of language has come from studies on unfortunate individuals who have suffered damage to the speech areas and have the condition known as *aphasia*, or difficulty in speaking and writing. In young children the effect of brain damage on language is dramatically different from the effect on adults. If the entire dominant hemisphere is destroyed, the child is completely aphasic but usually recovers over a period of months and ultimately develops almost normal language. No such dramatic recovery occurs in adults.

The final common path for speech begins at the lower face and mouth area of the primary motor cortex. This area sends its motor commands down the pyramidal tract to the motor neuron nuclei in the brain stem that control the movements of the larynx, tongue, and mouth (Figure 12-1; see also Chapter 9). Damage to this area causes muscular weaknesses and slurring of speech—it is hard to articulate sounds—but there is usually considerable recovery. There is no impairment in language comprehension, or in the ability to write if the motor hand area has been spared. The impairment is not in language but rather in articulating speech sounds because of lessened control over motor neurons.

The *supplementary motor area* (Figure 12-1) is an intriguing cortical region in humans and other primates. Electrical stimulation of it can produce complex movements, and it receives auditory and visual as well as somatic sensory input. Recent work indicates that it functions as a "supermotor" area. PET-scan studies (see Chapter 11) indicate that this area becomes more active when complex sequences of voluntary movements are made, such as counting aloud and sequences of finger movements. Even thinking about making finger movements causes it to light up, but internal speech does not. It is not a language area per se but is involved in the movements of speech. Removal of this area in the left hemisphere causes what is called global aphasia—complete loss of speech—but this loss is temporary, lasting only a few weeks. Recovery is virtually complete.

Broca's speech area lies in front of the motor cortex on the lateral part of the hemisphere (Figure 12-1). The basic problem with damage to Broca's area is in speaking—speech is non-fluent and not much speech is produced. Grammar is also impaired—the small parts of speech "to" and "the" are omitted, as are proper grammatical endings of words. However, there is no impairment of the ability to move the tongue as such. Broca's area damage is a speech impairment, and not just a motor impairment. It appears that key aspects of syntax may also be coded in Broca's area.

There is important evidence that comprehension of speech is also impaired by damage to Broca's area, particularly where meaning depends on syntax. Eric Warner gives a particularly clear example. Consider the following two sentences:

The apple that the boy is eating is crunchy.

The girl that the boy is chasing is tall.

In the first sentence, syntax is not needed to understand the meaning; boys eat apples but apples don't eat boys, and apples can be crunchy but boys are not. In the second sentence, either the girl or the boy could be chasing the other and either one could be tall. Only syntax gives us the information that the boy is chasing the girl and that the girl is tall. Patients with damage to Broca's area have no problem understanding sentences like the first one but have great difficulty understanding sentences like the second, where meaning depends critically on syntax.

Extensive damage to *Wernicke's area*, the posterior speech area, causes massive impairment in understanding and speaking language. Such patients can produce rapid, well-articulated sound and even proper phrases and sequences of words, but what they say is not language. The "speech" of such a person has the correct rhythm and general sound of normal speech but in fact conveys no information. These patients show essentially total failure to understand both spoken and written language, although basic hearing and vision are normal.

Norman Geschwind of Harvard University elaborated Carl Wernicke's earlier view of brain function in language in terms of the interconnections among the various sensory-receptive and association areas and the speech areas. Indeed, Geschwind has renamed the aphasias the *disconnection syndromes* to emphasize the importance of the connecting pathways. In brief, his view is as follows. Wernicke's area is the critical region for the conceptual formation and production of language. If a phrase is to be spoken, it originates in Wernicke's area, is transmitted by a fiber bundle called the *arcuate fasciculus* to Broca's area, where the correct sequence of articulations is aroused, and is then transmitted to the motor cortex to be spoken (Figure 12-2).

According to Geschwind, a word spoken by someone else projects from the primary auditory area (called *Heschl's gyrus* in humans) to Wernicke's area, where it is understood. If a written word is seen (Figure 12-2), it projects to the primary visual cortex (the striate cortex), then to a visual association area, then to a region called the *angular gyrus*, which is said to integrate visual and auditory information, and then to Wernicke's area to be understood. If a spoken word is to be spelled, information about the word travels from the auditory area to Wernicke's area, then to the angular gyrus, then back to Wernicke's area and on to Broca's area and the motor cortex. If a written word is to be spoken, it passes from the primary visual cortex to the visual association cortex and then on to the angular gyrus, to Wernicke's area, to Broca's area, and to the motor cortex. To further complicate the picture, auditory and visual information travels from one hemisphere to the other via the corpus callosum.

This rather complicated hypothesis about the brain mechanisms of speech was developed from a study of individuals showing very specific and selective disorders of speech and language function. A lesion limited to the arcuate fasciculus interconnecting Wernicke's area and Broca's area (Figure 12-2) produces what is called *conduction aphasia*. The individual has perfect comprehension of spoken and written language, but speech is severely abnormal and resembles that of individuals with damage to Wernicke's area, who speak fluently but make no sense. Repetition of spoken language is grossly impaired. Both Broca's and Wernicke's areas are normal, but Wernicke's no longer controls Broca's.

Many years ago the French neurologist Joseph Déjérine described a patient who had lost the ability to read and write but could understand spoken language and could speak. This disorder is called *alexia* (inability to read) with *agraphia* (inability to write). Autopsy revealed a lesion in the left angular

SPEAKING A HEARD WORD

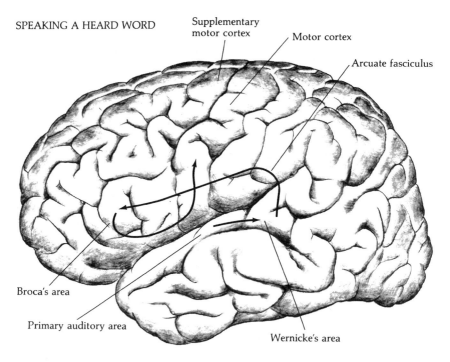

Supplementary motor cortex

Motor cortex

Arcuate fasciculus

Broca's area

Primary auditory area

Wernicke's area

SPEAKING A WRITTEN WORD

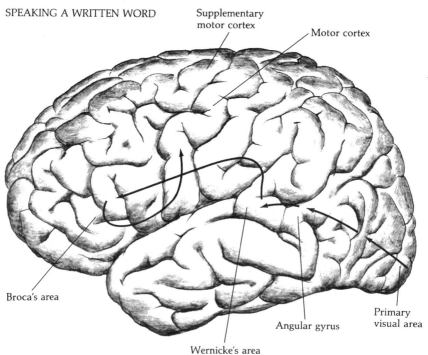

Supplementary motor cortex

Motor cortex

Broca's area

Wernicke's area

Angular gyrus

Primary visual area

Figure 12-2 *(Left)* The language areas of the brain and how they are thought to interact when a person speaks a heard word or a written word. Top: When a word is heard, the auditory sensation is received by the primary auditory cortex, but the word cannot be understood until the signal has been processed in Wernicke's area. If the word is to be spoken, some "representation" of it is transmitted from Wernicke's area to Broca's area through a bundle of nerve fibers called the arcuate fasciculus. In Broca's area, a "program" for articulation is activated and supplied to the face area of the motor cortex. The motor cortex in turn drives the muscles of the lips, the tongue, the larynx, and so on. Bottom: When a written word is read, the visual sensation is first registered by the primary visual cortex and then presumably relayed to the angular gyrus, where associations between the visual form of the word and the corresponding auditory pattern in Wernicke's area are thought to be formed. Speaking the word then draws on the same systems of neurons as speaking a heard word.

gyrus, the auditory–visual association area. The patient would have seen words and letters correctly but only as meaningless visual patterns, since the visual pattern must first be converted to the auditory form before the word can be understood. The auditory pattern of hearing a word must be transformed into the visual pattern before it can be spelled and rewritten. However, heard words could have been processed through the auditory cortex and Wernicke's area for understanding and thence to Broca's area for speech.

Another of Déjérine's patients awakened one morning to discover that he could not read. He was found to be blind in the right half of his visual field due to occlusion (blocking) of a cerebral artery, that is, a "stroke." The visual cortex of the left hemisphere was completely destroyed. This explains the halfblindness but not the inability to read. The patient could speak and comprehend spoken language. Vision in the right side of his visual field was normal. He could also write. Postmortem examination revealed that in addition to the destruction of the left visual cortex, the posterior region of the corpus callosum, which carries visual information between the hemispheres, was destroyed. Consequently, although visual information could get to the right visual cortex and association area, it could not cross to the left angular gyrus, the critical region for the integration of visual and auditory function, or to the left Wernicke's area (Figure 12-3).

The regions of cortex that control language function, particularly those in the posterior association cortex, Wernicke's area, and the angular gyrus, are indeed localized but relatively large. There are some hints in the literature that a fine-grained localization of language functions may exist, with different subregions of cortex involved in storing different aspects or categories of words. Elizabeth Warrington in London studied two dramatically illustrative

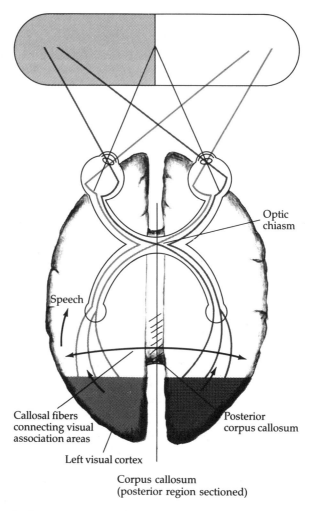

Figure 12-3 In Déjérine's patient who could not read but could speak and comprehend spoken language, the left primary visual cortex and the fibers of the posterior part of the corpus callosum interconnecting the visual association areas of the two hemispheres had been destroyed by a stroke.

cases. The patients had different areas of damage in the posterior speech regions but the exact extent of damage was not known. JBR was a young man who had suffered extensive brain damage as a result of encephalitis (brain infection). His aphasia was such that he was impaired in understanding and naming both abstract and concrete words. Within the category of concrete words, he was greatly impaired for names of living things and foods but not impaired for names of objects. VER was an elderly homemaker with severe aphasia following a major left-hemisphere stroke. She had almost complete loss of comprehension of words for objects, even common kitchen items of the utmost familiarity to her, but her performance on living things and foods was surprisingly good. These two patients showed complementary losses of certain categories of nouns.

George Ojemann of the University of Washington in Seattle has used the method of inactivating a small region of cerebral cortex by disruptive electrical stimulation in conscious patients undergoing brain surgery for the treatment of epilepsy. This transient disruption caused deficits in both comprehension and speech. The band of cortical tissue critically involved in language sweeps from Broca's area and the primary motor face area back around the Sylvian fissure to Wernicke's region. Disruption of Broca's area altered both mouth movements and identification of basic speech sounds (phonemes). Also, in the vicinity of Wernicke's area were regions where only naming or only reading was impaired and even sites that involved only syntax. Ojemann's results raise questions about the conventional views of Broca's and Wernicke's areas presented earlier. He found similar naming impairments with disruptive electrical stimulation in both areas. In Wernicke's area, he found several naming regions, but each is very small and localized—no more than 5 millimeters on a side. The existence and boundaries of Broca's and Wernicke's areas have been determined mostly from studying elderly patients who suffered brain damage from strokes. The organization, or perhaps the vulnerability, of the language areas may differ as a function of age. Ojemann's patients were relatively young. Another point to note is that Ojemann's patients all suffered from epilepsy—their brains were not normal.

Another finding by Ojemann was the existence of a separate area that was selective for short-term visual memory. This corresponded well to the region for short-term visual memory deduced from studies of brain-damaged patients by Warrington and Weiskrantz (see Figure 11-22).

Perhaps most striking are Ojemann's studies of people who are bilingual—people who can speak two languages fluently, for example, Greek and English. Stimulation in the central region of Broca's or Wernicke's area tended to disrupt language functions for both languages, but in some areas stimulation disrupted only Greek or only English (Figure 12-4). In short, different subregions of the language areas may be used when one learns a second language.

Another intriguing example of possible differential localization of language functions comes from studies of Japanese patients with brain injury. There are two forms of written Japanese, the picture-words (Kanji) derived from Chinese and a cursive alphabetic writing (Kana). It appears that brain damage can have differential effects on ability to read and write these two forms of writing. Depending on the region damaged, reading picture writing might be much more impaired than reading cursive writing, or vice versa.

Figure 12-4 Selective effects of stimulation inactivation of small regions of the cerebral cortex of the left hemisphere on ability to name objects in Greek (squares) and English (circles). Greek was the patient's second language. In this patient, inactivations were completely selective for language: sites that inactivated Greek did not inactivate ability to name objects in English, and vice versa.

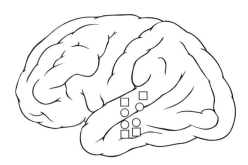

Imaging of Language in the Brain

The PET-scan method has added new complications to our understanding of brain substrates of language. Work by Michael Posner (now at the University of Oregon) and Marcus Raichle and associates at Washington University in St. Louis focused on words. They used the $H_2 15 O$ technique for measuring changes in regional blood flow and simply presented words or had subjects repeat words or associations with words for the 40-second recording period.

They used the *subtraction method* to reveal brain areas particularly involved in different aspects of language. Some explanation is in order about the subtraction method; it is an ingenious way of identifying regions of the brain that are particularly engaged in complex aspects of language function. To take a much simplified example, suppose we have divided the brain into a 2 x 2 spatial grid and use the PET-scan to determine increased activity in each of the four areas when subjects engage in language activities.

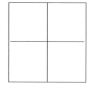

We wish to determine which of the four areas become active when the subject sees words, as opposed to simply seeing visual stimuli. We show the subject words on a screen and find that two squares in the grid image of the brain light up:

But in addition to seeing the words the subject is also seeing the screen (a form of visual stimuli). We now just show the subject the screen and find that only one square in the grid image of the brain lights up:

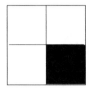

This is presumably the primary visual region of the cerebral cortex that will light up when any visual stimulation is given. We now subtract this image from the image we found when the subject looked at the screen with words, and obtain the following:

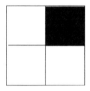

We conclude that this last image indicates the region of the brain that becomes selectively activated when people look at words, as opposed to simply looking at visual stimuli (i.e. the screen).

In sum, they had subjects look at a fixation point and subtracted this brain image from that when the subject was looking at words. Similarly, when the subject had to repeat the words aloud, the visual word-presentation images were subtracted. The same procedures were used with verbally presented words. Finally, in the semantic test the subjects had to respond with the most appropriate verb they associated with the presented nouns, for example, "cake"—"eat." The images for simple repeating of the nouns were subtracted from those for the associated spoken words.

Overall, the researchers found a number of regions of the cerebral cortex and cerebellar cortex to be activated in these tasks. When subjects simply looked at words, regions in the occipital cortex (visual areas) were activated, and when they simply heard words, auditory areas were active, as expected. When subjects had to repeat the words (mere presentation of words subtracted) a number of motor systems became active, including the primary and supplementary motor areas and the anterior cerebellum. In addition, a region in Broca's area was activated (Figure 12-5). The results held for both visual and auditory presentations of the words. Again, these results were not unexpected.

The most surprising results came from the semantic subtraction tasks. Here an area on the medial wall of the cerebral hemisphere, the *anterior*

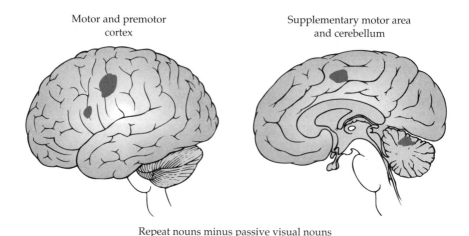

Motor and premotor cortex

Supplementary motor area and cerebellum

Repeat nouns minus passive visual nouns

Figure 12-5 Results of PET scan when subjects were repeating aloud nouns shown on a screen, subtracting presentations of the nouns without naming. The areas that were selectively activated by naming (dark areas) included the primary and supplementary motor areas, Broca's area, and the anterior cerebellum.

cingulate region, showed several foci of activity. This region is part of the prefrontal cortex. In addition there was a striking focus of activation in the right lateral cerebellum (Figure 12-6). Note that in this analysis, the images for the motor behavior itself, speaking the words, had been subtracted. The activation of frontal cortical and lateral cerebellar regions by the semantic task did not occur when the presented words were simply spoken. The implication is that hitherto unexpected regions of prefrontal cerebral cortex and lateral cerebellar cortex play a special role in semantics or meaning, the most complex aspect of language. These association regions of the cerebrum and cerebellum are the most recent to evolve and are much elaborated in the human brain.

Dyslexia and Stuttering

So far we have focused on the aphasias, the major deficits in language caused by extensive brain damage. Dyslexia is a much more common language disorder and can range from mild to severe. Dyslexic children have trouble learning to read and write. An unfortunate case of a dyslexic child who was killed in an accident and came to autopsy has been described. There was a clear abnormality in the pattern of arrangement of the neurons in a part of Wernicke's area. Although this is only one case, it raises the possibility that dyslexia may

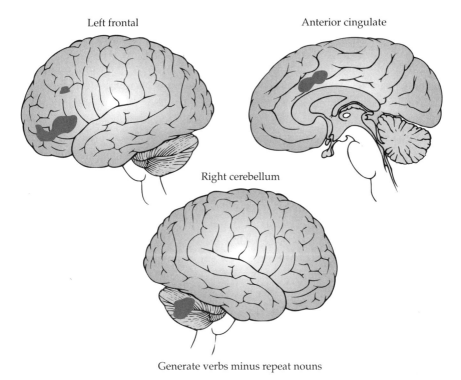

Generate verbs minus repeat nouns

Figure 12-6 PET scan when subjects had to respond with the most appropriate verbs when shown nouns. Images for just repeating the nouns (Figure 12-5) were subtracted. There were several foci of activation on the anterior cingulate gyrus (anterior medial wall of cerebral cortex—top right), the anterior lateral prefrontal cortex (top left), and the lateral cerebellar cortex (bottom). Note that these prefrontal and lateral cerebellar areas are the most recent regions of the brain to become elaborated in the evolution from apes to humans.

be due to brain abnormalities. Dyslexia is five times more common among boys than among girls, and males apparently have fewer fibers in the posterior part of the corpus callosum interconnecting the visual association areas of the two hemispheres. These pathways are essential for reading if there is also damage to one or the other visual cortex.

One final language difficulty worth noting is stuttering, which also occurs much more frequently in males than in females. We do not yet have any idea of possible brain abnormalities that may be involved. Folk wisdom says that stuttering results from forcing a left-handed child to be right-handed, but there are no real data on this possibility. An extensive study examined 2035 relatives of 397 unrelated stutterers. Results indicated clearly that it runs in families. It does not appear to be a single gene defect but may have significant heritability.

Connectionist Models of Language Acquisition

The field of neural networks burst on the scene in psychology and computer science just a few years ago and appears to be creating a revolution of sorts in our understanding of complex or cognitive processes in humans and other mammals. Neural networks are not real neural circuits but they have some similarities. The basic architecture of the artificial networks consists in nodes or neurons that connect to other nodes, much like a neuron synapses on another neuron (Figure 12-7). Each of these connections has a synaptic weight, ranging from 0 to 1 for excitatory connections and from 0 to -1 for inhibitory connections. These networks can learn; the synaptic weights can change with experience. In a typical network, the synaptic weights might initially be set at random between -0.5 and +0.5. Some kind of input is given to the network; the network processes the input and compares its output against the desired or correct output. The difference between the actual output and the correct output is the error. The "goal" of the network is to reduce this error to a negligible level over repeated trials. Some kind of error correcting-formula or algorithm is built into the network to accomplish this. The network is not real but rather is simulated on a computer (Figure 12-7). Actually, several neural networks have been built as complex transistor systems. A striking example is a transistor circuit model of the retina of the eye

Figure 12-7 Schematic illustrating a neural network. Arrows indicate excitatory connections and dots indicate inhibitory connections. This little network can account for many aspects of the perception of the Necker cube (as you look at the cube, it seems alternately to extend out from the page or into the page).

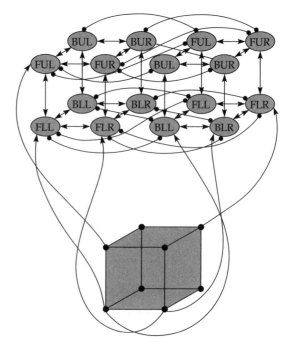

to detect motion, developed by Carver Meade at the California Institute of Technology.

Among the most interesting of the cognitive neural networks are those that have been developed to model the process of language acquisition. David Rumelhart and Jay McClelland, then at the University of California at San Diego, designed an initial network to learn the past tenses of verbs. The input to the network was simply verbs and their past tenses. The rules for forming past tenses were not put into the network; instead it had to learn these rules by example. The investigators fed verbs and their past tenses into the network in proportion to their frequency of usage in English. A key issue was how the network learned to form correct past tenses of regular and irregular verbs.

The astonishing result was that the network seemed to learn the past tenses of verbs much as young children do. It learned the general rules for forming regular past tenses before it had learned to form the past tenses of irregular verbs correctly. Thus, during the learning process it formed regular past tenses for irregular verbs, for example, "digged" rather than "dug." This result had profound implications for the nature of language. The network had no deep grammatical structure built into it. Rather, it formed the abstract rules for forming past tenses strictly from example; it learned the rules by "inference." If a simple neural network with a few hundred units can learn this way, so can the vastly complex human brain. Perhaps there is no deep language structure built into the brain.

Mark Seidenberg, now at the University of Southern California, and McClelland have elaborated this "past-tense" network into a much more general language acquisition network. This network generates learning outcomes in laboratory tasks, for example, responding quickly to frequently and infrequently used words, that correspond closely with the actual performance of people. Perhaps the most striking results occurred when Seidenberg and McClelland damaged the network by deleting some of the units. The network then performed just as though it had dyslexia!

A key current goal in artificial intelligence is to construct computer programs that can understand spoken language and respond (speak) appropriately. This goal has not yet been achieved but the Rumelhart–McClelland and Seidenberg–McClelland networks seem to indicate that it will someday be possible to have a meaningful conversation with a machine.

CONSCIOUSNESS

The nature of human consciousness or awareness has been among the most baffling of problems in philosophy and science. Each of us is convinced we have consciousness. However it cannot be measured directly but only from our descriptions of it. Except for language, it is not easy to infer consciousness from behavior; hence the many debates over the years about whether animals have consciousness. From an evolutionary perspective, it seems unlikely that only humans have consciousness; indeed this seems a most self-centered view. Evolution works in very small steps to change the physical characteristics of animals. Whatever consciousness is, we appear to have it in large measure, implying that it must have evolved gradually from small beginnings in simpler animals because it has adaptive advantages.

Consciousness is normally considered to be a part of the "mind." William James and many other psychologists have equated it more or less with short-term or working memory (see Figure 11-3). Your consciousness—what you are aware of at a given moment—is the content of your short-term or working memory. You are also of course aware of auditory, visual, and tactile sensations, particularly those you are attending to. Your awareness involves thinking about something or simply daydreaming, which includes implicit verbal processes (thinking in words) and images. Your awareness also extends back in time; you are aware of events that just happened and vaguely aware of experiences that occurred earlier. You are also aware to some degree of some aspects of experiences and knowledge that are more remote and are stored in long-term or permanent memory. Awareness includes the immediate situation, working memory, and some representations from long-term memory. Perhaps the most remarkable aspect of consciousness is its unitary and integrated character. Robert Doty at the University of Rochester expressed it well: "The digital discharges of widely dispersed neurons create the grainless panorama of three-dimensional colored space that the normal seeing eye conveys to the brain. (Doty, R. W. (1990). In John, E. R. (Ed.) *Machinery of the mind*. Boston: Birkhauser, pp. 3–13.)" But the mind includes much more than consciousness, namely, the vast repository of knowledge, experience, and skills stored in long-term memory that you are not aware of at any given moment but that can be called back into awareness from the "unconscious" mind.

Consciousness and the Cerebral Cortex

Evidence continues to grow that the essential neuronal substrate of consciousness is the cerebral cortex, together, of course, with its input and output connections to other brain structures. A striking example of this is blindsight, studied in detail by Larry Weiszkrantz of Oxford University. People whose primary visual areas of the cerebral cortex have been completely destroyed are completely blind, so far as they are aware. They have no conscious experience of any visual stimuli. If you were to present a spot of light to such a patient at various locations in the visual field and ask the patient to point to it, the response would be "What spot of light? I don't see anything." If you persist and tell the patient to point anywhere, the patient will point accurately to the light, wherever it may be, still denying any awareness of it. Such patients also avoid objects—walking through a room they walk around chairs and other objects, all the while insisting that they can't see anything. Clearly, some parts of the visual system are still functioning. From a behavioral point of view these patients can still "see" locations of objects. But they are completely unaware of it. So the visual areas of the cerebral cortex are essential for the awareness of seeing.

Thus, awareness of sensory stimuli requires the sensory areas of the cerebral cortex. Other aspects of consciousness also seem to have representations in the cerebral cortex. Damage to particular regions in the human cerebral cortex impair short-term visual or auditory memory, as we saw in Chapter 11 (Figure 11-22). HM provides another kind of example. He has normal short-term memory and relatively normal consciousness or awareness. Indeed, his cerebral cortex is mostly intact. However, his awareness is truncated in the past because his experiences are not stored in long-term memory. Recall how he described his own awareness—as though he had just awakened from a dream he could not remember.

Consciousness and the Split Brain

The most remarkable studies on brain substrates of human consciousness have been those of Roger Sperry and Michael Gazzaniga at the California Institute of Technology (Gazzaniga is now at the University of California, Davis). Sperry received a Nobel Prize in 1981. Certain patients suffer from a form of epilepsy that involves abnormal electrical activity on one side of the brain that spreads to the other side via the corpus callosum connecting the two hemispheres, producing severe seizures. In Figure 12-8, we are looking down on the top of the brain, the front of which is facing the top of the page. The two hemispheres have been separated to show the corpus callosum, a structure consisting of many millions of nerve fibers, each crossing from one hemisphere to the other. This massive transverse band of fibers extends perhaps half the length of the brain from front to back, interconnecting corresponding association regions of the cerebral cortex of the two hemispheres. Neurosurgeons found that they could help some epilepsy patients greatly by severing the nerve fibers of the corpus callosum.

The most surprising thing about this drastic surgical intervention in the human brain is that at first glance it seems to have no deleterious effects on the patients. Indeed, when the operation succeeds in abolishing the epileptic seizures, the patients are much improved. They show no loss of intelligence and none of the typical signs of brain damage, in spite of the fact that the two cerebral hemispheres have been disconnected.

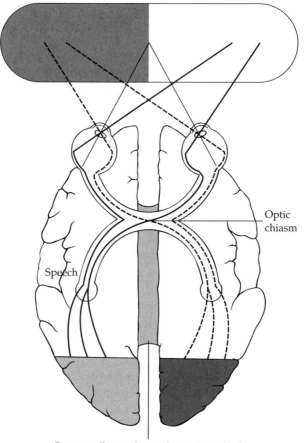

Optic
chiasm

Speech

Corpus callosum (cut in Sperry's studies)

Figure 12-8 Visual input to the left and right cerebral cortex in humans. The left half of each visual field (right half of each retina) projects to the right visual cortex, and vice versa. Visual association areas of the two hemispheres are interconnected through the corpus collosum. In Sperry's patients, the corpus collosum was sectioned.

Sperry's work on the split brain actually began some years ago in studies on animals with his student Ronald Myers. Sperry and Myers sectioned the corpus callosum in cats and monkeys and also cut the optic chiasm so that the left eye projected only to the left visual cortex and the right eye only to the right side (Figure 12-9). One eye could be covered and the open eye would communicate only with the hemisphere on its side of the brain. Suppose the animal was trained on a visual discrimination, say pressing a lever for food when horizontal stripes appeared, but not vertical stripes. If the animal was trained using only the right eye and right hemisphere of the brain, it had to

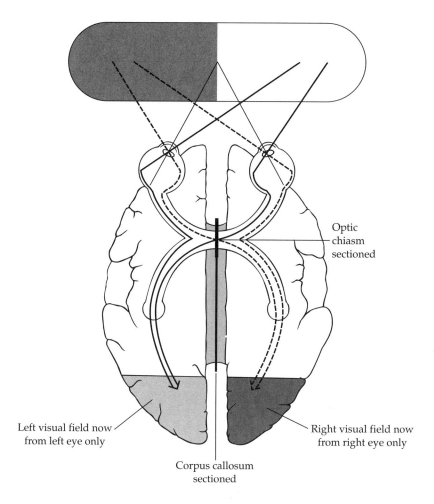

Optic
chiasm
sectioned

Left visual field now
from left eye only

Right visual field now
from right eye only

Corpus callosum
sectioned

Figure 12-9 In Sperry's studies on cats and monkeys, both the corpus callosum and the optic chiasm were sectioned so that the left eye went only to the left hemisphere and the right eye only to the right hemisphere (compare with Figure 12-8). He could then train the left and right hemispheres completely separately by covering the right or left eye.

learn all over again using only the left eye and left hemisphere. Interestingly, the two hemispheres within the same animal learned at essentially identical rates, whereas hemispheres from two different animals typically learned at different rates. If the optic chiasm was cut but the corpus callosum was left intact, the animal that had learned with one eye remembered perfectly when shifted to the other eye. Normally, the corpus callosum transfers the essential information and memories between the two hemispheres. When the callosum is cut, the two hemispheres can no longer transfer information back and forth.

Fear-conditioned responses like heart rate to a visual conditioned stimulus do transfer from one side of the brain to the other when the callosum and chiasm have been cut. It seems that basic "visceral" information can cross in lower pathways in the brain. However, more specific kinds of information, as in visual discrimination learning, do not.

In humans with a sectioned corpus callosum it is easy to access just the right or just the left hemisphere. (1) The left half of each eye projects to the left visual cortex and vice versa (Figure 12-8). By presenting information only to the left half of each eye (which is the right half of the visual field since the lens reverses images), information is projected only to the left hemisphere. (2) Somatic sensory input from the hands and motor control of the hands is crossed, left hand to right hemisphere and vice versa. The right hemisphere can receive tactile (touch) information from the left hand and control and communicate with the left hand, and the same for the left hemisphere and right hand. The output from each of the two hemispheres can be evaluated by measuring the actions of the hands in the absence of visual information—for example, by testing each hand behind a screen that blocks the patient's view of them (Figure 12-10). (3) The auditory system is bilateral—both hemispheres receive spoken information from each ear.

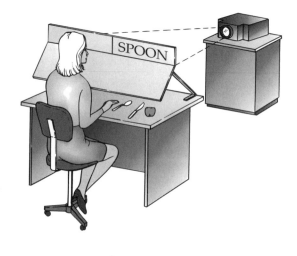

Figure 12-10 Experimental situation used to evaluate output from the two hemispheres in humans with the corpus callosum sectioned. When the subject's gaze is fixed on a dot marking the center of the visual field, the examiner flashes a word or a picture of an object on a translucent screen to either side of the fixation dot. As shown, the information projects to left hemisphere. Either a verbal (reading the flashed word) or a nonverbal (selecting the object named among the many objects on the table) response may be required. The objects are screened from the patient's view and can be identified only by touch.

The experimental test situation is shown in Figure 12-10. The patient (all patients were right-handed, and the speech area was in the left hemisphere) looked at a fixation point, and visual information—words, drawings, pictures—were flashed briefly to the left or right cerebral cortex. The patient could respond verbally or with movements of either hand behind the screen. Remember, the corpus callosum had been severed in these patients.

The first of the human split-brain studies began when Gazzaniga joined Sperry as a graduate student at Cal Tech. A neurosurgeon, Joseph Bogen, began a series of callosum sections on severely epileptic patients and the three collaborated, beginning with the first patient, WJ. The operation itself was a great success. The basic findings were seen quite clearly in WJ. Before the operation he integrated information between the two hemispheres freely in all modalities as do all normal humans. After the operation, WJ had two separate minds or mental systems, each with its own abilities and capacities to learn, remember, and experience emotion and behavior. As Gazzaniga put it: "WJ lives happily in Downey, California, with no sense of the enormity of the findings or for that matter any awareness that he had changed."

Let us consider the results more specifically. If a word was flashed to the left hemisphere, the patient could immediately say it and write it with his right hand. He appeared to be functioning normally. In marked contrast, if the word was flashed to the right hemisphere, the patient could neither say nor write it. In spite of this, it soon become apparent that the right hemisphere was quite capable of recognizing objects. The trick was to find a way for it to tell the experimenter. If, when a picture of a fork was flashed to the right hemisphere, the left hand was allowed to feel many different objects behind the screen, including a fork, it would immediately select the fork and hold it up. The right hemisphere was nonverbal but not incompetent. Having correctly identified the fork, the patient still could not say what it was. However, if the right hand was allowed to take the fork from the left hand, the patient immediately said "fork."

Actually, the right hemisphere did show some limited verbal comprehension. If simple words rather than pictures of objects were flashed to it, the patient could often identify the object by touching it with his left hand. Similarly, if an object like a pencil was placed in his left hand behind the screen, and a series of words, including "pencil," was flashed to the right hemisphere, the patient could correctly signal with his left hand the word "pencil." However, he still could not say the word. Compared to the left hemisphere, the right hemisphere was distinctly superior in spatial tasks such as arranging blocks or drawing a cube in three dimensions. Examples of drawings of simple designs made separately by each hand show this strikingly (Figure 12-11). In each case the picture was presented only to the appropriate hemisphere (right hemisphere for left hand and vice versa). The left-hand drawings are clearly superior, even though all the patients were right-handed.

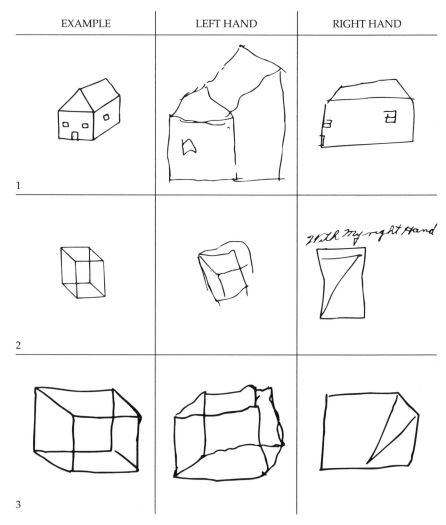

EXAMPLE	LEFT HAND	RIGHT HAND

1

2

3

Figure 12-11 Drawings made by three split-brained patients using the right hand and the left hand. The left-hand drawings are clearly superior to the right-hand ones for all three patients (who were all right-handed). These drawings illustrate the superiority of the right hemisphere in spatial or visual-constructional tasks.

Finally, emotional perception and responsiveness were handled quite well, although nonverbally, by the right hemisphere. Gazzaniga described an example of flashing a picture of a nude woman amidst a series of ordinary pictures to the left or right hemisphere of a female patient. When the picture was shown to the left hemisphere, the patient laughed and identified the picture. When it was shown to her right hemisphere she said she saw nothing but she laughed. When asked why she laughed, she said she did not know— "Oh, that funny machine."

One patient sometimes found his two hemispheres in conflict. One time, he found his left hand (nonverbal right hemisphere) struggling against his right hand when trying to put on his pants in the morning. As the right hand pulled them up, the left hand pulled them down. On another occasion, he was angry with his wife and his left hand grabbed at her but his right hand gripped the left in an attempt to hold it away.

Gazzaniga later studied one rather unusual split-brain patient who had good verbal ability in each hemisphere. The patient, Paul S., suffered early damage to the left hemisphere, and the right hemisphere developed considerable language comprehension. The left hemisphere apparently recovered its language function as well. After the split-brain operation, each hemisphere was quite verbal and could be communicated with separately using visual presentations to the left or right visual field. Although Paul's right hemisphere could understand, it could not speak; only the left hemisphere controlled his speech, but the right hemisphere could communicate in language by writing with Paul's left hand.

It started when Paul awoke from surgery. He was immediately able to understand many kinds of language in his right hemisphere. This ability was most unusual; all other patients had been able to comprehend language only with their dominant left hemisphere. Only patients LB and NG in the California series had shown evidence of right-hemisphere language, and then only some time after the operation. Moreover, Paul's language was a richer kind. His right hemisphere could not only understand the meaning of nouns (a skill the California patients had finally achieved), but he could also carry out verbal commands presented exclusively to his mute right half-brain. Even more startling was Paul's ability to write answers to questions asked of the right half-brain. Instead of wondering whether or not Paul's right hemisphere was sufficiently powerful to be dubbed conscious we were now in a position to ask Paul's right side about its view on matters of friendship, love, hate, and aspirations. "Who are you?" He writes: "Paul." "Where are you?" He writes: "Vermont." "What do you want to be?" He writes: "Automobile racer." When the left hemisphere was asked this same question, he wrote (with his right hand), "Draftsman."

When Paul first demonstrated this skill, my student, Joseph LeDoux, and I were in the middle of Vermont in our compact DelRey camping trailer that we had converted to a testing laboratory. Joseph and I just stared at each other for what seemed an eternity. A half-brain had told us about its own feelings and opinions, and the other half-brain, the talkative left, temporarily put aside its dominant ways and watched its silent partner express its views. I quickly grabbed the movie camera and we proceeded with more questions. Paul's right side told us about its favorite TV star, girlfriend, food, and other preferences. After each question, which Joseph and I had carefully lateralized to the right hemisphere through our testing techniques, we asked Paul what the question was. He (that is the left brain) shot back, "I didn't see anything." Then his left hand, which gains its major control from the right hemisphere, would pick up a pencil and proceed to write out the answer to our question. Paul is indeed unique. (Gazzaniga, M. S., Split-brain research: A personal history. *Cornell University Medical College Alumni Quarterly, 45,* 8–9, 1982.)

In sum, the right hemisphere is not simply inferior, it is different. The right hemisphere seems to have become specialized for spatial and synthetic tasks (and music) and the left for verbal, analytic, and sequential tasks, as we noted earlier in the context of hemispheric asymmetries. These hemispheric specializations are seen dramatically in patients with section of the corpus callosum. In the rest of us, where the two hemispheres of course function smoothly and normally together, it is also possible to detect these specializations. Joseph Hellige, at the University of Southern California, has demonstrated this in a number of test situations. If words or spatial objects are flashed to the right or left hemisphere, the subject responds more rapidly (faster reaction time) to words given to the left hemisphere and to objects given to the right hemisphere. The interested reader is urged to consult Hellige's recent book on the subject (see Suggested Readings).

Probing the Brain for Consciousness

A significant increase in our understanding of the nature of consciousness has come from some remarkable experiments by Benjamin Libet at the University of California, San Francisco. He worked with human patients who were undergoing neurosurgery (often done with local anesthetics, so the patients are conscious) or with patients who had stimulating electrodes permanently implanted in the somatic sensory thalamus (ventrobasal complex—see Chapter 8) to control otherwise intractable pain. Libet electrically stimulated the primary somatic sensory area of the cerebral cortex or the ventrobasal complex in the thalamus that projects to it. Both procedures produce activation of the somatic sensory cortex and the results were the same for both, so I will group them together in describing his experiments.

Libet used a stimulus train—repeated electrical pulses at various frequencies—to elicit sensations. If the cortical electrode was over the right thumb representation, the patient would report a tingling sensation in the thumb (this is how the body representation on the human somatosensory cortex was first mapped—see Figure 8-13). The minimum intensity of the electrical pulses necessary to just elicit a sensation was determined. At this intensity the duration of the stimulus train necessary to evoke sensation was about 0.5 seconds over a wide range of stimulus frequencies (15 per second to 120 per second). Single electrical pulses could not be detected; the pulses had to be repeated at a rate of at least 15 per second. So far, no surprises: neural activity in the cerebral cortex has to be recruited by repeated stimulation in order for a sensation to occur. We can easily detect a single electrical pulse to the skin because this results in repetitive activity in the neurons of the somatic sensory system projecting to the cerebral cortex. Again, no surprises.

But now comes an astonishing result (see Figure 12-12). When a single pulse is given to the skin, it takes 0.5 seconds for necessary activation of the sensory cortex to yield the sensation, but the subject refers the time of onset of the stimulus to the finger *backward* in time to about the time of its actual occurrence. Libet determined this by having the subject watch a fast real-time clock. After each trial the subject indicated when in real time the stimulus was delivered. Also shown in the figure is the field potential recorded from the

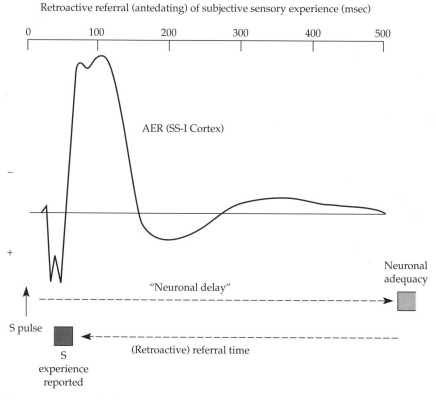

Retroactive referral (antedating) of subjective sensory experience (msec)

Figure 12-12 Comparison of reaction times and the averaged evoked response (AER) recorded from the cerebral cortex of area somatic sensory I to a very weak shock to the hand in awake human subjects. The AER is a field potential and presents the averaged activity of many thousands of neurons in the somatic sensory cortex. The initial sharp downward-going (+) AER at about 40 milliseconds represents the arrival of information about the shock to the hand region of somatic sensory cortex. The subject does not become "aware" of the stimulus until about 500 milliseconds after the weak shock. However, the subject refers the time of occurrence of the shock backward in time to the occurrence of the initial AER response at about 40 milliseconds after the shock. Sound confusing? See corresponding text.

scalp overlying the activated region of cortex (called an *averaged evoked response—AER*). Field potentials are generated by the coordinated activity of many thousands of neurons. The subject referred the occurrence of the stimulus back to the time of occurrence of the primary component of the AER that is generated very locally in somatic sensory cortex. But the actual time of onset of the sensation occurred half a second later, during the later afterpotentials of the AER that are believed to be generated over wide regions of the cerebral cortex.

Another question Libet addressed was whether subjects could behaviorally detect electrical stimulus trains to the sensory thalamus that were too short to be detected consciously. Sound confusing? His experiment was very simple. He used a stimulus train duration of about 0.3 seconds, which the subjects never reported feeling. A light was turned on and off twice in a row and the brain stimulus was given randomly during either the first or the second presentation of the light. The subject was simply required to choose either light on each trial and also to report whether or not any sensation was felt. Subjects chose the "correct" light well above chance, even though they did not report feeling any sensation. This result should remind you of the phenomenon of blind sight we noted earlier. Actually this result is not too surprising. I served as subject in absolute auditory threshold studies when I was a graduate student. When the sound was about at threshold intensity I was convinced I was just guessing on each trial whether or not the sound occurred. I could not "hear" it. But my performance was better than chance. The bottom line is that conscious awareness is not necessary for behavioral detection of stimuli.

CONCLUSION

In his Nobel address, Sperry argued forcefully that consciousness must be viewed as having an "integral causal control role in brain function and behavior." For many years, the behaviorist movement in psychology excluded consciousness from consideration as a part of psychology. The work of Sperry and many others who study brain function and behavior has changed that. In Sperry's words: "The mental forces of the conscious mind are restored in the brain of objective science from which they had long been excluded on materialist–behaviorist principles." But it is still true that the only way we can study consciousness is to measure behavior, verbal or otherwise, and *infer* consciousness. It cannot be measured directly.

Our own experience has always told us that much of our own behavior is the result of the operations and actions of our conscious mind. Indeed, surprises come only when we seem to behave for reasons not clear to our conscious mind—as in Freudian "unconscious" motives. Consciousness is an extraordinary system that serves to unify our sense impressions into a cohesive, ongoing experience of the world and combines this with our memories and knowledge to organize and direct our behavior.

There is every reasons to suppose that evolution has selected for consciousness. It is an extremely efficient and unitary way of running the very complicated machine that is our body and brain. This implies that humans are not the only conscious animals, as we noted earlier. Evidence points to the cerebral cortex as the neural substrate of consciousness. Perhaps the extraordinary expansion of the evolving human cerebral cortex over the past three million years occurred because it resulted in an increasing degree and depth of consciousness, which provided the competitive edge for the human race in the struggle for survival.

The nature, meaning, and "reality" of consciousness or awareness are questions that have been endlessly debated. Most scientists prefer to sidestep these large questions and treat consciousness as a product of the evolution of the brain. A questionnaire sent to many neuroscientists asked them to rank animals in terms of degree of consciousness. The results were just what might be expected: primates and possibly sea mammals ranked highest, then carnivores, then rodents, and so on. Serious doubt was expressed concerning the consciousness of flies and worms. The result of the questionnaire is of course merely opinion but here opinion corresponds rather closely with the evolution of the forebrain and cerebral cortex.

SUMMARY

Speech is the one species-typical behavior that sets the human species apart from all other animals. It would appear that speaking and understanding spoken language evolved apace with the evolution of *Homo sapiens*. Every child learns his or her native language seemingly without effort. From ages 2 to 8, the average child learns language at the astonishing rate of eight new words a day.

Natural language is speech; reading and writing are recently developed and unnatural skills. The brain evolved to its fully modern form long before writing was developed. The most elementary unit of speech is the phoneme, the smallest speech sound. Phonemes are combined into morphemes, the most elementary unit of meaning, usually words. The rules governing the sequence of words in a sentence are syntax, and the ways in which language conveys meaning is semantics.

Monkeys have developed impressive learned communication systems and apes can be taught sign and symbol languages. However, it is not yet clear whether "talking apes" exhibit syntax and "deep" grammatical structure, key properties of human language.

In most humans, the left hemisphere is specialized for language—structural differences are clear—and the left hemisphere "speech" area is larger than the corresponding area in the right hemisphere. An oversimplified view of the speech areas is that the posterior or Wernicke's area handles semantics and the anterior of Broca's area handles syntax. Damage to Wernicke's area results in fluent but meaningless speech and to Broca's area in abbreviated and ungrammatical but meaningful speech. Traditionally, Wernicke's area damage severely impairs speech understanding and damage to Broca's area does not; however Broca's area damage does impair understanding where syntax, the grammatical structure of a sentence, conveys meaning. Geschwind developed a theory of the organization of the language areas and their dysfunctions, termed the disconnection syndromes, that accounts for a wide range of impairments in, for example, reading, writing, understanding spoken speech. Recent work suggests that a number of localized areas in the cerebral cortex may have specialized functions in language, as in the patient whose cortical representations for English and Greek were differently localized. Imaging studies indicate that a number of localized brain regions become activated in semantic verbal tasks, including areas in the prefrontal cortex and in the lateral cerebellum. Finally, connectionist computational models of language acquisition have been developed that appear to display grammatical deep structure and exhibit typical symptoms of aphasia (Wernicke's area syndrome) when damaged.

Consciousness can be equated roughly with short-term and working memory—what a person is aware of at a given time. The cerebral cortex appears to be the essential substrate for consciousness. Complete destruction of the visual areas of the cortex (VI) results in blindsight; patients are completely unaware of any visual experience, yet they can localize objects in space even though they insist they cannot.

The classic studies of split-brain humans by Sperry, Gazzaniga, and others indicate that after section of the corpus callosum, the great band of nerve fibers that connect the two hemispheres, the two hemispheres appear to have separate "consciousness." The left hemisphere (the patients were right-handed) could verbally identify seen objects normally. The right hemisphere could identify objects in pictures by touch (with the left hand, projecting to the right hemisphere) but could not name them. A case was described where both disconnected hemispheres had verbal ability and the two hemispheres had different "personalities."

In studies employing electrical stimulation of the somatic sensory cortex, it was found that a threshold-level stimulus must be repeatedly given (over a wide range of frequencies) for about 0.5 seconds for the person to become consciously aware of it. Yet the person refers the experience backward in time to the actual onset of the stimulus.

It seems very likely that whatever consciousness is, humans have it in large measure and it is highly adaptive. Given this, it must follow that infrahuman animals also possess consciousness to varying degrees. It may be that the degree or complexity of consciousness in animals is proportional to the degree of elaboration of the cerebral cortex.

SUGGESTED READING AND REFERENCES

Books

Caplan, D. (1987). *Neurolinguistics and linguistic aphasiology.* Cambridge, MA: Cambridge University Press.

Churchland, P. S., and Sejnowski, T. J. (1992). *The computational brain*. Cambridge, MA: MIT Press.

Geschwind, N., and Galaburda, A. M. (1987). *Cerebral lateralization: Biological mechanisms, associations, and pathology*. Cambridge, MA: MIT Press.

Griffin, D. R. (1981). *The question of animal awareness: Evolutionary continuity of mental experience*. Los Altos, CA: William Kaufmann.

Hellige, J. (1993). *Hemispheric asymmetry: What's right and what's left?* Cambridge, MA: Harvard University Press.

Kolb, B., and Whishaw, I. Q. (1990). *Fundamentals of human neuropsychology* (3rd ed.). New York: W. H. Freeman.

Loftus, E. F., and Loftus, G. R. (1983). *Human memory*. Hillsdale, NJ: Erlbaum.

Olton, D. S., and Kesner, R. P. (1986). *Neurobiology of comparative cognition*. Hillsdale, NJ: Erlbaum.

Plum, F. (1988). *Language, communication, and the brain*. New York: Raven Press.

Popper, K. R., and Eccles, J. C. (1985). *The self and its brain*. New York: Springer-Verlag.

Posner, M. I. (1989). *Foundations of cognitive science*. Cambridge, MA: MIT Press.

Rumelhart, D. E., McClelland, J. L., and PDP Research Group. (1986). *Parallel distributed processing: Explorations in the microstructure of cognition*. Cambridge, MA: MIT Press.

Springer, S. P., and Deutsch, G. (1989). *Left brain, right brain* (3rd ed.). New York: W. H. Freeman.

Articles

Libet, B. (1989). Conscious subjective experience vs. unconscious mental functions: A theory of the cerebral processes involved. In Cotterill. R. M. J. (Ed.), *Models of brain function*. Cambridge: Cambridge University Press.

Mountcastle, V. B. (1986). The neural mechanisms of cognitive functions can now be studied directly. *Trends in Neuroscience, 9*, 505–508.

Petersen, S. E., and Fiez, J. A. (1993). The processing of single words studied with positron emission tomography. *Annual Review of Neuroscience*. In press.

Posner, M. I., Petersen, S. E., Fox, P. T., and Raichle, M. E. (1988). Localization of cognitive operations in the human brain. *Science, 240*, 1627–1631.

Seidenberg, M. S., and McClelland, J. L. (1989). A distributed, developmental model of word recognition and naming. *Psychological Review, 96*, 523–568.

Wanner, E. (1988). Language. In Lindzey, G., Thompson, R. F., and Spring, B. *Psychology*. New York: Worth, pp. 252–275.

Epilogue

It is perhaps appropriate in this Decade of the Brain to look into a crystal ball and try to discern the shape of things to come in the future of the brain sciences. While we have learned a great deal about neuron and brain, a perusal of this book makes very clear that much more is to be learned. We do not yet have answers to the "big" questions: What causes schizophrenia, Alzheimer's disease, drug addiction, neuroses, and most other brain disorders, and how can we cure them? How does the brain code and store memories? How is it that we see and perceive a seamless world? How is language coded in the brain? What is consciousness and how does it arise from the brain? It seems unlikely that satisfactory answers to these broad questions will be found in the next decade. But they will someday be found.

Molecular biology will increasingly dominate study of the basic processes of the neuron. Virtually everything a neuron does depends ultimately on the activity of genes in making more, fewer, or different proteins. Our knowledge of neuron-specific proteins and their genetic substrates is growing exponentially. We saw in Chapter 7 that different kinds of stress can induce a given neuron in the hypothalamus to alter gene expression and synthesis of different amounts and kinds of peptide hormones and neurotransmitters, exerting different actions on its target neurons. Our understanding of the molecular mechanisms of this "switching" process will advance rapidly. But the question of how this switching is induced, for example, by seeing a bear in the woods, will be much harder to answer. It is in this regard that the brain and liver differ. Both are made up of very similar cells with the same DNA. But from a functional point of view, if you have seen one liver cell, you have seen them all. The point is not that there are different types of nerve cells. Rather, it is the ways the nerve cells connect together and function to transmit and process information that determine which peptides the hypothalamic neuron will make. The patterns of connectivity and interactions among the neurons are what makes the brain unique. Analyses at the level of gene expressions per se can never tell us how seeing a bear leads to changes in gene expression in neurons in the hypothalamus.

Understanding of the biochemical mechanisms of hormone and neurotransmitter actions is increasing rapidly. The structures of virtually all hormones have been determined and their genes sequenced. In the next decade or so it is likely that the structures of most hormone and neurotransmitter receptors will be determined and their genes sequenced. This is among the most intensely active areas of research in neuroscience. We are also rapidly gaining an understanding of the "readout," the neural circuitry, from hypothalamus to the autonomic and somatic motor systems that result in organisms drinking and eating after being deprived of water and food. But I quoted Alan Epstein at the beginning of Chapter 7 to the effect that the primary reason higher animals drink and eat is because they *feel* thirsty and hungry. We have virtually no understanding of the neural substrates of these feelings at present except for their final actions on the hypothalamus. The neural basis of such feelings must involve activity in enormously complex neural circuitry.

Study of the brain substrates of learning and memory is at a most exciting stage. We are rapidly gaining an appreciation of the neural circuits and pathways that form the essential substrates for different forms of learning and memory. On the other hand, analysis of the basic mechanisms of synaptic plasticity, LTP and LTD, is proceeding rapidly. But these two approaches have yet to meet. At present LTP and LTD are mechanisms in search of phenomena and the various forms of learning and memory are phenomena in search of mechanisms. It is our fervent hope that the two will meet. The fundamental problem posed by Karl Lashley in 1929 remains: in order to analyze mechanisms of memory storage it is first necessary to localize the sites of storage in the brain. This is now close to being accomplished for simpler forms of learning: classical conditioning of fear (amygdala) and discrete behavioral responses (cerebellum). Only when this has been done can we build a tight causal chain from, for example, LTP in the amygdala or LTD in the cerebellum to the behavioral expression of memory. The problem is more severe in the hippocampus, a structure that prominently displays LTP and is clearly necessary for declarative/experiential storage (and/or retrieval) in humans and seemingly in other primates as well. Virtually nothing is known about the readout, the neural circuitry, from hippocampus to behavioral expression of memory.

To return to molecular biology, the bases of LTP, LTD, and other aspects of synaptic plasticity are likely to be understood in detail at the biochemical, structural, and genetic levels in the next decade or so. Assume for the moment that LTP and LTD are the mechanisms of memory storage in the mammalian brain. Having achieved all this, will we understand memory storage in the brain? The answer is clearly no. All LTP and LTD do is to increase or decrease transmission of information at the synapses where they occur. The nature of the memories so coded are determined entirely by the particular complex neural circuits in the brain that form the memories. Molecular–genetic analysis can someday tell us the nature of the *mechanisms* of memory storage and perhaps even the loci of storage, but it can never tell us *what* the memories are. Only a detailed characterization of the neural circuitries that code, store, and retrieve memories can do this.

Finally, current understanding of the more complex cognitive aspects of brain function—language, thought, and consciousness—is fragmentary. The new imaging techniques are telling us in increasing detail what regions of the brain become engaged in complex mental operations. Progress here will be rapid. But these processes are the product of the activity of the immensely complex circuitries of the brain. Understanding at this level of the neural networks will be slow to come. The relatively new field of mathematical–computational analysis of neural networks will be increasingly important. Even at our current level of understanding of neural circuitry essential for simple aspects of behavior, the circuits are far too complex to understand at a verbal–qualitative level. Only by constructing computational models of these circuits can we understand how they function at a quantitative level.

In sum, molecular analysis of neuron and synapse is proceeding rapidly. As all the genes in the human genome are sequenced, it is very possible that a wide range of brain disorders, particularly those that have a strong genetic component, will be understood, treated, and even cured. On the other hand, analysis of the immensely complex neural networks in the brain that subserve the wide range of behavioral phenomena from thirst to thought—all the important things the brain does—is slow going. There will be plenty of opportunities for employment in the study of the brain for many centuries to come.

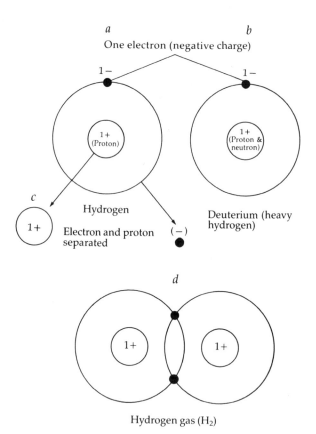

a   *b*
One electron (negative charge)

1−

1−

1+
(Proton)

1+
(Proton &
neutron)

c

Hydrogen

Deuterium (heavy
hydrogen)

1+

Electron and proton
separated

(−)

d

1+

1+

Hydrogen gas (H$_2$)

Appendix

A Tiny Bit of Chemistry, Physics, and Pharmacology

ATOMS AND MOLECULES

The world of modern physics is a strange and wondrous place. The nuclei of atoms are made up of quarks, with such properties as color, flavor, beauty, and charm. Both the quarks and the electrons that circle the nucleus have the properties of both particles and waves. But mastery of the esoteric field of particle physics is not necessary to understand something about atoms and electricity. An earlier model of the atom, the Bohr atom, is quite adequate for the purpose and much simpler. In this model the chemical elements are made up of atoms, and atoms consist of a nucleus made up of protons and neutrons and a circling "planetary" system of electrons. Each electron has a unit negative charge. Exactly what that means is not entirely clear, but the electron's charge is the smallest unit of negative charge that exists. A proton has a unit positive charge equal and opposite to the negative charge of the electron and also has considerable mass, whereas the electron has virtually no mass (actually, it has about one

Figure A-1 (a) An atom of ordinary hydrogen has a nucleus consisting of a proton and one electron that spins around it. (b) A much rarer form of hydrogen, heavy hydrogen or deuterium, has a neutron and a proton in its nucleus. (c) The electron and proton of hydrogen can be separated to form pure negative and positive charges. (d) In gaseous form, two hydrogen atoms share their electrons and form a covalent molecule, H_2. In this way each of the atoms acquires the full complement of two electrons in its shell.

thousand eight hundred thirty-sixth the mass of a proton). Neutrons have about the same mass as protons, but they have no charge: they are electrically neutral.

The common form of hydrogen, the simplest element, has just one proton in the nucleus and one electron "spinning" around it (Figure A-1). A rarer form of hydrogen, deuterium, has a proton and also a neutron in the nucleus, giving it a mass twice that of ordinary hydrogen (Figure A-1). If the hydrogen atom's electron is separated from its nucleus, the two entities represent a unit negative charge and a unit positive charge (Figure A-1). Electricity itself is simply the movement of electrons in a conducting medium such as metal or water. Good conductors have many electrons that are relatively free and so can move away from their atoms. When electricity is flowing in a wire, a given electron only travels a very short distance: it "bumps," or transfers its energy to, another electron, and a series of electron bumpings down the wire transfers the electric current. Because electrons have virtually no mass, electricity travels almost as fast as light, 186,000 miles per second (300,000 kilometers per second).

Atoms combine to form chemical molecules or compounds by sharing or exchanging electrons. The element hydrogen exists in nature as a gas made up of hydrogen molecules, each molecule consisting of two hydrogen atoms. A hydrogen molecule is formed when two hydrogen atoms each share their electron with the other atom, forming a complete first "shell" (Figure A-1). In the model of the atom we are using, atoms have successive shells of electrons. The first shell can hold only two electrons. Atoms have a strong tendency to complete their outermost shell, even if it means losing some electrons or gaining some that don't belong to them. In hydrogen gas, the atoms combine in pairs to share their electrons so that each of the two atoms constituting a hydrogen molecule has its full complement of two electrons. When electrons are fully shared by atoms, the combination is called a covalent compound.

The next two shells of electrons after the first shell each require eight electrons to be complete. In general, atoms that have all but one electron needed to fill the outermost shell, or have only one electron in the outermost shell, are the most reactive chemically. Hydrogen, with only one electron, is highly explosive; it was used with disastrous consequences in the German zeppelin the Hindenburg in 1937. Helium has two protons in its nucleus and a complete first shell of two electrons, and it is extremely unreactive; it will not explode and is used in present day blimps and dirigibles.

The carbon atom forms the basis of all organic molecules, the molecules that make up living organisms. It has just six protons in the nucleus (and six neutrons in the commonest form) and therefore six electrons (Figure A-2). The first shell is complete, with two electrons, but the outer shell is half full, with only four electrons. Thus carbon can share its four electrons with other elements very easily, but it does not readily give them up entirely or take away electrons from other atoms or molecules (Figure A-2). The covalent (electron-sharing) property of carbon is at the root of all life. Covalent compounds form stable molecular shapes. Carbon not only binds easily with other atoms and molecules but also forms such stable compounds that tend to keep their shape. This is a key aspect of living systems. For example, the genetic material in all cells, the DNA, must have a stable structure and a stable shape, since the information that directs the cell's entire repertoire of activities is encoded in the

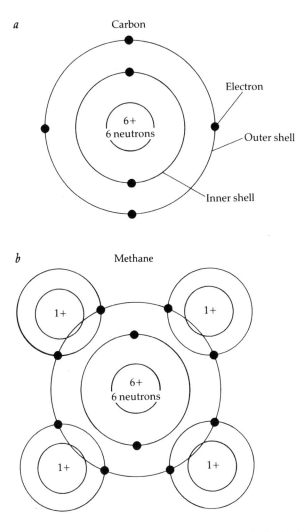

Figure A-2 The carbon atom has only four electrons in its outer shell, which requires eight to be complete, and so carbon shares electrons with other atoms to form covalent compounds (*a*). In methane gas, a carbon atom shares electrons with four hydrogen atoms, forming a covalent compound (*b*). In this way the carbon atom completes its outer shell by adding four electrons to it, and the hydrogens complete their shells by adding one electron each to them.

sequence of the nucleic acid building blocks that constitute the DNA molecule, and the shape of the entire molecule has much to do with the transmission of that information. If the nucleic acids changed places too easily or form one compound into another, or the entire DNA molecule changed too much in shape, the DNA could not transmit information accurately enough to keep the cell going.

IONS

Elements that are highly reactive do not share electrons, but rather give them up or take them and so form instead of molecules separate elemental atoms with electric charge; these are called ions. Table salt (sodium chloride) is a common example of an ionic compound. Each sodium and chloride ion exists as a separate ion, not as a sodium chloride molecule. Ionic compounds tend to form crystals, such as table salt crystals, because the ions form weak bonds with other ions. Ionic compounds are easily dissolved in water to form solutions of ions surrounded by water molecules. In general, atoms that form ions easily are either short one or two electrons in their outermost shell or have only one or two electrons in an outermost shell that requires, say, eight to be completed. Sodium, with a total of 11 electrons, has only one electron in its outer shell, which it gives up easily to form the sodium ion with a charge of +1: the sodium ion has one more positively charged proton in the nucleus than electrons circling it (Figure A-3). Chlorine gas needs 1 electron to complete its outermost shell, which needs eight electrons to be filled. It takes this electron up, becoming a chloride ion with a net charge of −1; it has one more electron than protons. Sodium is a highly toxic, explosive metal in its atomic form and chlorine gas a deadly poison. They are extremely reactive and so do not exist in the atomic form for very long outside the chemistry laboratory. These two poisons combine explosively as ions to form table salt, a very stable compound essential for life (Figure A-3).

Several ions are directly involved in the activities of the neuron: sodium, with a charge of +1 (Na^+), chloride, with a charge of −1 (Cl^-), potassium, with a charge of +1 (K^+), and calcium, with a charge of +2 (Ca^{2+}). Protein molecules in solution in the interior of the cell tend to acquire electrons and form negative ions, which accounts for the negative charge on the inside of the cell membrane relative to the zero charge of the tissue fluids outside them. The negative charge inside is maintained because these proteins are too large to pass through the cell membrane.

IONS AND ELECTRICITY: THE NERVE IMPULSE

When a nerve impulse occurs, channels in the cell membrane briefly open and ions, mostly sodium, move into the cell (see Chapter 2). Electricity is the movement of charged particles and ions have charge, so that during the nerve impulse electricity flows. One must be careful to distinguish between the movement of ions across the neuron membrane and the electricity that flows inside and outside the membrane when this occurs. When ions move across the cell membrane, this is a movement of positively charged particles, such as Na^+, K^+, or Ca^{2+}, or of negatively charged ones, such as Cl^-. But these ion movements, which generate electricity inside and outside the cell, are much slower than the speed of electricity itself, which is the movement of electrons.

The movement of the charged particles generates an electric field. The inside and outside of the neuron membrane are fluids that conduct electricity relatively well.

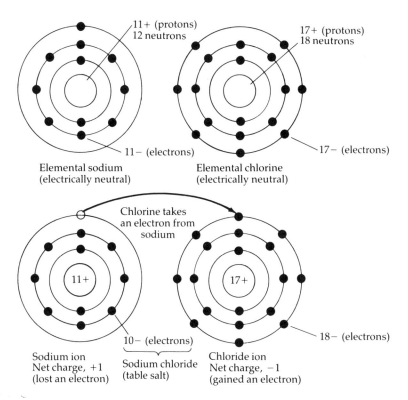

Figure A-3 Formation of ionic compounds. Atomic forms of sodium and chlorine (top drawing). Sodium has only one electron in its outermost shell and chlorine has seven. The shell needs eight electrons to be complete. Consequently, sodium and chlorine are highly reactive elements and combine explosively to form sodium chloride (table salt). In the process chlorine takes the outermost electron away from the sodium (bottom drawing). Chlorine is now an ion, chlor*ide*, with a net negative charge (−1) and sodium is an ion with a net positive charge (+1).

When positively charged ions move in, electrons try to move in (positive charge tries to move out) to complete the electrical circuit (Figure A-4). But the sodium ions are only moving in, and only when their gates are open. At this point in the action potential, ions cannot move out at all (actually there is a much smaller outward movement of potassium ions, as we saw in Chapter 2, but we can neglect that here).

The flow of electricity (movement of electrons) occurs at close to the speed of light, as we noted. The membrane of a nerve fiber, however, has a relatively high degree of resistance to the flow of electricity, and so not many electrons get through it. The transatlantic telephone cable works in much the same way. A voltage difference is established between the wire inside the cable and the neutral sea water outside. Electricity cannot flow across the cable to any appreciable extent because it is covered by a heavy layer of electrical insulation that has a high degree of resistance to

a

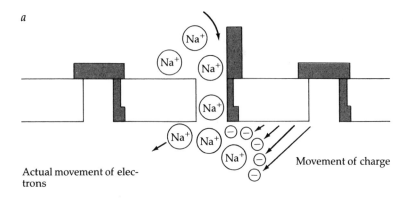

Actual movement of elec-
trons

Movement of charge

b

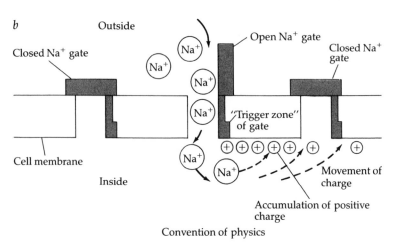

Outside

Closed Na⁺ gate

Open Na⁺ gate

Closed Na⁺
gate

"Trigger zone"
of gate

Cell membrane

Inside

Movement of
charge

Accumulation of positive
charge

Convention of physics

Figure A-4 Movement of electric charge when a Na⁺ channel gate opens and Na⁺ moves into the axon through the channel. (*a*) Electrons move away from the inner surface of the membrane toward the positively charged sodium ions. A given area of the inner surface of the membrane becomes less negatively charged by an amount depending on how close it is to the inrushing sodium ions. (*b*) The movement of electricity is shown according to convention in physics, with positive charge accumulating on the inside of the axon membrane.

electricity. Consequently, electricity flows along the inner wire of the cable all the way from New York to London and completes the circuit.

Some confusion may be caused by the way the movement of electricity is described in physics. Electricity was studied long before it was known that it is actually the movement of electrons, and early workers thought it flowed from positive to negative. In fact, electricity does the opposite: negatively charged electrons flow from a negative region to a positive one. However, the original way of describing electricity has stuck, and so electricity is always referred to as flowing from positive to negative.

Since we have seen that nerve fibers and transatlantic cables conduct electricity in much the same way, and that the electricity generated by the sodium ions moving in through the membrane travels at the speed of electricity, why is a synapse at the end of the axon not almost instantaneously activated? Why does the nerve impulse travel so slowly, at rates from about a mile (1.6 kilometers) per hour to something under 200 miles (322 kilometers) per hour? Part of the reason is that the amount of electricity flowing decreases rapidly the further away it gets from its "generator," which is the little region on the axon where the sodium gates are open and sodium ions are moving in (Figure A-4). The amount of electricity also decreases with distance in the transatlantic cable, but much less so because its inside wire cable is a much better conductor than the axoplasm of the axon.

When sodium ions move in through the membrane, they form a positively charged region and electrons flow to them away from the membrane just next to where the sodium ions are moving in (Figure A-4a). The electron flow is greatest right at the point where the sodium ions move in, and so the membrane is the most positive near the next (closed) sodium gate. According to convention in physics, when the positively charged sodium ions move in through the membrane, positive charge (electricity) tries to move out (Figure A-4b). But the result is the same whichever way one describes it. The inside of the membrane just next to the open sodium channel becomes a little less negative than at rest. When the inside of the membrane at the closed sodium channel just next to the open one becomes enough less negative, say, changes from -70 millivolts to -60 millivolts, the electrical switch on its closed gate is activated and pops open, and so on down the axon.

The speed at which electrons move from the inside of the membrane toward the incoming sodium ions (Figure A-4a) is the speed of electricity in the conducting fluid of the interior of the axon, close to the speed of light. But it takes much longer than that for the next Na^+ channel to pop open. Why? The cell membrane has one other electrical property: capacitance. A capacitor (also called a condenser) is simply two conducting surfaces separated by an insulator; in electrical circuits it is two plates of metal or metal foil separated by air, paper, glass, or some other insulator (Figure A-5). If a source of electricity such as a battery is connected to a condenser, charge will accumulate on the two plates until a steady state is reached (Figure A-5). Electrons actually accumulate on the plate connected to the negative pole of the battery and leave the plate connected to the positive pole, but it is usually shown as positive charges accumulating on one plate and negative charges on the other.

When the switch in a circuit like the one shown in Figure A-5 is closed, electricity flows briefly until the condenser is fully charged and stops. If the switch is then opened, the charge remains on the condenser until it is discharged by connecting the two plates with a conductor such as a wire. The key point about a capacitor is the rate at which charge accumulates. This rate is very much slower than the speed of electricity. There are capacitors that take seconds to reach full charge. The rate of charge accumulation is determined by the capacitance C of the capacitor and the resistance of the circuit. In an ideal circuit with no resistance, the capacitor would charge instantaneously. The circuit in Figure A-5 has no resistance, but actually the wire would have some. The greater the resistance in the circuit, the slower the rate of charge.

As we said, the neuron membrane acts like a capacitor. The two conducting fluid mediums inside and outside the membrane act like plates and the membrane itself has a relatively high resistance and acts as an insulator. Return now to Figure A-4. Sodium

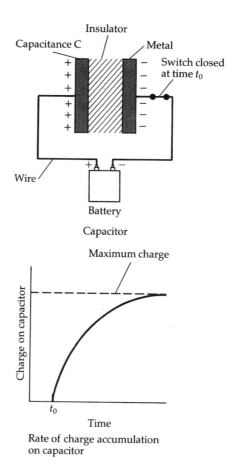

Rate of charge accumulation
on capacitor

Figure A-5 Left: An ordinary capacitor connected to a battery. When the switch is closed at time t_0, opposite charges accumulate on the two metal plates of the capacitor. (Actually, electrons accumulate on the plate attached to the negative pole of the battery, leaving the plate attached to the positive pole.) Right: The rate of accumulation of charge (electrons) on the capacitor after the circuit switch is closed at time t_0. The time required for the charge to approach maximum can range from almost instantaneous to seconds, depending on the capacitance (c) of the capacitor and the resistance of the circuit.

ions have moved in at the open gate and electricity is flowing: (positive charge is accumulating on) the inside of the membrane at the next gate, which is closed. But the rate at which positive charge accumulates under the closed gate is determined by the capacitance and resistance of the membrane, and so this occurs much more slowly than the rate at which electrons move toward the inrushing Na^+ ions, which occurs at the speed of electricity. It will take a relatively long time for the positive charge to accumulate to the point where the threshold for triggering open the channel gate is reached, but because the distance is very short, it still occurs in a fraction of a millisecond. The rate at which charge can accumulate on the inner surface of the membrane determines the speed of the nerve impulse. This rate is determined by the capacitance of the membrane, which in turn is determined by the resistance of the membrane and its size or surface area. This is why larger-diameter axons conduct faster.

We have used the term "electricity" a little loosely. Electricity really refers to the amount of charge, or rather charged particles involved: the number of electrons. Technically this is called *charge* and is measured in units called coulombs. One coulomb consists of about 6×10^{18} electrons. But we are usually more interested in how many electrons are flowing over a given period of time, rather than just how many are involved. This is *current (I)*, the number of coulombs per second, and is measured in terms of amperes, or A. One ampere is one coulomb of electrons flowing per second, or 6×10^{18} electrons flowing per second. When describing an electrical circuit or the nerve impulse, it is easy to fall into the bad habit of referring to the "flow of current." Current does not flow; it is the measure of the flow of electrons.

Any real electrical circuit, be it in a computer or a neuron, has some resistance. The conductors, wires, or intracellular and extracellular fluids are not perfect and have resistance. About the simplest electrical circuit is shown in Figure A-6. It is just a battery, a source of electrons, connected by a wire. But the wire has some resistance, symbolized by R, and measured in units of ohms.

Electricity has another property called *voltage (V)*. It refers to how much energy is available. In a battery, chemical work has been done to separate positive and negative charges. The more charges are separated, the more energy is required and hence the more energy is available from the battery. Technically, the amount of energy is the number of electrons times the voltage, or $q \times V$. Energy is usually symbolized by J, for joules (in the English system expressed in foot-pounds). So $J = Vq$ or $V = J/q$, the basic definition of voltage.

To return to our simple circuit, the battery has a given voltage that is fixed. When we close the switch, electrons flow through the wire (that has resistance) from the negative pole to the positive pole. Voltage (V in volts) is the energy available from the battery, and current (I in amps) is the rate of flow of electrons through the wire that has some resistance (R in ohms).

In Chapter 3 we used the analogy of water flowing through a hose. Voltage is equivalent to the water pressure, resistance is equivalent to the resistance of the hose to the flow of water—a small-diameter hose has more resistance than a large-diameter hose—and current is equivalent to the rate of flow of water from the hose, for example, the number of gallons per minute of water that flows out of it.

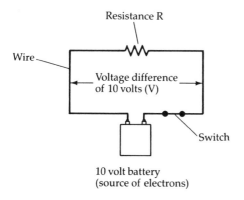

Resistance R

Wire

Voltage difference of 10 volts (V)

Switch

10 volt battery (source of electrons)

Figure A-6 A very simple electrical circuit having a battery of a given voltage V, a switch and a resistance R. The current I in the circuit is given by the expression $V = IR$ or $I = V/R$.

In basic electrical circuits (as in Figure A-6), the voltage, resistance, and current are related by the simple expression Ohm's law: $V = IR$. (The same type of expression holds for water flowing out of a hose.) Suppose in our simple circuit that the battery is a 10-volt battery and the wire has a resistance of 5 ohms. The current is thus determined: $V = IR$, $10 = I \times 5$, $I = 10/5 = 2$ A. If the resistance of the wire were higher, say 20 ohms, the current would be $I = 10/20 = 0.5$ A.

If we add a condenser to our simple electrical circuit and make the resistor variable, it becomes a "model" of the neuron membrane (Figure A-7), with a battery (the resting potential due to the distributions of ions inside and outside maintained by the energy-using ion pump and the closed and open ion channels), a resistance and a capacitance. In the resting state there is no current across the membrane. However, when the sodium gates open, positive charge moves into the membrane (actual positive charge, the Na^+ ions), and an electric current develops that begins to increase the positive charge on the inside of the membrane just next to the open sodium channels. The capacitance of the membrane charges until the threshold is reached, triggering the opening of the closed sodium channel at that point on the membrane, and so on down the membrane.

The problem Hodgkin and Huxley faced when trying to measure the ionic currents during the action potential is that everything changes. The voltage is easy to measure with electrodes inside and outside the axon membrane, but both the current and the resistance are changing. When sodium gates open, the resistance of the membrane drops and it also drops when the fewer closed potassium channels open. As we noted in Chapter 3, Hodgkin and Huxley developed a voltage clamp system that uses feedback to hold the voltage constant and so they could measure the charging currents, which in turn enabled them to determine the changes in resistance. Actually, what is usually expressed is the conductance, which is simply 1 over the resistance ($1/R$), its reciprocal. Each different kind of ion has its own conductance or permeability value, as we indicated in the Goldman equation in Chapter 3. During the

Figure A-7 A simplified electrical circuit that is a model of the circuit formed by the neuron membrane. R is the resistance for each type of ion involved (sodium, potassium and chloride) and is variable (arrow); for example, during the initial phase of the action potential the resistance of the membrane to sodium ions moving in decreases rapidly from high to low. The membrane also has a capacitance C. A more detailed equivalent circuit would have a separate variable resistor for each type of ion involved and some leakage resistance as well.

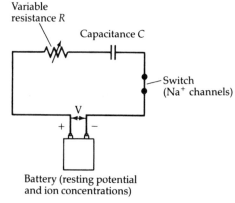

Simple model of the neuron membrane

action potential, the conductances for sodium and potassium change, resulting in ionic currents and the flow of electrons.

A somewhat more detailed circuit than that shown in Figure A-7 is needed to describe the nerve action potential accurately, but although each ion type has its own resistance and there is some leakage of ions across the membrane, the neuron membrane circuit is basically like the circuit in Figure A-7. By working out this "equivalent" circuit, Hodgkin and Huxley were able to write the differential equations for the circuit and hence for the neuron membrane. With the measurements of the ionic currents, they were able to solve the differential equations and predict with extraordinary accuracy all aspects of the nerve action potential. (This was in the days before computers and Huxley solved the equations in about two weeks of intense effort using extremely laborious numerical approximation methods.)

RECEPTOR PHARMACOLOGY

If any one key concept underlies our current understanding of how the nervous system works, it is that neurons (and the cells releasing hormones) communicate by releasing chemical transmitter substances that attach to specific receptors on neurons and other cells (see Chapters 4 through 6). By virtue of its shape and other properties, a given transmitter molecule fits into its receptor like a key fits into a lock (Figure A-8).

A transmitter molecule is said to bind to its receptor (see Chapter 4). But this sort of binding is very different from the two types of binding, covalent and ionic, that occur when atoms combine to form molecules. The binding forces are very much weaker for transmitters and receptors. These bonds depend on the molecular shape of the transmitter and receptor and what regions of them are hydrophobic or hydrophilic (that is, are not or are attracted to water) and what regions of them tend to have a negative or positive charge; the receptor will have hydrophobic and hydrophilic regions matching those of the transmitter, and complementary, or opposite, regions of charge.

Since the forces that bind transmitter molecules to receptor molecules are very weak, a given transmitter molecule will attach only briefly to the receptor and then let go. The rate of binding, or association, is symbolized by a constant and so is the rate of unbinding or dissociation (Figure A-8). The tendency of transmitter to bind to its receptor is called its *affinity*. In general, most receptor molecules are on the outside surface of the cell membrane and there are only so many per cell. When all the receptors on a membrane are occupied by transmitter molecules, they are said to be saturated. In a mixture of receptors and transmitter molecules either in the brain or in a test tube, the process of binding and unbinding is continuous. With fixed concentrations of both receptors and transmitter to begin with, a steady-state equilibrium is soon reached in which the net concentration of free transmitter and bound transmitter is constant.

In general, transmitter molecules tend to attach to membranes in a nonspecific way as well as attaching in a very specific way to their receptors. A major problem in pharmacology is in distinguishing transmitter-receptor binding from nonspecific binding. Typically, transmitter-receptor binding is characterized by a high affinity of the transmitter for the receptor and a low capacity of receptors for the transmitter, in other

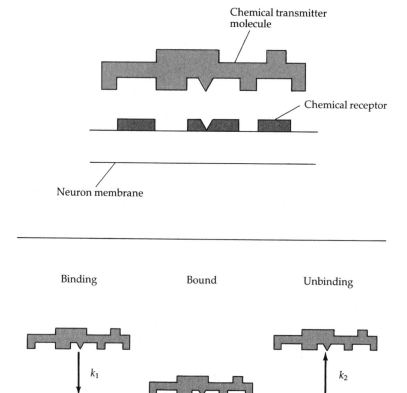

Figure A-8 Top: The key and lock notion of how transmitter and drug molecules fit receptor molecules. In addition to shape, some parts of the transmitter and receptor molecules have regions that attract or repel water and complementary regions of electric charge. All these properties can loosely be called the shape. Bottom: Transmitter molecule binding to its receptor (left), the bound state (middle) and unbinding (right). The rate of binding (k_1) is not necessarily the same as the rate of unbinding (k_2), or dissociation.

words, not much transmitter is needed to saturate the receptors. In contrast, non-specific binding is characterized by a low affinity and is virtually unsaturable.

These considerations apply just as well to the action of a drug on a receptor. The main reason such drugs as heroin, LSD, and cocaine have powerful actions on the brain, mind, and behavior in very small doses is that they fool receptors into accepting them as the natural transmitter; at least parts of the drug molecules are similar in shape and other properties to those of the transmitter molecule. A striking example of this is the close resemblance of one end of the morphine molecule to a part of the natural brain opioid substance met-enkephalin (see Chapter 6 and Figure 6-2). A transmitter molecule or drug that attaches to a receptor is called a ligand (L).

The rates of binding and unbinding of a ligand and receptor can be determined, whether the binding is high or low affinity and whether there is only one kind of binding or more than one. Known concentrations of a receptor and a transmitter or drug are mixed together in a test tube and the final steady-state, or equilibrium, concentrations of bound and unbound ligand are determined. Typically, a fixed known concentration of receptors is mixed with varying concentrations of the ligand (drug or transmitter), which is radioactively labeled, and the final concentration of ligand that remains unbound is measured. From this steady-state concentration of free ligand and ligand-receptor complex can be determined.

A useful way of looking at receptor-ligand binding is to calculate the fraction of the receptors that are bound to, or occupied by, the ligand, usually symbolized by r. The following paragraphs show algebraically how the value of r can be obtained and its use in describing binding. Readers who are not fond of algebraic relations may skip to the final paragraph of this section.

Given a ligand L and a receptor R the binding process can be described as

$$L + R \xrightarrow{k_1} LR$$

where LR is the receptors that have bound the ligand and k_1 is the association rate constant.

For unbinding, or dissociation

$$LR \xrightarrow{k_2} L + R$$

where k_2 is the dissociation rate constant. The above equations can be combined as follows:

$$L + R \underset{k_2}{\overset{k_1}{\leftrightarrow}} LR$$

The ratio of the association and dissociation constants, k_2/k_1, defines the dissociation equilibrium constant Kd:

$$Kd = \frac{k_2}{k_1} = \frac{[L][R]}{[LR]}$$

The brackets stand for concentrations; for example, $[L]$ is the concentration of ligand present.

The fraction of the receptors bound, symbolized r, is simply the ratio of the bound receptors to the total receptors R_t or

$$r = \frac{[LR]}{[R_t]}$$

The total number of receptors present is

$$[R_t] = [R] + [LR] \quad \text{and} \quad [R] = [R_t] - [LR]$$

Thus

$$Kd = \frac{[L]([R_t] - [LR])}{[LR]}$$

Solving for [LR]:

$$[LR]Kd = [L][R_t] - [L][LR]$$
$$[LR]Kd + [L][LR] = [L][R_t]$$
$$[LR]([L] + K_d) = [L][R_t]$$
$$[LR] = \frac{[L][R_t]}{[L] + K_d}$$

Since

$$r = \frac{[LR]}{[R_t]}, \quad r = \frac{[L]}{[L] + K_d}$$

The point of all these calculations is to get an expression for r in terms that can be measured.

If $r/[L]$ is plotted against r, a straight line will result if there is only one type of binding sites, for example, high-affinity ones (Figure A-9). Such plots, which are very useful, are called Scatchard plots. The x intercept of the straight line is the number of binding sites per molecule and the y intercept is $1/K_d$, which gives an easy way of determining K_d. Most importantly, if there are two different types of binding sites, for example, high-affinity sites and low-affinity ones, the Scatchard plot will give two straight lines of different slopes (Figure A-9).

Molecular Biology — Proteins and Genes

The field of neuroscience has developed to the point where it must now join forces with molecular biology. Some of the most basic questions about neuron and brain can be answered only at the level of the gene. Genes provide the information necessary to make peptides and proteins in cells. These in turn are responsible for the structure and functioning of neurons and their synaptic connections, not to mention the development of the body and brain from a single fertilized egg cell. Although estimates are vague, there may upwards of 100,000 genes in human chromosomes. Of these, some 30,000 to 50,000 are active only in cells in the brain. At present, only a few of these have been characterized (sequenced).

A key question in neuroscience and in the first few chapters of this book concerns identification of proteins, particularly chemical receptors in brain cells—see the discussion of the ACh receptor protein in Chapter 4. We use this question as the illustration here.

Proteins are simply long chains of amino acids (peptides are shorter chains), and there are only 20 standard amino acids. Amino acids are small molecules containing

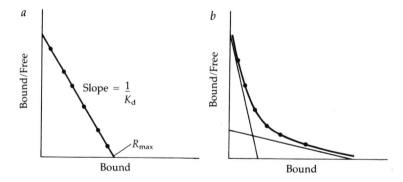

Figure A-9 Scatchard plots of the binding of ligand to a receptor. The ordinate is the ratio of bound to free ligand, or $r/(L)$, and the abscissa is the amount bound, r. (See text for details.) In (a) there is only one type of binding site, as shown by the straight-line plot, but in (b), both high- and low-affinity binding sites are suggested by the fact that the plot is not a straight line but has a break.
(After J. R. Cooper, F. E. Bloom, and R. H. Roth, *The Biochemical Basis of Neuropharmacology*, 3d ed., New York: Oxford University Press, 1978.)

carbon (C), an amino group (NH_2), a carboxyl group (COOH), and a variable side chain (R):

$$
\begin{array}{c}
NH_2 \\
| \\
R - CH \\
| \\
HO - C = 0
\end{array}
$$

Cells in our body can manufacture some amino acids, but others, the essential amino acids, must be obtained from the protein foods we eat.

If we know the exact sequence of the amino acids a protein comprises we know the protein and can make it. The chemical properties of the protein derive from the sequence of amino acids and some complications—the various other attached molecules, such as carbohydrates, and the three-dimensional shape of the protein molecule (see Figure 4-9, the three-dimensional shape of the ACh receptor). If we know the amino acid sequence of the protein, then we know the sequence of nucleotides in the gene that made it (with some complications).

Most readers have seen the diagrams of the DNA double helix, the basic structure of genes. All genes are composed of only four molecules, nucleic acids, arranged in particular sequences. Each nucleic acid is a combination of a sugar molecule (2-deoxyribose in DNA and ribose in RNA) and a nitrogenous base. DNA nucleic acids use four bases: adenine (A), guanine (G), cytosine (C), and thymine (T); RNA also uses four but substitutes uracil (U) for thymine. DNA consists of a chain of nucleic acids linked together by phosphate groups. The actual molecular structures of the nucleic acids are not needed for our brief discussion here, but they are given in any biology text.

The key point here is that the sequence of nucleic acids in a gene determines the sequence of amino acids in the protein the gene "makes." In fact, it takes a sequence of three nucleic acids to specify one amino acid, and these triplets (called "codons") do not overlap. Since DNA has four different nucleic acids, a maximum of 64 different sequences taken three at a time are possible. But only 20 different amino acids are actually made. (If two nucleic acids determined an amino acid, only 16 different amino acids would be made—four items taken two at a time—so at least three are needed). Actually, several different codons can code for the same amino acid; for example, there are six different triplet codons for the amino acid leucine.

Messenger RNA (mRNA) provides the intermediate steps between the genes (DNA) and the manufacture of the protein. A strand of DNA in a gene makes an identical strand of RNA, except that mRNA substitutes uracil (U) for thymine (T). As examples, the mRNA codon G-C-U specifies and "makes" the amino acid alanine, U-G-C specifies cystine, and so on for the twenty amino acids. (The reader with some background in biology will realize that this paragraph vastly oversimplifies volumes of knowledge of molecular biology.)

Thanks to the extraordinary technology that molecular biologists have developed, it is now possible to make large amounts of specific sequences of nucleic acids, even if only tiny amounts are initially available. The most recent breakthrough in technology (in 1988) is termed the polymerase chain reaction (PCR) which, among other things, made use of bacteria that live only in a geyser in Yellowstone Park and can tolerate boiling water.

Let us now return to the nicotinic ACh receptor. As described in Chapter 4, the electric organ of the torpedo fish is very rich in this receptor. Further, cobra venom toxin binds specifically to this receptor so the toxin is radiolabeled and infused into the electric organ. The protein containing the label can then be purified. Once we have the pure receptor protein (actually several protein subunits) its amino acid sequence can be determined directly using modern instrumentation, which is difficult, or, using molecular biology techniques, the corresponding mRNA and then DNA can be identified. We can also prepare antibodies specific to the protein by injecting the protein into a rabbit. This antibody helps to identify the mRNA and can also be used to determine the distribution of the receptor protein in the brain. The mRNA can be implanted in bacterial clones and a large amount of the receptor molecule made. We can also insert the mRNA in a frog egg and it will make the receptor and incorporate it into the egg membrane, where it reconstitutes the receptor sodium ion channel, which can be studied in "pure culture."

We have glossed over the actual steps whereby the amino acid sequence of the protein is determined and the correct mRNA prepared; the procedures are very complex in detail. In a piece of real brain tissue, thousands of proteins are present. The job of separating and identifying them and their mRNA and DNA precursors remains a forbidding and largely unaccomplished task. Present knowledge is limited to a few hundred brain-specific proteins. But the field moves very rapidly.

Glossary

Absolute Refractory Period The *spike* phase of an action potential during which further stimulation *cannot* produce another spike. See *Relative Refractory Period*.

Acetylcholine (ACh) A neurotransmitter abundant in the nervous system and specifically released at *neuromuscular junctions*.

Acetylcholinesterase (AChE) The enzyme responsible for the breakdown and inactivation of *acetylcholine* in the synaptic cleft.

Action Potential The all-or-none rapid change in electrical potential which is propagated down an axon conducting information along the extent of the neuron.

Adenosine Triphosphate (ATP) A primary source of energy for cells. When ATP is broken down to adenosine diphosphate (ADP) energy is released. ATP can also be converted to cAMP, a second messenger in the nervous system. See *Cyclic Adenosine Monophosphate (cAMP)*.

Adenyl Cyclase The enzyme which converts ATP to cAMP. See also *Adenosine Triphosphate*.

Adrenal Cortex The portion of the adrenal gland (an *endocrine gland* located near the kidney) which secretes testosterone and stress-related hormones in both males and females.

Adrenal Medulla The central part of the adrenal gland (surrounded by *adrenal cortex*) consisting of *chromaffin cells* which release epinephrine and norepinephrine in response to arousal of the sympathetic nervous system (stress).

Afferent Directed toward a stucture. Neural fibers "afferent" to the central nervous system relay sensory information (*sensory neurons*).

Afterpotential The slower phase of an action potential, following the spike, when the voltage drops below the resting potential level and then levels off, returning to resting potential. See *Relative Refractory Period*.

Agonist A drug which simulates the effect of a particular neurotransmitter or acts to enhance that transmitter's effect. See also *Antagonist*.

Aldosterone A hormone produced by *adrenal cortex* which regulates the body content of basic ions by increasing their absorption by the kidneys.

Alzheimer's Disease A progressive degenerative disorder associated with aging which affects cognitive processes, memory, language, and perception. Characteristic pathology includes senile placques and tangles. Acetylcholine neurons in the *nucleus basalis* of the forebrain are also affected, but the cause of the disease is as yet undetermined.

AMPA Receptor One type of *glutamate* receptor in the brain associated with sodium-potassium channels. See also *NMDA Receptor*.

Amygdala A group of nuclei located in the anterior temporal lobe which have been implicated in emotion and memory.

Antagonist A drug which inhibits or counteracts the effect of a particular neurotransmitter. See also *Agonist*.

Anterograde Amnesia Inability to store any new memories since the onset of the amnesia. Memories prior to the amnesia are retrievable. See also *Retrograde Amnesia*.

Antibodies Proteins produced by the body and circulated through the bloodstream to attack foreign substances.

Antidromic An action potential travelling up the axon, opposite to the normal direction, from a point of electrical stimulation somewhere along the axon. See *orthodromic*.

Aphasia A disorder of language. (e.g., *Wernicke's aphasia, Broca's aphasia* and *conduction aphasia*).

Association Cortex Areas of cortex integrating multi-sensory information and motor commands.

Associative Learning Behavior in which responses to stimuli are dependent on the relationships (associations) between different stimuli. Examples are *classical conditioning* and *instrumental learning*.

Astrocyte Glial cell within the central nervous system which forms the *blood–brain barrier* .

Auditory Cortex Area of cerebral cortex receiving auditory information. Located on the upper surface of the temporal lobe embedded in the Sylvian fissure.

Autonomic Nervous System Made up of the *Sympathetic Nervous System* and *Parasympathetic Nervous System* divisions these peripheral neural connections control internal organs and glands responsible for basic vegetative functions.

Autoreceptors Protein molecules, in the membrane of axon terminals, which recognize transmitters released by that neuron and regulate the amount of transmitter released.

Axon Elongated fiber extending from the cell body of a neuron by which information is transmitted from the cell body to terminal endings.

Axoplasmic Transport The movement of substances up and down an axon propelled by certain proteins along *microtubules* running the length of the axon.

Basal Ganglia Caudate nucleus, putamen, globus pallidus; a group of nuclei involved in the control of movement.

Basilar Membrane Contains hair cell receptors which are connected to auditory nerve fibers projecting to auditory nuclei in the brainstem. Critical for the coding of auditory information.

Benzodiazepines A group of drugs effective in treating panic attack and anxiety due to their tranquilizing effect.

Betz Cells The largest cells in cerebral cortex. Located in *motor cortex* their projections make up the *pyramidal tract.*

Binocular Vision When the visual fields of two eyes partially overlap.

Bipolar Depression Also called "manic-depressive disorder." A condition of major depression where the individual has experienced at least one episode of mania, or wild, intense euphoria.

Blood–Brain Barrier A barrier produced by astrocytes between the brain and cells in capillary walls so that only selected substances pass between them.

Broca's Aphasia Language disorder affecting speech production and *syntax*. Involves lateral frontal cerebral cortex (Broca's speech area).

Capacitance The storage of electrical charge; rate of accumulation depends, in part, on *resistance*.

Caudate Nucleus Largest nucleus of the *basal ganglia*. Involved in the inhibition of movement.

Cell Body Also known as "soma," this part of the neuron contains the nucleus and other organelles necessary for sustaining normal cell function.

Cell Membrane A thin lipid bilayer surrounding the organelles and substances which make up a cell and separating them from external surroundings.

Central Nervous System (CNS) The brain and spinal cord.

Cerebellum Structure overlying the pons involved in sensory-motor coordination.

Cerebral Cortex The brain's outermost layer of gray matter (cell bodies).

Cerebrum Structures overlying the brainstem including cerebral cortex, the basal ganglia and the limbic system.

Chemical Messenger See *neurotransmitter chemicals.*

Chemically Gated Ion channel openings controlled by transmitters or second messengers.

Cholinergic Of or relating to acetylcholine.

Circumventricular Organs Neuronal cell groups lying outside the blood–brain barrier, lining the ventricles and serving as bridges between substances in the cerebrospinal fluid unable to cross the barrier and targets within the brain (e.g., subfornical organ, area postrema).

Classical Conditioning An *associative learning* procedure popularized by Pavlov in which a neutral *conditioned stimulus* (CS) is paired with a response eliciting *unconditioned stimulus*. With repeated pairing the CS comes to evoke a *conditioned response* resembling the *unconditioned response*.

Cochlea A fluid filled coiled tube connecting the middle ear to the *basilar membrane*.

Complex Neuron Neuron in primary visual cortex responding to the image of an edge of a particular orientation falling on the retina. See also *Hypercomplex Neuron.*

Conduction Aphasia A disorder resulting from the disruption of connections between *Broca's* and *Wernicke's Areas*. Symptoms resemble Wernicke's Aphasia and individuals have difficulty repeating spoken language.

Cones Photoreceptors primarily concentrated in the *fovea* of the retina which are sensitive to color. Important for acute detail vision these cells are inactive in the dark. See also *Rods*.

Consciousness One's immediate awareness. See *Working Memory*.

Consolidation A term used to describe the transition of information from *working memory* to *long-term memory*.

Corpus Callosum A large bundle of fibers interconnecting the two cerebral hemispheres.

Corpus Striatum The major nuclei of the basal ganglia, the caudate nucleus, putamen, and globus pallidus.

Cortisol A stress related hormone released by the *adrenal cortex* causing the breakdown of complex proteins (stored energy) to glucose (usable energy) and increases blood pressure.

Cranial Nerves Grouped fibers that carry information to and from the brain and head. See also *Peripheral Nerves*.

Cyclic Adenosine Monophosphate (cAMP) A *second messenger* produced when adenosine triphosphate (ATP) is converted by the enzyme adenyl cyclase.

Declarative Memory One type of long-term memory refering to the learning of "what." Memory for facts or general knowledge. This classification encompasses *episodic* and *semantic* memories. See also *Procedural Memory*.

Dendrite Treelike processes extending from the cell body of a neuron which receive information from other neurons.

Dendritic Spines Tiny mushroom shaped extensions of dendrites which form synapses with axon terminals of other neurons.

Depolarization A change in membrane potential reducing the negativitity and rendering the cell more excitable.

Dopamine (DA) A major neurotransmitter in the brain distrubuted via three different systems all originating in brainstem structures. Implicated in *schizophrenia*, *Parkinson's disease*, and *reward*. See also *Medial Forebrain Bundle*.

Dorsal A term used to describe the direction "posterior" or "in back" (for an upright animal) or "on top" (based on a four-legged position).

Dorsal Bundle A group of noradrenergic fibers arising in the locus ceruleus and projecting to higher brain structures.

Dynamic Equilibrium The state achieved when ions are distributed such that there is no net ionic movement.

Efferent Directed away from a stucture. Neural fibers "efferent" to the central nervous system control muscles (*motor neurons*) and glands.

Electrotonic Current A graded current strongest at its point of origin and weakening as it travels.

Endocrine Glands Organs which secrete hormones directly into the bloodstream.

Endoplasmic Reticulum (ER) A system of membrane-bounded channels in the cytoplasm of a neuron cell body. See also *Nissl bodies*.

Endorphins Endogenous (secreted by the brain or pituitary) opiates which act like morphine.

Episodic Memory One type of long-term memory which references time. Memories for specific events, places, or situations that occured in the past. See also *Semantic Memory*.

Estrogen Sex hormone primarily produced in the ovaries and associated with the formation of female secondary sex characteristics (e.g., breast development, broad hips, etc.).

Excitatory Postsynaptic Potential (EPSP) A graded potential representing the sum of small depolarizations.

Exocrine Glands Organs which secrete hormones into ducts found on the skin (e.g., sweat) and body cavities (e.g., digestive).

Exocytosis The process by which membrane bound materials are released from a cell. The vesicular membrane fuses with the cell membrane and opens toward the outside spilling its contents into the extracellular space. This is the process of neurotransmitter release into a synapse.

Explicit Memory Awareness of one's ability to retrieve stored information. See *Implicit Memory*.

Extrapyramidal Motor System The basal ganglia, pontine nuclei, cerebellum and areas of reticular formation which control movement (traditionally, involuntary movement).

Fast Nerve Fibers Small myelinated fibers which transmit pain information at about 5–30 m/sec. Also known as A-fibers and associated with sharp pain. See *Slow Nerve Fibers*.

Fiber Tracts Bundles of neuronal axons within the central nervous system. See also *Nerves*.

First Messenger Refers to chemical messengers which are involved in the first step of neural activation by affecting receptors on the cell membrane. See also *Second Messenger*.

Fovea The center of the retina densely packed with *cones*. Important for detail and color vision.

Frequency Referring to sound, the number of oscillations of a sound wave per second.

Frequency Theory Theory of auditory perception which states that the *frequency* with which auditory nerve fibers fire codes the frequency of the sound.

G-Protein A protein in the cell membrane which, when activated, initiates activation of second messenger systems.

GABA (gamma-amino butyric acid) The primary fast inhibitory neurotransmitter in the brain.

Ganglia A collection of neural cell bodies located outside the central nervous system.

Ganglion Cells The final output of the retina to the brain. These are the first cells in the visual pathway to produce an action potential.

Gap Junction The very tight synaptic connection of electrical synapses. See *Synapse*.

Glia Non-neuronal cells thought to provide structural support and "housekeeper" functions, such as clearing away excess or debris materials. See also *Schwann Cell, Astrocyte* and *Oligodendrocyte*.

Globus Pallidus One of the nuclei of the *basal ganglia*. This structure has an excitatory role in the control of movement by the *extrapyramidal system*.

Glutamate The primary fast excitatory neurotransmitter in the brain.

Glycine The primary fast inhibitory neurotransmitter in the spinal cord.

Golgi Apparatus A complex of membranes which package secretory substances produced by the endoplasmic reticulum into *vesicles*.

Golgi Tendon Organ A stretch receptor at the tendon-muscle junction. See also *Spindle Organs*.

Gonadotropin-Releasing Hormone (GnRH) A hypothalamic hormone which activates release of sex hormones (FSH and LH) from the anterior pituitary gland.

Gray Matter Areas of the central nervous system consisting mostly of neural cell bodies. Tissue appears gray in color.

Habituation The decrease in a response as a result of repeated exposure to the stimulus. See also *Sensitization* and *Non-Associative Learning*.

Hair Cells Auditory receptors located in the *basilar membrane*.

Haloperidol An antipsychotic drug used to treat schizophrenia. Binds to dopamine receptors.

Heroin A synthetic faster acting form of *morphine* which is able to cross the blood-brain barrier.

Hippocampus A structure of the limbic system implicated in spatial mapping and memory. See also *Long-Term Potentiation*.

Homeostasis The process of maintaining body substances and functions at optimal levels. Often viewed as a balancing process.

Hormones Chemical substances, typically released into the bloodstream by endocrine glands, which have an effect on a distant organ.

Hypercomplex Neuron Neuron in primary visual cortex responding to particular forms and sizes of objects. See also *Complex Neuron*.

Hyperpolarization A change in membrane potential *increasing* the negativity inside the cell and rendering the cell less excitable.

Hypersensitivity Theory A theory proposed to explain the opposite effects of withdrawal and addiction. The theory suggests that the brain and body are trying to maintain a constant state (see *homeostasis*) by counteracting drug effects. When the drug is withdrawn the system is in a hypersensitive state until it regresses to normal.

Hypothalamus Group of nuclei functioning as a master control system for the autonomic and endocrine systems making interconnections to many brain regions.

Iconic Memory Very short lasting (max < second) visual memory.

Implicit Memory Not being aware of one's ability to call on a stored past experience. See *Explicit Memory*.

Induction The process of development which under underlies the differentiation and fate of cells which will form the nervous system.

Inferior Olive Brainstem structure sending sensory *climbing fiber* projections to the cerebellum.

Inhibitory Postsynaptic Potential (IPSP) A graded potential representing the sum of small hyperpolarizations.

Instrumental Learning A form of *associative learning* in which the subject can control the occurence of the stimuli by the response it performs (in contrast to *classical conditioning*).

Interneuron A neuron which connects two other neurons. Usually very short and contained to a particular region of the nervous system (local connections).

Ion Channels Openings in the cell membrane formed by specialized protein molecules which permit or prevent certain ions from passing through the membrane. See also *Semipermeable*.

Ions Atoms which have an electric charge.

Lateral Geniculate Body A bilateral nucleus of the thalamus which receives projections from the retina via the *optic tract* and, in turn, projects the visual information to visual cortex.

Lateral Hypothalamus (LH) A nucleus of the hypothalamus involved in sensory behavior and reward. Lesions cause animals to stop eating and experience sensory neglect (see also *ventromedial hypothalamus*). Stimulation seems to be pleasurable and increases the frequency of behaviors associated with the stimulation (see also *medial forebrain bundle*).

Learned Helplessness The result of prolonged exposure to inescapable aversive stimulation characterized by elevated activity in *adrenal cortex* and long-term deficits on other tests.

Lemniscal System The pathway involved in relaying sensory information about touch, pressure and joint position to cortex.

Ligand A substance which binds to a receptor.

Limbic System A group of nuclei involved in emotion and motivation. Structures include the amygdala, hippocampus, adjacent cortex, septal nuclei, and parts of the thalamus and hypothalamus.

Lipid Bilayer A descriptive term for the basic structure of cell membranes: Two layers of phospholipids arranged so that the hydrophilic fatty acid "heads" face the inside and outside of the cell while the hydrophobic glyceride "tails" face each other.

Locus Ceruleus A group of bluish colored neurons in the brainstem which contain the brain's richest supply of norepinephrine.

Long-Term Memory Stored memories transferred from *working memory*. Believed to have a limitless capacity and endurance, but items must be retreived and temporarily transferred to working memory while being accessed. See also *Working Memory*.

Long-Term Potentiation (LTP) The phenomena where repeated electrical stimulation of input pathways to the hippocampus produces an increase in the excitability of hippocampal neurons which persists for an extended period of time. See *NMDA Receptor*.

Long-Term Depression (LTD) The phenomena where cumulative activation of inputs to the Purkinje neurons of the cerebellum produces a decrease in the excitability of these neurons. See *Metabotropic Receptor*.

Medial Preoptic Nucleus A nucleus of the hypothalamus which controls secretion of GnRH and may be responsible for the direction of sexual development (male or female). See also *Gonadotrophin-Releasing Hormone*.

Medial Forebrain Bundle (MFB) Major dopaminergic fiber bundle closely associated with different hypothalamic nuclei and critically involved in the brain's reward system. Stimulation of the MFB can replace biological rewards such as food, water, and sex.

Medulla Lower portion of the brainstem containing several vital autonomic nuclei and fiber tracts connecting the brain and spinal cord.

Membrane Potential See *Potential Difference*.

Mesencephalon See *Midbrain*.

Metabotropic Receptor One type of glutamate receptor. Involved in long-term depression.

Microtubules Tiny tubes running the length of the axon along which *axoplasmic transport* takes place.

Midbrain Area anterior to the brainstem consisting of the *tectum* dorsally and the *tegmentum* ventrally.

Mitochondria Organelle within a cell body responsible for producing energy necessary for cell function. Mitochondria have their own DNA and can reproduce within the cell.

Monoamine Oxidase (MAO) An enzyme which breaks up monoamine transmitters in the synaptic cleft.

Monoamines Norepinephrine, dopamine, and serotonin; A class of neurotransmitters containing one amino group.

Morpheme Combinations of *phonemes* which are the smallest unit of meaning in a language. In English, for example, these would include one syllable words as well as the appendage "s" which carries the meaning "plural."

Motor Neuron Neuron which relays efferent information from the central nervous system to control activity of skeletal muscles, smoooth muscles, and glands.

Motor Cortex The area of cerebral cortex just anterior to the central sulcus in the frontal lobes which is involved in the control of movement. See also *Betz Cells*.

Motor Unit A single motor meuron and the muscle fibers it innervates.

Muscarinic Receptor Type of acetylcholine receptor found in the autonomic nervous system. These receptors respond to the poison "muscarine." See also *Nicotinic Receptor*.

Myasthenia Gravis A disease in which the body produces *antibodies* against acetylcholine receptors. Symptoms include varying degrees of muscular weakness due to receptor destruction at *neuromuscular junctions*.

Myelin A thin sheath of fatty substance which surrounds axon fibers and enhances conduction velocity. See also *Schwann Cell*, *Astrocyte* and *Oligodendrocyte*.

Negative Feedback A regulatory mechanism by which activation of a particular neural signal produces a relay signal back to the point of origin of the signal and serves to diminish the activation. For example, see *Testosterone*.

Nernst Equation A mathematical calculation which predicts the *potential difference* across a membrane once *dynamic equilibrium* has been reached.

Nerve Growth Factor A particular chemical which supports the development of neurons of the *sympathetic ganglia* and increases nerve cell division.

Nerves Bundles of neurons axons outside the CNS. See also *Fiber Tracts*.

Neural Plate Ectodermal cells which differentiate first and develop into neural tissue.

Neural Tube The elongated hollow crevis which forms as the result of the *neural plate* folding over as it grows eventually pinching together to form a tube. This tube will develop into the brain and spinal cord.

Neurite The early stage of an axon while still the developing outgrowth of a neuron cell body.

Neuromuscular Junction A synapse formed between the axon terminal of a *motor neuron* and a skeletal muscle fiber.

Neuron Basic building block of the nervous system; specialized cell for integration and transmission of information.

Neurotransmitter Chemicals Substances released from an axon terminal into a synapse. Neurotransmitters diffuse across the synapse to cause excitation or inhibition of the adjacent neuron.

Nicotinic Receptor Type of acetylcholine receptor found at neuromuscular junctions. Also recognizes and responds to nicotine. See also *Muscarinic Receptor*.

Nissl Bodies Clumps of *endoplasmic reticulum* which pick up thionine from histological stains thereby marking neural cell bodies.

NMDA Receptor One type of glutamate receptor critically involved in *long-term potentiation*.

Node Also known as "Node of Ranvier." Unmyelinated portions along the length of the axon between adjacent glial cells.

Non-Associative Learning Behaviors considered to be primitive forms of learning in which the response is *not* based on relationships (associations) between stimuli. Examples are *habituation* and *sensitization*.

Noradrenergic Containing norepinephrine.

Norepinephrine (NE) A major neurotransmitter found in the brain and peripherally in the sympathetic division of the autonomic nervous system. Also called "noradrenalin."

Nucleus Accumbens A nucleus in the forebrain which recieves dopaminergic inputs and is part of a system which produces feelings of pleasure and rewarding sensations.

Nucleus 1. Organelle within a cell which encases the genetic instructions for cell function, the DNA. 2. A grouping of neural cell bodies within the central nervous system.

Nucleus Basalis A major source of cholinergic neurons to the hippocampus and cerebral cortex, this nucleus of the basal forebrain degenerates in individuals with Alzheimer's disease.

Occipital Cortex Posterior region of cerebral cortex receiving visual information.

Ocular Dominance Column The primary visual cortex is arranged in such a way that there are columns of orientation-specific cells receiving input from one preferred eye. Adjacent columns receive alternating visual information from each eye.

Off-Center/On-Surround Opposite of *On-Center/Off-Surround.*

Oligodendrocyte Glial cell which wraps its processes around CNS neurons to form myelin.

On-Center/Off-Surround Refering to the receptive field of one type of ganglion cell in the retina. A spot of light in the center of the receptive field will excite this neuron, but light on the periphery will inhibit the neuron. See also *Off-Center/On-Surround.*

Opioids Peptide substances found in the brain or pituitary gland which act like *opium.*

Opium An extract of the opium poppy used to relieve pain and induce a pleasurable feeling.

Optic Chiasm Visible on the base of the brain, the point where the two optic nerves cross over.

Optic Nerves The second cranial nerve, made up of fibers from retinal ganglion cells carrying visual information to the brain.

Optic Tracts See *Optic Nerves* and *Fiber Tracts.*

Organelles The structures within a cell (e.g., nucleus, mitochondria).

Orthodromic An action potential travelling down the axon, in the normal direction, from the point of electrical stimulation. See antidromic.

Oxytocin One of 2 hormones secreted by neurons in the posterior pituitary. See also *Vasopressin.*

Parasympathetic Nervous System Part of the autonomic nervous system involved in self-sustaining and restorative functions of the relaxed state. See also *Sympathetic Nervous System.*

Parietal Lobe Upper middle region of cerebral cortex receiving somatosensory information from the skin and body.

Parkinson's Disease Movement disorder involving dopaminergic cells of substantia nigra. Symptoms include tremors, repetitive movements, and difficulty initiating movements.

Patch Clamp A technique used to study the activity of single channels in which a tight seal is made between a glass pipette tip and a "patch" of cell membrane.

Pavlovian Conditioning See *Classical Conditioning.*

Peptide A short chain of amino acids.

Peptides A class of hormones, peptides are chains of amino acids which serve as the building blocks of proteins.

Periaqueductal Gray (PAG) A region in the brainstem surrounding the cerebral aqueduct which is involved in the sensation and control of pain. Especially associated with slow pain.

Peripheral Nerves Grouped fibers that carry information to and from the spinal cord. See also *Cranial Nerves.*

Phoneme The smallest possible distinguishable unit of a language. In English this usually corresponds to a letter of the alphabet. See also *Morpheme.*

Pineal Gland A small gland situated at the top of the brainstem which is involved in cyclic behaviors such as the female reproductive cycle and sleeping and waking.

Pinocytosis The reverse of *exocytosis.* The process by which substances (e.g., neurotransmitters) are taken back into a cell. The membrane surrounds the substance and pinches off on the inside of the cell to form a *vesicle.*

Pitch The psychological perception of the frequency of a tone.

Pituitary Gland Attached to the base of the brain and primarily controlled by the hypothalamus, this master endocrine gland releases a variety of hormones which act on other glands throughout the body. **Anterior:** The glandular portion of the pituitary which secretes hormones directly into the bloodstream via the *portal system.* **Posterior:** Secretes oxytocin and vasopressin from neuron terminals into the bloodstream.

Place Theory Theory of auditory perception which states that a particular frequency is coded by the activation of hair cells in a particular location on the *basilar membrane.*

Pons Anterior portion of the brainstem recognized by crosswise fibers connecting the cerebellum and brainstem.

Pontine Nuclei A group of nuclei located in the pons which receive descending motor cortical input and input from sensory systems and send *mossy fiber* projections to the cerebellum.

Portal System The blood vessels supplying the hypothalamus and anterior *pituitary gland.*

Posterior Nucleus A nucleus of the thalamus involved in relaying information about fast pain to the cerebral cortex. See also *Ventrobasal Complex.*

Postsynaptic After the synaptic cleft. Typically a dendrite or cell body.

Potential Difference The voltage difference of the inside of a cell relative to the outside (e.g., −70 mV indicates more negative electrical potential on the inside of the cell than on the outside). Also called *membrane potential.*

Precentral Cortex The area of cerebral cortex immediately in front of the central sulcus. Also known as *motor cortex* because of its role in controlling movement.

Presynaptic Before the synaptic cleft. Usually an axon terminal.

Procedural Memory One type of long-term memory referring to the learning of motor skills, or "how." See *Declarative Memory.*

Purkinje Cell Principle neuron in the cerebellar cortex and exclusive conveyor of information to other brain structures; in particular to cerebellar deep nuclei and vestibular nuclei. The output of Purkinje cells is inhibitory.

Putamen One of the *basal ganglia* nuclei.

Pyramidal Motor System A system for control of movement (traditionally, voluntary movement) made up of long axon fibers originating in cerebral motor cortex.

Pyramidal Tract The bundle of fibers extending from Betz cells in motor cortex and projecting to cranial motor nuclei and motor regions of the spinal cord.

Quantum The smallest amount of a neurotransmitter ever released; One " packet" of neurotransmitter substance.

Raphe Nucleus A group of nuclei distributed along the midline of the brainstem.

Receptor A protein molecule typically embedded within the cell membrane which recognizes and binds a particular *chemical messenger.*

Red Nucleus Nucleus in the midbrain involved in the control of movement. The red nucleus receives inputs from the cerebellum and motor cortex and projects to the spinal cord.

Relative Refractory Period The *afterpotential* phase of an action potential when another spike can occur but requires stronger stimulation than normal. See also *Absolute Refractory Period.*

Resistance (R) The ease or difficulty with which charged particles or ions move through a substance. The unit of resistance is an Ohm (R = V/I).

Resting Potential The potential difference across the membrane when there is dynamic equilibrium, approximately −70 mV inside relative to outside.

Retina A layer of photoreceptors and neurons lining the back of the eye.

Retinal A chemical found in rods in the form 11-cis-retinal which changes shape to all-trans-retinal when a photon of light hits the rod.

Retrograde Amnesia Loss of memory for events preceding the onset of the amnesia. See also *Anterograde Amnesia.*

Rhodopsin A photosensitive chemical found in rods which consists of *retinal* and the protein opsin. See *Retinal.*

Rods Photoreceptors distributed throughout the retina, but more densely outside the fovea. Very sensitive to light and sense shades of gray. Important for night vision. See also *Cones.*

Schizophrenia A general label for a group of related psychoses in which the primary symptoms include loss of contact with reality, disordered thought, and hallucinations. See also *Haloperidol.*

Schwann Cell Glial cell which wraps its processes around peripheral neurons to form myelin.

Second Messenger Refers to a substance (e.g., cAMP) which produces a transmitter like action from within the postsynaptic cell. Such an action usually results from changes within a cell following activation by a *first messenger.* See also *G-Protein.*

Semantic Memory One type of long-term memory refers to knowledge, facts, or meaning without any reference to "when" it was learned. See also *Episodic Memory.*

Semantics The *meaning* of language once it has been assembled.

Semipermeable A characteristic of cell membranes such that certain ions are permitted to pass through the membrane freely while others, usually large protein ions, are not.

Sensitization The increase in a response as a result of exposure to a typically strong stimulus. See also *Habituation* and *Non-Associative Learning*.

Sensory Neuron Neurons carrying information from the skin, muscles, and joints to the spinal cord (central nervous system). The cell bodies are located outside the CNS in *ganglia*.

Septal Nuclei A group of nuclei located between the anterior portions of the lateral ventricles. Part of the *limbic system* and a major source of cholinergic projections.

Serotonin (5-HT) A neurotransmitter involved in depression, sleep, and regulation of body temperature.

Set Point The optimum value within a system which homeostatic regulatory mechanisms try to maintain. Deviations from the set point trigger homeostatic mechanisms. See *Homeostasis*.

Short-Term Memory A short-term memory lasting about 10 seconds with a limited capacity of 7 ±2 items. Information can be maintained by continuous rehearsal. See also *Working Memory*.

Slow Nerve Fibers Tiny diameter unmyelinated fibers which transmit pain information at 0.5–2 m/sec. Also known as C-fibers and associated with dull pain. See *Fast Nerve Fibers*.

Smooth Muscle Muscle under control of the autonomic nervous system (non-striated), found, for example, in the the walls of blood vessels and in the digestive tract. Smooth muscle can function without neural input.

Somatic Nerves Peripheral nerves which connect to skeletal muscles and to sensory receptors in skin and muscle.

Spatial Summation The cumulative action of several different synapses on one neuron to increase its chances of firing.

Spike The short phase of the action potential characterized by a rapid change from the −70 mV resting potential to a +50 mV peak potential and return to resting potential. See *Absolute Refractory Period*.

Spindle Organs Made up of intrafusal fibers these organs relay information about the degree of stretch in a muscle back to the spinal cord.

Steroids A class of hormones, which does not contain amino acids, derived from cholesterol (see also peptides). Steroid receptors are located within the target cell rather than on the membrane surface. Associated with stress and sexual functions.

Striate Cortex Primary visual area of occipital cortex.

Striated Muscle Muscles typically involved in "voluntary" movements and dependent on neural input.

Subplate Neuron A special type of neuron which guides cells and developing fibers destined for cortex and dies out as cortex is established.

Substantia Nigra A group of darkly stained neurons located in the *tegmentum*. These dopamine-containing neurons project to the *basal ganglia* and are implicated in the regulation of movement. See also *Parkinson's Disease*.

Superior Olive Structure in the brainstem receiving auditory information from both ears and detecting time-of-arrival differences critical for locating the source of the sound.

Supersensitivity Refers to the increase in number of receptors post-synaptically as a result of low transmitter availability.

Suprachiasmatic Nucleus (SCN) A nucleus of the hypothalamus recently identified as the source generator of cyclic biological rhythms.

Supraoptic Nucleus A hypothalamic nucleus involved in regulating thirst and drinking by detecting fluid levels based on cell size or shrinkage.

Sympathetic Ganglia A series of ganglia lying next to the spinal cord which receive cholinergic (ACh) motor inputs and send noradrenergic (NE) fibers to synapse on target organs of the *sympathetic nervous system*.

Sympathetic Nervous System Part of the autonomic nervous system involved in arousal during emergency situations. Works in opposition to the *Parasympathetic Nervous System*.

Synapse The communication point between the axon terminal of one neuron and the dendrite or cell body of another neuron. **Chemical:** A synapse where communication is achieved by chemical signals. **Electrical:** A synapse where communication is achieved by inducing an electric field in the postsynaptic cell (see *Gap Junction*).

Synaptic Cleft A tiny space between communicating neurons at a synapse.

Synaptic Terminals Specialized endings of axon branches which form synapses with adjacent cells.

Syntax The innate as well as learned *rules* for assembling a language. For example, grammar. See *Broca's Aphasia.*

Tardive Dyskinesia A movement disorder characterized by uncontrollable movements of the face and neck due to an overactive dopamine system often resulting from treatment with antipsychotic drugs.

Tectum The roof of the midbrain made up of the superior and inferior colliculi.

Tegmentum The floor of the midbrain containing nuclei such as the *substantia nigra* and *red nucleus* involved in the control of movement.

Temporal Summation The cumulative action over time of sub-threshold depolarizations occurring in rapid succession to one another can build up an EPSP which will reach threshold and result in an action potential.

Testosterone Sex hormone primarily produced in the testes of males and associated with the formation of male secondary sex characteristics (e.g., facial hair, deep voice, etc.). Testosterone also decreases the release of *gonadotrophin-releasing hormone* (*negative feedback*).

Thalamus A large group of nuclei situated anterior to the midbrain and above the hypothalamus. Serves as the final relay station for sensory information being projected to cerebral cortex.

Threshold A minimum value which must be reached in order for something to occur. In the case of an action potential, the membrane potential which must be reached for an action potential to occur.

Tympanic Membrane Eardrum. First structure affected in the perception of auditory stimuli.

Vasopressin One of 2 hormones secreted by neurons in the posterior pituitary. See *Oxytocin.*

Ventral A term used to describe the direction "anterior" or "in front" (for an upright animal) or "on the bottom" (based on a four-legged position).

Ventral Bundle A group of noradrenergic fibers arising from several brainstem cell groups near the locus ceruleus and projecting to reticular formation and hypothalamus.

Ventrobasal Complex A nucleus of the thalamus involved in relaying information about fast pain, touch, and pressure (*lemniscal system*) to the cerebral cortex. See also *Posterior Nucleus.*

Vesicles Membrane bound packets produced by the Golgi apparatus, tansported down the axon and clustered within terminals at a synapse. Vesicles in a neuron terminal contain neurotransmitters.

Voltage Clamp A technique which holds membrane potential constant while ionic currents across the membrane are measured.

Voltage Gated A channel which is either open or closed to the passage of ions depending on the voltage across the membrane.

Wernicke's Aphasia Language disorder affecting language comprehension and production of semantically correct (meaningful) language. Involves lateral parietal and superior temporal cortex (Wernicke's Area).

White Matter Areas of the central nervous system consisting mostly of neural fibers. Myelination make tissue appear white in color.

Working Memory Intermediate time course memory ranging from *short-term memory* to a period of minutes. Often equated with *consciousness.*

Sources of Illustrations

Figure 1-1 Micrograph by C. Gilbert and T. N. Wiesel. From C. F. Stevens, The neuron. In *The Brain* [a *Scientific American* book], San Francisco: W. H. Freeman and Company, 1979.

Figure 1-4 After W. J. H. Nauta and M. Feirtag, The organization of the brain. In *The Brain* [a Scientific American book], San Francisco: W. H. Freeman and Company, 1979.

Figure 1-5 After R. F. Thompson, *Introduction to Physiological Psychology*, New York: Harper & Row, 1975.

Figure 1-6 After E. R. Kandel and J. H. Schwartz, *Principles of Neural Science*, New York: Elsevier/North-Holland, 1981.

Figure 1-7 After S. W. Ranson and S. L. Clark, *Anatomy of the Nervous System*, 9th ed., Philadelphia: W. B. Saunders, 1953.

Figure 1-8 After R. F. Thompson, *Introduction to Physiological Psychology*, New York: Harper & Row, 1975.

Figure 1-9 After R. F. Thompson, *Introduction to Physiological Psychology*, New York: Harper & Row, 1975.

Figure 2-1 Micrograph courtesy of Judith Thompson.

Figure 2-3 From L. L. Iversen, The chemistry of the brain. In *The Brain* [a *Scientific American* book], San Francisco: W. H. Freeman and Company, 1979.

Figure 2-4 From C. P. Stevens, The neuron. In *The Brain* [a *Scientific American* book], San Francisco: W. H. Freeman and Company, 1979.

Figure 2-5 From C. P. Stevens, The neuron. In *The Brain* [a *Scientific American* book], San Francisco: W. H. Freeman and Company, 1979.

Figure 2-6 From L. L. Iversen, The chemistry of the brain. In *The Brain* [a *Scientific American* book], San Francisco: W. H. Freeman and Company, 1979.

Figure 2-8 Adapted from J. E. Dowling, *Neurons and Networks: An Introduction to Neuroscience*. Cambridge, MA: Harvard University Press, 1992.

Figure 2-9 After R. M. Julien, *A Primer of Drug Action*, New York: W. H. Freeman and Company, 1981.

Figure 3-1 Based on the Singer–Nicholson model. After S. L. Wolfe, *Biology of the Cell*, 2nd ed., Belmont, CA: Wadsworth Publishing Company, 1981.

Figure 3-10 (top) From L. Stryer, *Biochemistry*, 2nd ed., New York: W. H. Freeman and Company, 1988.

Figure 4-1 From C. P. Stevens, The neuron. In *The Brain* [a *Scientific American* book], San Francisco: W. H. Freeman and Company, 1979.

Figure 4-9 From J. E. Dowling, *Neurons and Networks: An Introduction to Neuroscience*. Cambridge, MA: Harvard University Press, 1992.

Figure 4-10 From L. Stryer, *Biochemistry*, 2nd ed., New York: W. H. Freeman and Company, 1988.

Figure 4-12 Courtesy of Michael Baudry.

Figure 4-15 After J. R. Cooper, F. E. Bloom, and R. H. Roth, *The Biochemical Basis of Neuropharmacology*, 6th ed., New York: Oxford University Press, 1991.

Figure 4-16 After H. Mohler and J. G. Richards, Benzodiazepine receptors in the central nervous system. In E. Costa, ed., *The Benzodiazepines: From Molecular Biology to Clinical Practice*, New York: Raven Press, 1983.

Figure 4-17 After W. Haefely, P. Pole, L. Pieri, R. Schaffner, and J.-P. Laurent, Neuropharmacology of benzodiazepines: Synaptic mechanisms and neural basis of action. In E. Costa, ed., *The Benzodiazepines: From Molecular Biology to Clinical Practice*, New York: Raven Press, 1983.

Figure 5-1 Micrograph by Heuser and Salpeter. From C. F. Stevens, The neuron. In *The Brain* [a *Scientific American* book], San Francisco: W. H. Freeman and Company, 1979.

Figure 5-4 After J. T. Coyle, D. L. Price, and M. R. DeLong, *Science* 219: 1184–1190, 1983.

Figure 5-6 From J. R. Cooper, F. E. Bloom, and R. H. Roth, *The Biochemical Basis of Neuropharmacology*, 6th ed., New York: Oxford University Press, 1991.

Figure 5-8 From R. F. Thompson, *Introduction to Physiological Psychology*, New York: Harper & Row, 1975.

Figure 5-9 After J. R. Cooper, F. E. Bloom, and R. H. Roth, *The Biochemical Basis of Neuropharmacology*, 6th ed., New York: Oxford University Press, 1991.

Figure 5-10 After J. R. Cooper, F. E. Bloom, and R. H. Roth, *The Biochemical Basis of Neuropharmacology*, 6th ed., New York: Oxford University Press, 1991.

Figure 5-11 After L. L. Iversen, The chemistry of the brain. In *The Brain* [a *Scientific American* book], San Francisco: W. H. Freeman and Company, 1979.

Figure 5-12 After J. R. Cooper, F. E. Bloom, and R. H. Roth, *The Biochemical Basis of Neuropharmacology*, 3rd ed., New York: Oxford University Press, 1978.

Figure 5-14 After J. R. Cooper, F. E. Bloom, and R. H. Roth, *The Biochemical Basis of Neuropharmacology*, 6th ed., New York: Oxford University Press, 1991.

Figure 5-15 After J. R. Cooper, F. E. Bloom and R. H. Roth, *The Biochemical Basis of Neuropharmacology*, 3rd ed., New York: Oxford University Press, 1978.

Figure 6-1 After S. H. Snyder, *Scientific American* 236(3):44–56, 1977.

Figure 6-2 After S. H. Snyder, *Scientific American* 236(3):44–56, 1977.

Figure 6-3 After J. R. Cooper, F. E. Bloom, and R. H. Roth, *The Biochemical Basis of Neuropharmacology*, 6th ed., New York: Oxford University Press, 1991.

Figure 6-4 After S. H. Snyder, *Scientific American* 236(3):44–56, 1977.

Figure 6-5 After L. L. Iversen, The chemistry of the brain. In *The Brain* [a *Scientific American* book], San Francisco: W. H. Freeman and Company, 1979.

Figure 6-6 From R. F. Thompson, *Introduction to Physiological Pharmacology*, New York: Harper & Row, 1975.

Figure 6-7 After S. Reichlin, *Neural Control of the Pituitary Gland: Normal Physiology and Pathophysiologic Implications*, The Upjohn Company, 1978.

Figure 6-8 After M. B. Carpenter and J. Sutton, *Human Neuroanatomy*, 8th ed., Baltimore, MD: Williams & Wilkins, 1983.

Figure 6-9 After D. T. Krieger and J. C. Hughes, eds., *Neuroendocrinology*, Sunderland, MA: Sinauer Associates, 1980.

Figure 6-10 From R. M. Berne and M. N. Levy, *Physiology*, 2nd ed., St. Louis, MO: C. V. Mosby Company, 1988.

Figure 6-11 After A. J. Vander, J. H. Sherman, and D. S. Luciano, *Human Physiology: The Mechanisms of Body Functions*, 3d ed., New York: McGraw-Hill, 1980.

Figure 6-12 From E. R. Kandel and J. H. Schwartz, *Principles of Neural Science*, New York: Elsevier/North-Holland, 1981.

Figure 7-2 From E. R. Kandel and J. H. Schwartz, *Principles of Neural Science*, New York: Elsevier/North-Holland, 1981.

Figure 7-3 L. W. Swanson, Biochemical switching in hypothalamic circuits mediating responses to stress. In *Progress in Brain Research*, 87, 181–200, 1991.

Figure 7-4 Modified from R. F. Thompson, *Introduction to Physiological Psychology*, New York: Harper & Row, 1975.

Figure 7-5 G. M. Shepherd, *Neurobiology*, 2nd ed., New York: Oxford University Press, 1988.

Figure 7-6 L. W. Swanson, Biochemical switching in hypothalamic circuits mediating responses to stress. In *Progress in Brain Research*, 87, 181–200, 1991.

Figure 7-8 Modified from D. T. Krieger and J. C. Hughes, eds., *Neuroendocrinology*, Sunderland, MA: Sinauer Associates, 1980.

Figure 7-9 Modified from I. Zucker, Motivation, biological clocks, and temporal organization of behavior. In E. Satinoff and P. Teitelbaum, eds., *Handbook of Behavioral Neurobiology*, New York: Plenum Press, 1983.

Figure 7-10 (*a*) Modified from D. H. Hubel and T. N. Wiesel, Brain mechanisms of vision. In *The Brain* [a *Scientific American* book], San Francisco: W. H. Freeman and Company, 1979. (*b*) From R. Y. Moore, Central neural control of circadian rhythms. In W. F. Ganong and L. Martini, eds., *Frontiers in Neuroendocrinology*, Vol. 5, New York: Raven Press, 1978.

Figure 7-11 After E. Hartman, *The Biology of Dreaming*, Springfield, IL: Charles C. Thomas, 1967.

Figure 7-12 After A. J. Vander, J. H. Sherman, and D. S. Luciano, *Human Physiology: The Mechanisms of Body Function*, 3d ed., New York: McGraw-Hill, 1980.

Figure 7-13 N. R. Carlson, *Physiology of Behavior*, 4th ed., Boston: Allyn and Bacon, 1991.

Figure 7-14 After D. T. Krieger and J. C. Hughes, eds., *Neuroendocrinology*, Sunderland, MA: Sinauer Associates, 1980.

Figure 7-15 After N. R. Carlson, *Physiology of Behavior*, 4th ed., Boston: Allyn and Bacon, 1991.

Figure 8-1 After P. F. Lindsay and D. A. Norman, *Human Information Processing: An Introduction to Psychology*, 2nd ed., New York: Academic Press, 1977.

Figure 8-2 After P. H. Lindsay and D. A. Norman, *Human Information Processing: An Introduction to Psychology*, 2nd ed., New York: Academic Press, 1977.

Figure 8-3 After L. Stryer, *Biochemistry*, 3d ed., New York: W. H. Freeman and Company, 1988.

Figure 8-4 (*a*) After T. N. Cornsweet, *Visual Perception*, New York: Academic Press, 1970. (*b*) After J. E. Dowling, *Neurons and Networks: An Introduction to Neuroscience*, Cambridge, MA: The Belknap Press of Harvard University Press, 1992.

Figure 8-6 Modified from D. H. Hubel and T. N. Wiesel, Brain mechanisms of vision. In *The Brain* [a *Scientific American* book], San Francisco: W. H. Freeman, 1979.

Figure 8-7 From D. H. Hubel amd T. N. Wiesel, Brain mechanisms of vision. In *The Brain* [a *Scientific American* book], W. H. Freeman and Company, 1979.

Figure 8-8 After S. W. Kuffler and J. G. Nicholls, *From Neuron to Brain*, Sunderland, MA: Sinauer Associates, 1977.

Figure 8-9 After S. W. Kuffler and J. G. Nicholls, *From Neuron to Brain*, Sunderland, MA: Sinauer Associates, 1977.

Figure 8-10 Modified from D. H. Hubel and T. N. Wiesel, *Journal of Neurophysiology*, **28:** 229–289, 1965.

Figure 8-12 After J. E. Dowling, *Neurons and Networks: An Introduction to Neuroscience*, Cambridge, MA: The Belknap Press of Harvard University Press, 1992.

Figure 8-13 After C. N. Woolsey, W. Penfield, H. Jasper, and N. Geschwind, various publications.

Figure 8-14 After G. M. Shepard, *Neurobiology*, New York: Oxford University Press, 1983.

Figure 8-15 Modified from W. I. Welker, *Brain Behavior and Evolution*, **1:** 253–336, 1973.

Figure 8-16 After T. A. Woolsey and H. van der Loos, *Brain Research*, **17:** 205–242, 1970.

Figure 8-17 After P. H. Lindsay and D. A. Norman, *Human Information Processing: An Introduction to Psychology*, 2nd ed., New York: Academic Press, 1977.

Figure 8-18 Top: After G. L. Rasmussen and W. F. Windle, eds., *Neural Mechanisms of the Auditory Vestibular Systems*, Springfield, IL: Charles C. Thomas, 1960. Bottom: After P. H. Lindsay and D. H. Norman, *Human Information Processing: An Introduction to Psychology*, 2nd ed., New York: Academic Press, 1977.

Figure 8-19 Modified from R. F. Thompson, *Introduction to Physiological Psychology*, New York: Harper & Row, 1975.

Figure 8-20 After P. H. Lindsay and D. H. Norman, *Human Information Processing: An Introduction to Psychology*, 2nd ed., New York: Academic Press, 1977.

Figure 9-1 A. P. Georgopoulos, A. B. Scwartz, and R. E. Kettner, Neuronal population coding of movement direction. In *Science*, *233*, 1416–1419, 1986.

Figure 9-2 Modified from R. F. Thompson, *Foundations of Physiological Psychology*, New York: Harper & Row, 1967.

Figure 9-4 After A. J. Vander, J. H. Sherman, and D. S. Luciano, *Human Physiology: The Mechanisms of Body Function*, 3d ed., New York: McGraw-Hill, 1980.

Figure 9-5 After W. Bloom and D. W. Fawcett, *A Textbook of Histology*, 10th ed., Philadelphia: W. B. Saunders, 1975.

Figure 9-6 After H. E. Huxley. In A. L. Lehninger, *Biochemistry: The Molecular Basis of Cell Structure and Function*, 2nd ed., New York: Worth, 1975.

Figure 9-7 After A. J. Vander, J. H. Sherman, and D. S. Luciano, *Human Physiology: The Mechanisms of Body Function*, 3d ed., New York: McGraw-Hill, 1980.

Figure 9-8 Top: After A. J. Vander, J. H. Sherman, and D. S. Luciano, *Human Physiology: The Mechanisms of Body Function*, 3d ed., New York: McGraw-Hill, 1980. Bottom: After A. L. Lehninger, *Biochemistry: The Molecular Basis of Cell Structure and Function*, 2nd ed., New York: Worth, 1975.

Figure 9-10 Modified from R. F. Thompson, *Foundations of Physiological Psychology*, New York: Harper & Row, 1967.

Figure 9-11 Modified from R. F. Thompson, *Foundations of Physiological Psychology*, New York: Harper & Row, 1967.

Figure 9-12 After R. R. Llinas, *Scientific American*, *232* (1), 56–71, 1975.

Figure 9-13 After E. R. Kandel and J. H. Schwartz, *Principles of Neural Science*, New York: Elsevier/North-Holland, 1981.

Figure 9-14 In F. O. Schmitt and F. G. Worden, eds., *The Neurosciences: Third Study Program*, Cambridge, MA: MIT Press, 1974.

Figure 9-15 Top: After C. N. Woolsey in H. F. Harlow and C. N. Woolsey, eds., *Biological and Biochemical Bases of Behavior*, Madison, WI: University of Wisconsin Press, 1958. Bottom: Modified from N. Geschwind, Specializations of the human brain. In *The Brain* [a *Scientific American* book], San Francisco: W. H. Freeman and Company, 1979.

Figure 9-17 After E. V. Evarts, Brain mechanisms in movement. In *Progress in Psychobiology* [a *Scientific American* book], San Francisco: W. H. Freeman and Company, 1976.

Figure 9-18 Modified from E. V. Evarts, Brain mechanisms of movement. In *The Brain* [a *Scientific American* book], San Francisco: W. H. Freeman and Company, 1979.

Figure 10-1 From W. M. Cowan, The development of the brain. In *The Brain* [a *Scientific American* book], San Francisco: W. H. Freeman and Company, 1979.

Figure 10-2 After A. S. G. Curtis, *Journal of Embryology and Experimental Morphology* 10:410–422, 1962.

Figure 10-3 From W. M. Cowan, The development of the brain. In *The Brain* [a *Scientific American* book], San Francisco: W. H. Freeman and Company, 1979.

Figure 10-4 From D. H. Hubel, The brain. In *The Brain* [a *Scientific American* book], San Francisco: W. H. Freeman and Company, 1979.

Figure 10-5 From R. F. Thompson, *Introduction to Physiological Psychology*, New York: Harper & Row, 1975.

Figure 10-8 After J. E. Dowling, *Neurons and Networks: An Introduction to Neuroscience*, Cambridge, MA: The Belknap Press of Harvard University Press, 1992.

Figure 10-9 After D. Purves and J. W. Lichtman, *Principles of Neural Development*, Sunderland, MA: Sinauer Associates, 1985.

Figure 10-11 After A. Ghosh and C. J. Shatz, Involvement of subplate neurons in the formation of ocular dominance columns. In *Science*, 255, 1441–1443, 1992.

Figure 10-13 After T. A. Woolsey, D. Durham, R. M. Harris, D. J. Simons and K. L. Valentino, Somatosensory development. In *Development of Perception*, Vol. 1, New York: Academic Press, pp. 269–292, 1981.

Figure 10-14 From E. L. Bennett, M. C. Diamond, D. Krech, and M. R. Rosenzweig, *Science*, 146, 610–619, 1964.

Figure 10-15 After A. Brun, An overview of light and electron microscopic changes. In B. Reisberg, ed., *Alzheimer's Disease*, New York: The Free Press, 1983.

Figure 11-1 After E. Loftus, *Memory*, Reading, MA: Addison-Wesley, 1980.

Figure 11-2 (*a*) From G. Sperling, The information available in brief visual presentations. In *Psychological Monographs*, 74, 498, 1960. (*b*) From L. R. Petersen and M. J. Petersen, Short-term retention of individual verbal items. In *Journal of Experimental Psychology: Learning, Memory, and Cognition* **58**: 193–198, 1959.

Figure 11-3 After S. Sternberg, High speed scanning in human memory. In *Science*, 153, 652–654, 1966.

Figure 11-4 After E. R. Hilgard, R. L. Atkinson, and R. C. Atkinson, *Introduction to Psychology*, 7th ed., New York: Harcourt Brace Jovanovich, 1979.

Figure 11-5 After R. A. Rescorla, Pavlovian conditioning: Its not what you think it is. In *American Psychologist, 43*, 151–160, 1988.

Figure 11-6 Adapted from R. A. Rescorla, Behavioral studies of Pavlovian conditioning. In *Annual Review of Neuroscience, 11*, 329–352, 1988.

Figure 11-7 From E. R. Kandel, *Cellular Basis of Behavior*, San Francisco: W. H. Freeman and Company, 1976.

Figure 11-8 Based on E. R. Kandel, *Cellular Basis of Behavior*, San Francisco: W. H. Freeman and Company, 1976.

Figure 11-9 After O. A. Smith et al., *Federation Proceedings*, **39**(8):2487–2494, 1980.

Figure 11-10 From M. Davis, J. M. Hitchcock, and J. B. Rosen, A neural analysis of fear conditioning. In I. Gormezano and E. A. Wasserman, eds., *Learning and Memory: The Behavioral and Biological Substrates*, Hillsdale, NJ: Lawrence Erlbaum, pp. 153–181, 1992.

Figure 11-11 Adapted from M. Davis, J. M. Hitchcock, and J. B. Rosen, A neural analyses of fear conditioning. In I. Gormezano and E. A. Wasserman, eds., *Learning and Memory: The Behavioral and Biological Substrates*, Hillsdale, NJ: Lawrence Erlbaum, pp. 153–181, 1992.

Figure 11-12 From D. A. McCormick and R. F. Thompson, Cerebellum: Essential involvement in the classically conditioned eyelid response. In *Science, 223*, 296–299, 1984.

Figure 11-13 From J. E. Steinmetz, D. G. Lavond, D. Ivkovich, C. G. Logan, and R. F. Thompson, Disruption of classical eyelid conditioning after cerebellar lesions: Damage to a memory trace system or a simple performance deficit? In *Journal of Neuroscience,12*, 4403–4426, 1992.

Figure 11-15 From J. L. McGaugh and K. C. Liang, Hormonal influences on memory: Interaction of central and peripheral systems. In B. E. Will, P. Schmitt, and J. C. Dalrymple-Alford, eds., *Brain plasticity, learning and memory*, New York: Plenum Press.

Figure 11-16 After J. M. McGaugh, Affect, neuromodulatory systems and memory storage. In S. A. Christonson, *Handbook of Emotion and Memory: Current Research and Theory*, Hillsdale, NJ: Lawrence Erlbaum, pp. 245–268, 1992.

Figure 11-17 After M. Mishkin, A memory system in the monkey, *Phil. Trans. R. Soc. Lond.* **B298**:85–95, 1982.

Figure 11-18 (*a*) Adapted from M. Mishkin and T. Appenzeller, The anatomy of memory. In *Scientific American, 256*, 62–71, 1987; (*b*) L. R. Squire, *Memory and Brain*, New York: Oxford University Press, 1987; (*c* and *d*) S. E. la-Morgan, L. B. Squire, and M. Mishkin, The neuroanatomy of amnesia: amygdala–hippocampus versus temporal stem. In *Science, 218*, 1337–1339, 1982.

Figure 11-19 Rabbit: After J. O. O'Keefe and L. Nadel, *The Hippocampus as a Cognitive Map*, Oxford: Clarendon Press, 1978. Human: Modified from N. Geschwind, Specializations of the human brain. In *The Brain* [a *Scientific American* book], San Francisco: W. H. Freeman and Company, 1979.

Figure 11-20 After E. R. Kandel and J. H. Schwartz, *Principles of Neural Science*, New York: Elsevier/North-Holland, 1981.

Figure 11-21 Based on G. M. French and H. F. Harlow, Variability of delayed-reaction performance in normal and brain damaged rhesus monkeys. In *Journal of Neurophysiology* **25**: 585–599, 1962.

Figure 11-22 From E. K. Warrington and L. Weiskrantz, An analysis of short-term and long-term memory defects in man. In J. A. Deutsch, ed., *The Physiological Basis of Memory*, New York: Academic Press, pp. 365–396, 1973.

Figure 12-1 After N. Geschwind, Language and the brain. In *Scientific American*, *226*, 76–83, 1972.

Figure 12-2 Scheme developed by N. Geschwind. Illustration modified from N. Geschwind, Specializations of the human brain. In *The Brain* [a *Scientific American* book], San Francisco: W. H. Freeman and Company, 1979.

Figure 12-3 After R. F. Thompson, *Introduction to Physiological Psychology*, New York: Harper & Row, 1975.

Figure 12-4 Adapted from G. A. Ojemann and O. D. Creutzfeldt, Language in humans and animals: Contribution of brain stimulation and recording. In *Handbook of Physiology: The Nervous System*, Vol. 5, Bethesda, MD: American Physiological Society, 1987.

Figure 12-5 From S. E. Petersen and J. A. Fiez, The processing of single words studied with positron emission tomography. In *Annual Review of Neuroscience*, 1993.

Figure 12-6 From S. E. Petersen and J. A. Fiez, The processing of single words studied with positron emission tomography. In *Annual Review of Neuroscience*, 1993.

Figure 12-7 From D. E. Rumelhart, J. L. McClellan, and PDP Research Group, *Parallel Distributed Processing: Explorations in the Microstructure of Cognition*, Cambridge, MA: MIT Press, 1986.

Figure 12-11 Courtesy of Michael S. Gazzaniga.

Figure 12-12 B. Libet, Conscious subjective experience vs. unconscious mental functions: A theory of the cerebral processes involved. In R. M. J. Cotterill, ed., *Models of Brain Function*, Cambridge: Cambridge University Press, 1989.

Index

Note: Page numbers in *italics* indicate illustrations; page numbers followed by t indicate tables.